# Peripheral Arterial Disease

*Guest Editor*

SANJAY RAJAGOPALAN, MD

# CARDIOLOGY CLINICS

www.cardiology.theclinics.com

*Consulting Editor*
MICHAEL H. CRAWFORD, MD

August 2011 • Volume 29 • Number 3

SAUNDERS an imprint of ELSEVIER, Inc.

**W.B. SAUNDERS COMPANY**
*A Division of Elsevier Inc.*

1600 John F. Kennedy Blvd. • Suite 1800 • Philadelphia, PA 19103-2899

http://www.theclinics.com

**CARDIOLOGY CLINICS Volume 29, Number 3**
**August 2011 ISSN 0733-8651, ISBN-13: 978-1-4557-1091-1**

Editor: Barbara Cohen-Kligerman
Developmental Editor: Donald E. Mumford



*Cardiology Clinics* (ISSN 0733-8651) is published quarterly by Elsevier Inc., 360 Park Avenue South, New York, NY 10010-1710. Months of issue are February, May, August, and November. Business and Editorial Offices: 1600 John F. Kennedy Blvd., Ste. 1800, Philadelphia, PA 19103-2899. Customer Service Office: 3251 Riverport Lane, Maryland Heights, MO 63043. Periodicals postage paid at New York, NY and additional mailing offices. Subscription prices are $282.00 per year for US individuals, $458.00 per year for US institutions, $139.00 per year for US students and residents, $345.00 per year for Canadian individuals, $569.00 per year for Canadian institutions, $400.00 per year for international individuals, $569.00 per year for international institutions and $196.00 per year for Canadian and international students/residents. To receive student/resident rate, orders must be accompanied by name of affiliated institution, data of term, and the *signature* of program/residency coordinator on institution letterhead. Orders will be billed at individual rate until proof of status is received. Foreign air speed delivery is included in all *Clinics* subscription prices. All prices are subject to change without notice. **POSTMASTER:** Send address changes to *Cardiology Clinics*, Elsevier Health Sciences Division, Subscription Customer Service, 3251 Riverport Lane, Maryland Heights, MO 63043. **Customer Service: 1-800-654-2452 (U.S. and Canada); 314-447-8871 (outside U.S. and Canada). Fax: 314-447-8029. E-mail: journalscustomerservice-usa@elsevier.com (for print support); journalsonlinesupport-usa@elsevier.com (for online support).**

*Reprints.* For copies of 100 or more, of articles in this publication, please contact the Commercial Reprints Department, Elsevier Inc., 360 Park Avenue South, New York, NY 10010-1710. Tel.: 212-633-3812; Fax: 212-462-1935; E-mail: reprints@elsevier.com.

*Cardiology Clinics* is also published in Spanish by McGraw-Hill Interamericana Editores S. A., P.O. Box 5-237, 06500, Mexico D. F., Mexico; in Portuguese by Reichmann and Alfonso Editores Rio de Janeiro, Brazil; and in Greek by Dimitrios P. Lagos, 8 Pondon Street, GR115-28 Ilissia, Greece.

*Cardiology Clinics* is covered in *MEDLINE/PubMed (Index Medicus), Excerpta Medica, The Cumulative Index to Nursing and Allied Health Literature* (CINAHL).

# Contributors


## CONSULTING EDITOR

**MICHAEL H. CRAWFORD, MD**
Professor of Medicine, University of California, San Francisco; Lucie Stern Chair in Cardiology and Chief of Clinical Cardiology, University of California, San Francisco Medical Center, San Francisco, California

## GUEST EDITOR

**SANJAY RAJAGOPALAN, MD, FACC, FAHA**
John W. Wolfe Professor of Cardiovascular Medicine; Section Director, Vascular Medicine; Co-Director, Cardiovascular CT and MR Program, The Ohio State University, Columbus, Ohio

## AUTHORS

**SALMAN M. AZAM, MD**
Cardiovascular Medicine Fellow, Harrington-McLaughlin Heart and Vascular Institute, University Hospitals Case Medical Center, Cleveland, Ohio

**BARRY A. BORLAUG, MD**
Assistant Professor of Medicine, Mayo Clinic and Foundation, Rochester, Minnesota

**ROBERT D. BROOK, MD**
Associate Professor of Medicine, Division of Cardiovascular Medicine, University of Michigan, Ann Arbor, Michigan

**QUINN CAPERS IV, MD**
Assistant Professor of Medicine; Associate Dean for Admissions; Director, Peripheral Vascular Interventions, Division of Cardiovascular Medicine, The Ohio State University Medical Center, The Ohio State University College of Medicine, Columbus, Ohio

**TERESA L. CARMAN, MD**
Director, Vascular Medicine, Harrington-McLaughlin Heart and Vascular Institute, University Hospitals Case Medical Center; Assistant Professor of Medicine, Division of Cardiovascular Medicine, Case Western Reserve University School of Medicine, Cleveland, Ohio

**KEVIN COHOON, MD, RPVI**
Cardiology Fellow, Division of Cardiology, Loyola University, Chicago, Illinois

**ROBERT S. DIETER, MD, RVT**
Associate Professor, Vascular and Endovascular Medicine, Interventional Cardiology, Loyola University Medical Center; Director of Vascular Medicine and Peripheral Vascular Interventions; Medical Director, Cardiovascular Collaborative; Associate Chief of Cardiology, Chicago, Illinois

**SANJAY GANDHI, MD, FACC, FAHA, FSCAI**
Section of Vascular Medicine, Cardiology Division, Massachusetts General Hospital, Boston, Massachusetts

**LEANNE GROBAN, MD**
Associate Professor of Anesthesiology, Section of Cardiothoracic Anesthesia, Wake Forest University Health Sciences Center, Winston-Salem, North Carolina

**AKHILESH JAIN, MD**
Fellow, Vascular and Endovascular Surgery, Section of Vascular Surgery, Yale University School of Medicine, New Haven, Connecticut

**DAVID A. KASS, MD**
Abraham and Virginia Weiss Professor of Cardiology, Johns Hopkins Medical Institutions, Baltimore, Maryland

**DALANE W. KITZMAN, MD**
Professor of Medicine, Sections of Cardiology and Geriatrics, Department of Internal Medicine, Wake Forest University Health Sciences, Winston-Salem, North Carolina

**GEORGETA MIHAI, PhD**
Research Assistant Professor, Division of Cardiovascular Medicine, Department of Internal Medicine, The Ohio State University, Columbus, Ohio

**PATRICK MURRAY, MD**
Professor of Medicine, Section of Nephrology, University of Chicago, Chicago, Illinois

**ARAVINDA NANJUNDAPPA, MD, FACC, FSCAI, RVT**
Associate Professor of Surgery and Medicine, Division of Vascular Surgery, West Virginia University, Charleston, West Virginia

**JOHN PHILLIPS, MD**
Fellow in Interventional Cardiovascular Medicine, Division of Cardiovascular Medicine, The Ohio State University Medical Center, The Ohio State University College of Medicine, Columbus, Ohio

**RICHARD J. POWELL, MD**
Professor of Surgery, Section of Vascular Surgery, Dartmouth Hitchcock Medical Center, Lebanon, New Hampshire

**SANJAY RAJAGOPALAN, MD, FACC, FAHA**
John W. Wolfe Professor of Cardiovascular Medicine; Section Director, Vascular Medicine; Co-Director, Cardiovascular CT and MR Program, The Ohio State University, Columbus, Ohio

**MADHAV V. RAO, MD**
Fellow, Section of Nephrology, University of Chicago, Chicago, Illinois

**RAHUL SAKHUJA, MD, MPP, MSc**
Section of Vascular Medicine, Cardiology Division, Massachusetts General Hospital, Boston, Massachusetts

**ORLANDO P. SIMONETTI, PhD**
Associate Professor of Internal Medicine and Radiology; Director of Cardiovascular Imaging Research, Division of Cardiovascular Medicine, Departments of Internal Medicine and Radiology, The Ohio State University, Columbus, Ohio

**DAVID PAUL SLOVUT, MD, PhD**
Division of Cardiology, Department of Cardiovascular and Thoracic Surgery, Montefiore Medical Center, Bronx, New York

**PAALADINESH THAVENDIRANATHAN, MD, FRCPC**
Cardiologist and Multimodality Imaging Fellow, Division of Cardiovascular Medicine, College of Medicine, The Ohio State University, Columbus, Ohio

**DEEPTHI VODNALA, MD**
Medical Resident, Michigan State University, East Lansing, Michigan

**MICHAEL C. WALLS, MD**
Cardiovascular Imaging Fellow, Division of Cardiology, The Ohio State University, Columbus, Ohio

**CLYDE W. YANCY, MD**
Professor of Medicine, Section of Cardiology, Baylor Heart and Vascular Institute, Baylor University Medical Center, Dallas, Texas

# Contents

**Foreword** ix

Michael H. Crawford

**Preface: Peripheral Arterial Disease** xi

Sanjay Rajagopalan

**Diagnostic Approach to Peripheral Arterial Disease** 319

Salman M. Azam and Teresa L. Carman

This article discusses diagnostic imaging techniques used in the evaluation and management of patients with peripheral arterial disease (PAD). Along with a complete vascular examination, noninvasive physiologic testing is used for the initial evaluation of patients with suspected PAD. Duplex ultrasonography provides information on the degree of stenosis or occlusion within a vessel and allows assessment of the vessel wall and plaque morphology. Angiographic imaging techniques should be reserved for determining the optimal endovascular or surgical approach for patients requiring revascularization. Together, all available diagnostic modalities contribute to successful evaluation and management of patients with PAD.

**Advances in CT Angiography for Peripheral Arterial Disease** 331

Michael C. Walls, Paaladinesh Thavendiranathan, and Sanjay Rajagopalan

Multidetector CT scan (MDCT) has revolutionized the diagnosis of peripheral arterial disease. The most recent generation of CT scan systems increases the number of detector arrays, which allows further increases in volume coverage and acquisition of large volumes rapidly. These have provided advantages in vascular imaging. The introduction of dual-source scanners has allowed the possibility of tissue characterization in CT scans. This article briefly discusses the basic principles of MDCT and provides an overview of its application in vascular diseases.

**Noncontrast MRA for the Diagnosis of Vascular Diseases** 341

Georgeta Mihai, Orlando P. Simonetti, and Paaladinesh Thavendiranathan

The association between gadolinium-based contrast agents and neprogenic systemic fibrosis has helped propel noncontrast angiography techniques to center stage in the MR evaluation of vascular disease, especially in individuals with intrinsic renal diseases. Although balanced steady-state free precession, phase contrast, and time-of-flight sequences are currently being revisited and improved, new noncontrast angiographic methods have been created and are under development: ECG-gated 3D partial-Fourier fast spin echo (FSE) and 3D variable flip angle FSE (SPACE). All of these are attempts to develop noncontrast methods that offer equal or superior vascular diagnosis as compared with contrast-enhanced MR angiography.

**Advances in Percutaneous Therapy for Upper Extremity Arterial Disease** 351

Quinn Capers IV and John Phillips

Upper extremity arteries are affected by occlusive diseases from diverse causes, with atherosclerosis being the most common. Although the overriding principle in managing patients with upper extremity arterial occlusive disease should be cardiovascular risk reduction by noninvasive and pharmacologic means, when target organ ischemia produces symptoms or threatens the patient's well-being, revascularization is necessary. Given their minimally invasive nature and successful outcomes, percutaneous catheter-based therapies are preferred to surgical approaches. The fact that expertise in these techniques resides in not one but several disciplines (vascular surgery, radiology, cardiology, vascular medicine) makes this an area ripe for multidisciplinary collaboration to the benefit of patients.

**Medical Management of the Patient with Intermittent Claudication** **363**

Deepthi Vodnala, Sanjay Rajagopalan, and Robert D. Brook

Intermittent claudication (IC) due to peripheral arterial disease (PAD) causes substantial impairment in quality of life, and is strongly associated with increased cardiovascular morbidity and mortality. The overall medical approach to management focuses on reducing cardiovascular events, preventing progression of underlying PAD (eg, limb loss), and improving symptoms. Aggressive secondary prevention strategies (eg, statins and smoking cessation) are of critical importance. Cilostazol treatment should be considered for those with persistent IC symptoms despite exercise and risk factor control. Management of IC requires a comprehensive approach toward symptomatic relief of pain with strategies that prolong life and prevent limb loss.

**Recent Advances in Percutaneous Management of Iliofemoral and Superficial Femoral Artery Disease** **381**

Sanjay Gandhi, Rahul Sakhuja, and David Paul Slovut

Tremendous advances have been made in the endovascular treatment of lower-extremity arterial occlusive disease. New technology has enabled operators to successfully revascularize patients with complex arterial occlusive disease. This article summarizes the latest advances in endovascular therapy of aortoiliac and femoral arteries and reviews the clinical outcomes and costs associated with the use of these treatments.

**Percutaneous Management of Chronic Critical Limb Ischemia** **395**

Aravinda Nanjundappa, Akhilesh Jain, Kevin Cohoon, and Robert S. Dieter

Critical limb ischemia (CLI) is primarily a disease of advanced atherosclerosis but may occur in the setting of other causes. It is essential for the treating physician to understand the complexity of patients with CLI and the appropriate and emerging treatment approaches in this patient population. The authors provide a comprehensive review of the percutaneous endovascular management of CLI in this article.

**Update on Biological Therapies for Critical Limb Ischemia** **411**

Richard J. Powell

Gene and stem cell therapies have been shown to be safe and well tolerated. Early trial results using these therapies have had promising results on important clinical end points such as wound healing, ischemic pain, and major amputation. Despite this, there have been no pivotal trials to date that have proved the benefit of biological therapy, although there are numerous pivotal trials in progress or about to initiate enrollment. Persistent obstacles exist with current study designs that complicate the ability to successfully perform clinical critical limb ischemia trials.

**Perspectives on Optimizing Trial Design and Endpoints in Peripheral Arterial Disease: A Case for Imaging-Based Surrogates as Endpoints of Functional Efficacy** 419

Sanjay Rajagopalan and Georgeta Mihai

Surrogate endpoints are important for validation of mechanism, early proof of concept, and the rational design of clinical trials for regulatory approval of drugs. The recent failure of several drugs in peripheral arterial disease (PAD) and in atherosclerosis highlights the importance of understanding drug effect and is a clarion call for better endpoints. This review focuses on aspects relating to the current state of surrogate endpoints in PAD and reviews emerging endpoints using imaging approaches that may have the potential of improving study design in PAD.

**Special Articles**

**Management of Heart Failure with Renal Artery Ischemia** 433

Madhav V. Rao, Patrick Murray, and Clyde W. Yancy

With improved treatment, patients are surviving longer with impaired ventricular function. Hypertension results in ventricular remodeling in many patients. More than 5 million people have heart failure and are likely to have one or more co-existent diseases associated with aging, one of which is chronic kidney disease (CKD). Renal artery stenosis is fraught with varying opinions. Nephrologists, cardiologists, and interventional radiologists all manage these diseases with different strategies. This article outlines renovascular disease as it relates to CKD, the pathophysiology of development of renovascular disease and effects leading to congestive heart failure, treatment modalities, and outcomes of treatment regimens.

**Ventricular–Vascular Interaction in Heart Failure** 447

Barry A. Borlaug and David A. Kass

Nearly half of all patients who have heart failure have preserved ejection fraction (HFpEF). Patients who have HFpEF tend to be older, female, and hypertensive, and characteristically display increased ventricular and arterial stiffening. In this article, we discuss the pathophysiology of abnormal ventriculoarterial stiffening and how it affects ventricular function, cardiovascular hemodynamics, reserve capacity, and symptoms. We conclude by exploring how novel treatment strategies targeting abnormal ventricular–arterial interaction might prove useful in the treatment of patients who have HFpEF.

**Exercise Intolerance** 461

Dalane W. Kitzman and Leanne Groban

Exercise intolerance is the primary symptom of chronic diastolic heart failure. It is part of the definition of heart failure and is intimately linked to its pathophysiology. Further, exercise intolerance affects the diagnosis and prognosis of heart failure. In addition, understanding the mechanisms of exercise intolerance can lead to developing and testing rational treatments for heart failure. This article focuses on the fundamental principles of exercise physiology and on the assessment, pathophysiology, and potential treatment of exercise intolerance in diastolic heart failure.

**Index** 479

# Cardiology Clinics

## FORTHCOMING ISSUES

*November 2011*

**Left Ventricular Assist Devices**
John A. Elefteriades, MD, and
Donald M. Botta Jr, MD,
*Guest Editors*

*February 2012*

**Computed Tomography Imaging in 2012**
Jagat Narula, MD, PhD,
Stephan Achenbach, MD, and
Takeshi Kondo, MD, PhD, *Guest Editors*

*May 2012*

**Faces of Right Ventricular Failure**
James A. Goldstein, MD, and
Jonathan D. Rich, MD,
*Guest Editor*

## RECENT ISSUES

*May 2011*

**Catheterization Hemodynamics**
Michael J. Lim, MD,
*Guest Editor*

*February 2011*

**Prevention of Cardiovascular Disease: A Continuum**
Prakash Deedwania, MD, *Guest Editor*

*November 2010*

**Hypertension and Hypertensive Heart Disease**
George A. Mensah, MD, FACC, FACP, FACN,
*Guest Editor*

## ISSUES OF RELATED INTEREST

*Heart Failure Clinics,* July 2011 (Vol. 7, No. 3)
**Cardio-oncology Related to Heart Failure**
Daniel J. Lenihan, MD, and Douglas B. Sawyer, MD, PhD, *Guest Editors*
Available at: http://www.heartfailure.theclinics.com/

*Cardiac Electrophysiology Clinics,* June 2011 (Vol. 3, No. 2)
**Arrhythmogenic Cardiomyopathy**
Domenico Corrado, MD, PhD, Cristina Basso, MD, PhD, and
Gaetano Thiene, MD, *Guest Editors*
Available at: http://www.cardiacep.theclinics.com/

# Foreword

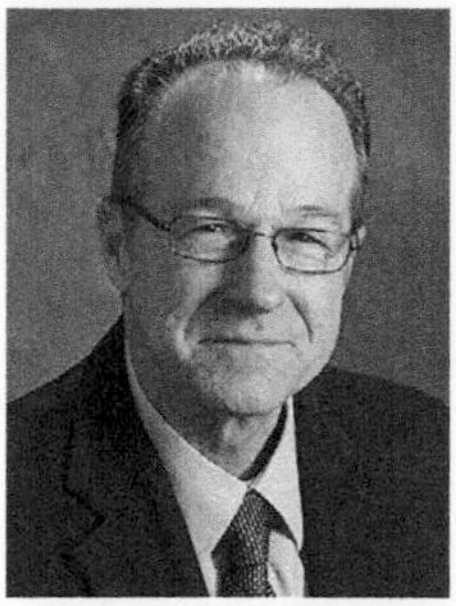

Michael H. Crawford, MD
*Consulting Editor*

I was delighted when Dr Rajagopalan agreed to guest edit an issue of *Cardiology Clinics* on peripheral vascular disease. A lot has happened in the 9 years since the previous issue on this topic. Because there has been such an explosion in knowledge, this issue is focused on peripheral arterial disease (PAD). Among the first articles in the issue is one on the diagnosis of PAD using CT angiography, which has largely replaced invasive angiography. Another article discusses MR angiography, which could be considered an emerging diagnostic modality. The impact of these new imaging techniques on therapeutic trial design in PAD is discussed in another article. The articles on the diagnostic approach to PAD, medical management of intermittent claudication, and biological therapies for critical limb ischemia are of particular interest to clinicians. The remainder of the issue is devoted to percutaneous invasive therapies for femoral artery, upper limb arteries, and critical limb ischemia. In parallel with coronary disease, percutaneous treatment approaches are replacing traditional surgical procedures for the management of PAD. This undoubtedly explains why interest in PAD among invasive cardiologists has increased. However, as this issue emphasizes, the management of PAD is inherently multidisciplinary, involving radiologists, vascular surgeons, and cardiologists, and Dr Rajagopalan has assembled such a multidisciplinary team of experts for this issue.

Another feature of this issue is a reprinting of some articles published in *Heart Failure Clinics* that have relevance to vascular disease. Renal artery stenosis can complicate the management of heart failure and can be treated percutaneously. Ventriculovascular interactions are an important component of diastolic heart failure, which can be aggravated by PAD. Finally, exercise intolerance in heart failure has a peripheral vascular component that needs to be considered. Thus, this issue has something for every physician caring for patients with heart and vascular disease.

Michael H. Crawford, MD
Division of Cardiology, Department of Medicine
University of California
San Francisco Medical Center
505 Parnassus Avenue, Box 0124
San Francisco, CA 94143-0124, USA

E-mail address:
crawfordm@medicine.ucsf.edu

Cardiol Clin 29 (2011) ix
doi:10.1016/j.ccl.2011.06.001
0733-8651/11/$ – see front matter 

# Preface
# Peripheral Arterial Disease

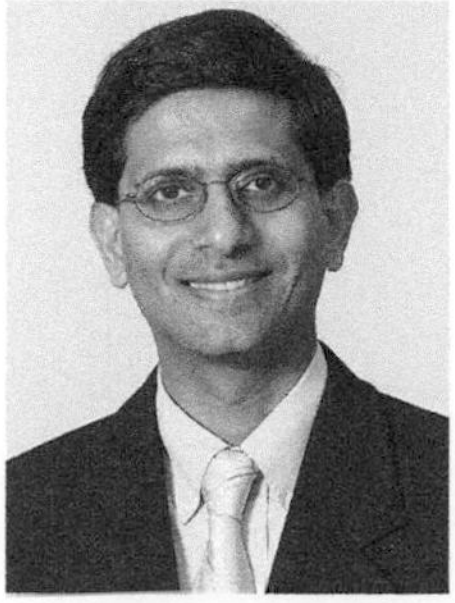

Sanjay Rajagopalan, MD
*Guest Editor*

The last decade has seen a tremendous surge of interest in peripheral arterial disease (PAD). The prevalence of multiple risk factors, chronic nature of disease, the nonspecificity of symptoms, and lack of adequate treatment options have all contributed to the large burden of disease, which is frequently unrecognized. The last issue of *Cardiology Clinics* devoted exclusively to peripheral vascular disease was published 9 years ago, 2 months after 9/11. Since that time, the world has quite literally changed. We have seen advertising campaigns from pharmaceutical companies about "seeing your doctor if you have PAD" come and go, and we have witnessed advances that have informed us about natural history, diagnosis, and new treatments. New guidelines for the treatment of PAD have been endorsed by many societies including the American Heart Association, American College of Cardiology, and the Society for Vascular Medicine and Biology. This information wave has resulted in the creation of a cadre of superbly trained vascular physicians. Thus, rather than a dearth of information that was the case in 2002, there is a surfeit of information. Some may legitimately argue about the true need for yet another monograph on PAD in this environment of information overload.

At a time when there is plethora of information from multiple sources, the need for resources like the *Clinics* is more important than ever. *Cardiology Clinics* has always been about distilling information and presenting topics in a format that is well suited to the practicing physician. This issue continues this tradition and, rather than representing the repository of all that you need to know, presents "just what you need to know" on practical aspects of PAD management. In contrast to the 2002 issue, which covered aortic disease, carotid artery disease, and vasospastic disorders, this issue focuses on PAD alone, as there is so much to cover. Once again, in keeping with the multidisciplinary nature, a group of experts from cardiology, vascular surgery, and vascular medicine have made this issue possible. An aspect that has been troublesome for many passionate about vascular diseases is the lack of suitable pharmacologic treatments for vascular disorders. This is addressed in a separate article where I discuss the trials and tribulations and some of the encouraging signals emanating from the world of imaging science (no pun intended for all).

I would like to thank the contributing authors and Barbara Cohen-Kligerman, whose help and patience throughout the issue was much appreciated.

Sanjay Rajagopalan, MD
Cardiovascular CT and MR Program
The Ohio State University
473 West 12th Avenue, Suite 200, DHLRI
Columbus, OH 43210, USA

E-mail address:
sanjay.rajagopalan@osumc.edu



Cardiol Clin 29 (2011) xi
doi:10.1016/j.ccl.2011.05.002
0733-8651/11/$ – see front matter 

# Diagnostic Approach to Peripheral Arterial Disease

Salman M. Azam, MD[a], Teresa L. Carman, MD[b,c,*]

**KEYWORDS**

- Peripheral arterial disease • Vascular imaging
- Diagnostic testing • Angiography • Noninvasive testing

The peripheral arterial system includes all noncardiac arteries: the thoracic and abdominal aortas and their branches extending to visceral organs and both upper and lower extremities as well as the extracranial vessels. Although the awareness of peripheral arterial disease (PAD) has increased in the past decade, PAD remains underdiagnosed and undertreated. The development of PAD guidelines has helped increase awareness and define diagnostics and treatment strategies in PAD.[1,2] Atherosclerotic disease is the most common cause of PAD, but nonatherosclerotic vascular disease may cause similar symptoms and must be considered in patients presenting with vascular insufficiency. The differential diagnosis of patients presenting should therefore include entrapment syndromes at the thoracic outlet or popliteal fossa, cystic adventitial disease, fibromuscular dysplasia, endofibrosis of the iliac artery, embolism, thromboangiitis obliterans (Buerger disease), and vasculitis, such as Takayasu arteritis or giant cell arteritis.[3] Musculoskeletal syndromes associated with arthritis, compartment syndrome, myositis, or pseudoclaudication may also present in a similar fashion.

From epidemiologic studies, approximately 12% of the adult population has PAD. At younger ages, PAD is more prevalent in men than in women; however, with advancing age, gender distribution is equal.[4] Disease prevalence increases with advancing age and cardiovascular risk factors. In one study, lower extremity PAD was identified in 29% of patients older than 70 years or patients older than 50 years with a history of smoking or diabetes.[5] Patients older than 70 years in the National Health and Nutrition Examination Survey and patients older than 65 years in the Framingham Heart Study had an increased risk of developing PAD, with a prevalence of 4.3% in patients older than 40 years compared with 14.5% in patients older than 70 years.[6] African Americans and Hispanics have an increased risk of PAD compared with Caucasians.

Most patients with lower extremity PAD are asymptomatic, whereas others may experience nondescript leg symptoms. Typical symptoms associated with PAD include claudication, ischemic rest pain, ischemic ulcerations, and gangrene. Compared with age-matched controls, patients with asymptomatic PAD have poorer functional performance and quality of life as well as smaller calf muscle area and greater calf muscle fat.[7] In general, patients perform poorly on health-related quality-of-life questionnaires and have an increased rate of depression. These patients are at risk for recurrent hospitalizations, revascularizations, as well as limb loss.[2,8,9] More importantly, patients with PAD have a higher rate

The authors have nothing to disclose.

[a] Harrington-McLaughlin Heart and Vascular Institute, University Hospitals Case Medical Center, 11100 Euclid Avenue, Mailstop LKS 5038, Cleveland, OH 44106, USA
[b] Vascular Medicine, Harrington-McLaughlin Heart and Vascular Institute, University Hospitals Case Medical Center, 11100 Euclid Avenue, Mailstop LKS 5038, Cleveland, OH 44106, USA
[c] Division of Cardiovascular Medicine, Case Western Reserve University School of Medicine, OH, USA
* Corresponding author. Vascular Medicine, Harrington-McLaughlin Heart and Vascular Institute, University Hospitals Case Medical Center, 11100 Euclid Avenue, Mailstop LKS 5038, Cleveland, OH 44106.
*E-mail address:* teresa.carman@uhhospitals.org

Cardiol Clin 29 (2011) 319–329
doi:10.1016/j.ccl.2011.04.004

of all-cause mortality and are at an increased risk of cardiovascular events, including myocardial infarction (MI), stroke, and cardiovascular death, compared with those without PAD.[10–13] This finding highlights the importance of early diagnosis of PAD and institution of treatment, both to limit progression of PAD and reduce the risk of cardiovascular and all-cause mortalities.

## DIAGNOSIS OF PAD

A thorough history taking and physical examination is the first step in diagnosing PAD before undertaking diagnostic testing. Any history of PAD, transient ischemic attack, or stroke, prior diagnostic studies, as well as interventions such as carotid endarterectomy, percutaneous stenting, or peripheral bypass surgery assist with formulating the next step in the evaluation of the patient. The initial evaluation should include an assessment of the patient's functional status and living situation, risk factors, and comorbidities, such as cardiac, pulmonary, or renal diseases, which may influence the diagnostic and/or therapeutic strategy, and gauge any decline in the patient's activity level.[14] This evaluation allows the clinician to establish a preliminary diagnosis and determine the most appropriate treatment. Most interventions are performed electively in patients with PAD, whereas more-urgent intervention may be required in the setting of critical limb ischemia.

Many patients with PAD are asymptomatic, and although patients do not have symptoms with their activities of daily living, they may have functional impairment on formal testing.[3] PAD may not present with classic claudication symptoms, and properly phrasing questions to obtain pertinent information from the patient is essential. Atypical symptoms of PAD include lower extremity discomfort or fatigue that begins during exertion but is not reproducible with the same level of exertion and may require a longer period of time to resolve. Classic symptoms include pain, discomfort and heaviness, tiredness, cramping, and burning sensation in the muscles of the calf, hip, thigh, or buttocks, which is reproducible with a similar level of activity such as walking and disappears after several minutes of rest. The same symptoms recur once walking is resumed. The Rose Angina and Claudication Questionnaire and the Edinburgh Claudication Questionnaire can be used to assist clinicians with screening patients for PAD at the time of the initial history taking and physical examination.[15,16] Critical limb ischemia includes symptoms of rest pain or tissue loss. Rest pain is characterized by pain in the toes or distal forefoot with elevation, which is relieved when the limb is dependent. Tissue loss includes the presence of ischemic ulcerations or frank gangrene.

Physical examination includes measurement of blood pressure in both arms, cardiac auscultation for heart rate and rhythm, auscultation for carotid, subclavian, abdominal, and femoral artery bruits, abdominal palpation for signs of aortic aneurysm, palpation of peripheral pulses in all 4 extremities; and inspection of the 4 extremities to assess for any signs of PAD.[14] A blood pressure difference of more than 15 mmHg between the 2 arm cuff measurements indicates innominate, subclavian, or axillary artery disease. The presence of arterial bruits warrants further investigation. One meta-analysis involving 17,295 patients showed that the yearly MI rate and cardiovascular death were 2 times greater in patients with carotid bruits than that in those without carotid bruits.[17] Peripheral pulses should be described as bounding (3+), normal (2+), diminished (1+), or absent.[7] Widened arterial pulsations in the femoral or popliteal artery should be noted, which may indicate the presence of a peripheral aneurysm. Careful inspection of the extremities should include observation for ulcerations, calluses, tinea pedia, trophic skin changes, infection, and pallor on elevation or temperature changes relative to the proximal and/or contralateral limb.

Noninvasive diagnostic testing should support the clinical diagnosis of PAD and supplement a thorough history taking and physical examination. In addition, noninvasive testing is useful to document the severity of disease, provides a baseline for follow-up, and can help predict the potential for ulcer/wound healing. Of the available noninvasive diagnostic tests, only the ankle-brachial index (ABI), segmental pressure measurement, and pulse volume waveform analysis can provide physiologic information about perfusion of the extremities. Other noninvasive imaging techniques can assist with planning endovascular or surgical treatment.

### *Continuous Wave Doppler*

The most basic assessment of arterial flow is performed using continuous wave Doppler (CWD). CWD may be used in the office or at the bedside to provide a qualitative assessment of arterial vascular flow. The audible Doppler signal is quantified in terms of strength and phasicity. CWD can neither determine the depth of the vessel nor assess the direction of flow. In a high-resistance vascular bed, such as the lower extremity, the normal Doppler signal is triphasic. A triphasic signal has 3 audible components: forward flow of systole, early reverse flow of diastole, and late forward flow of diastole.[14] In a low-resistance vascular bed, such as the internal carotid artery or lower extremity after exercise, the Doppler signal demonstrates continuous forward flow and is biphasic because of the lack of diastolic reversal. The Doppler probe is also used for measuring segmental pressures and the ABI.

### *ABI*

The ABI is an addition to the physical examination and is considered the single best initial screening test in patients with suspected PAD. The ABI correlates well with the severity of obstruction; however, it is poorly correlated with functional impairment because of PAD.[3] The ABI is easy to perform and can be done at the bedside. A handheld CWD and a manual blood pressure cuff are the only required equipments. The Doppler probe is placed over the arterial signal. The blood pressure cuff is inflated until the arterial signal disappears, the cuff is slowly deflated, and the pressure at first return of an audible signal is recorded. The ABI is calculated as the ratio of highest ankle systolic pressure, from either the dorsalis pedis or posterior tibial artery, to the highest arm systolic pressure recorded over the brachial artery. An ABI of between 0.91 and 1.3 is considered normal. An ABI of 0.71 to 0.90 indicates mild obstruction, 0.41 to 0.70 is consistent with moderate obstruction, and 0.00 to 0.40 denotes severe obstruction.[18,19] A low ABI, consistent with arterial occlusive disease, is an independent predictor of increased mortality.[10,20–24] Patients with an ABI less than 0.90 have a 5-year mortality approaching 25% and are twice as likely to have a history of MI, angina, and heart failure as patients with ABI greater than 1.00.[23,25,26] An ABI greater than 1.30 suggests the presence of medial calcinosis and noncompressibility of the vessels. This situation is most commonly encountered in patients with diabetes or renal failure. An ABI greater than 1.40 has been associated with increased cardiovascular and all-cause mortalities.[10]

In patients with ABI greater than 1.3 and suspected medial calcinosis, the toe-brachial index (TBI) is a better assessment of underlying vascular disease because the digital vessels of the toes are often spared from the process and accurate pressure measurements can be obtained. A 2-cm cuff is placed at the toe, and a photoplethysmography (PPG) sensor is placed at the tip. A TBI less than 0.7 is considered abnormal. TBIs can be used to predict healing of wound and foot amputation sites. An open wound is unlikely to heal in patients with an absolute toe pressure of less than 30 mm Hg.

In patients with a normal resting ABI but typical symptoms of claudication, exercise or treadmill ABI can be helpful in unmasking the presence of PAD. In the absence of PAD, treadmill exercise increases blood flow to the extremities; as such, the ABI increases slightly and remains elevated for several minutes. In patients with proximal PAD, exertional vasodilation of the lower extremity vascular bed increases blood velocity across the stenosis and decreases blood pressure distally, resulting in decreasing ABI and a slower return to baseline. Exercise testing also allows an objective assessment of symptom limitation in patients with claudication. This testing allows clinicians to better formulate individualized therapeutic exercise programs. Motorized treadmills and standard fixed load or graded protocols are used in most laboratories. However, alternative forms of exercise such as active pedal plantar flexion, stair climbing, hallway walking, or a 6-minute walk test can also be used.[2,27,28] For patients in whom standard supine ABI testing is not possible, a protocol to measure seated ABIs has been validated and can be used to assess for PAD as well.[29]

The ABI alone does not provide information about the level of obstruction. Segmental blood pressure measurement assists in anatomic localization of obstruction and can help predict wound healing as well as limb survival. Segmental blood pressures may be performed using a 3- or 4-cuff method. In the 3-cuff method, appropriately sized blood pressure cuffs are placed at the level of the upper thigh, proximal calf, and ankle. In the 4-cuff method, a fourth cuff is placed at the level of the distal thigh. Similar to the ABI measurement, the cuff is pressurized to occlude the artery, and using a Doppler probe, the first return of audible Doppler signal is recorded. Each cuff isolates the arterial segment proximal to the cuff. The pressure at the ankle should be similar to the brachial pressure, and the pressure at the thigh is usually slightly higher. A pressure decrease between cuff segments of more than 20 mm Hg indicates obstructive disease. This noninvasive test may be useful for anatomic localization of obstructive disease and may assist in planning further imaging or intervention (**Fig. 1**). Both the ABI and segmental blood pressures are useful in monitoring the success and patency of therapeutic interventions. Although generally well tolerated, some patients may find the inflation pressure required to occlude the thigh cuff uncomfortable. In addition, segmental blood pressures may be inaccurate with extensively developed collateral flow.

### *Pulse Volume Recording*

Air plethysmography (APG) and PPG are other noninvasive techniques used to assess PAD. These techniques require an appropriately sized blood pressure cuff, a transducer, and a recording

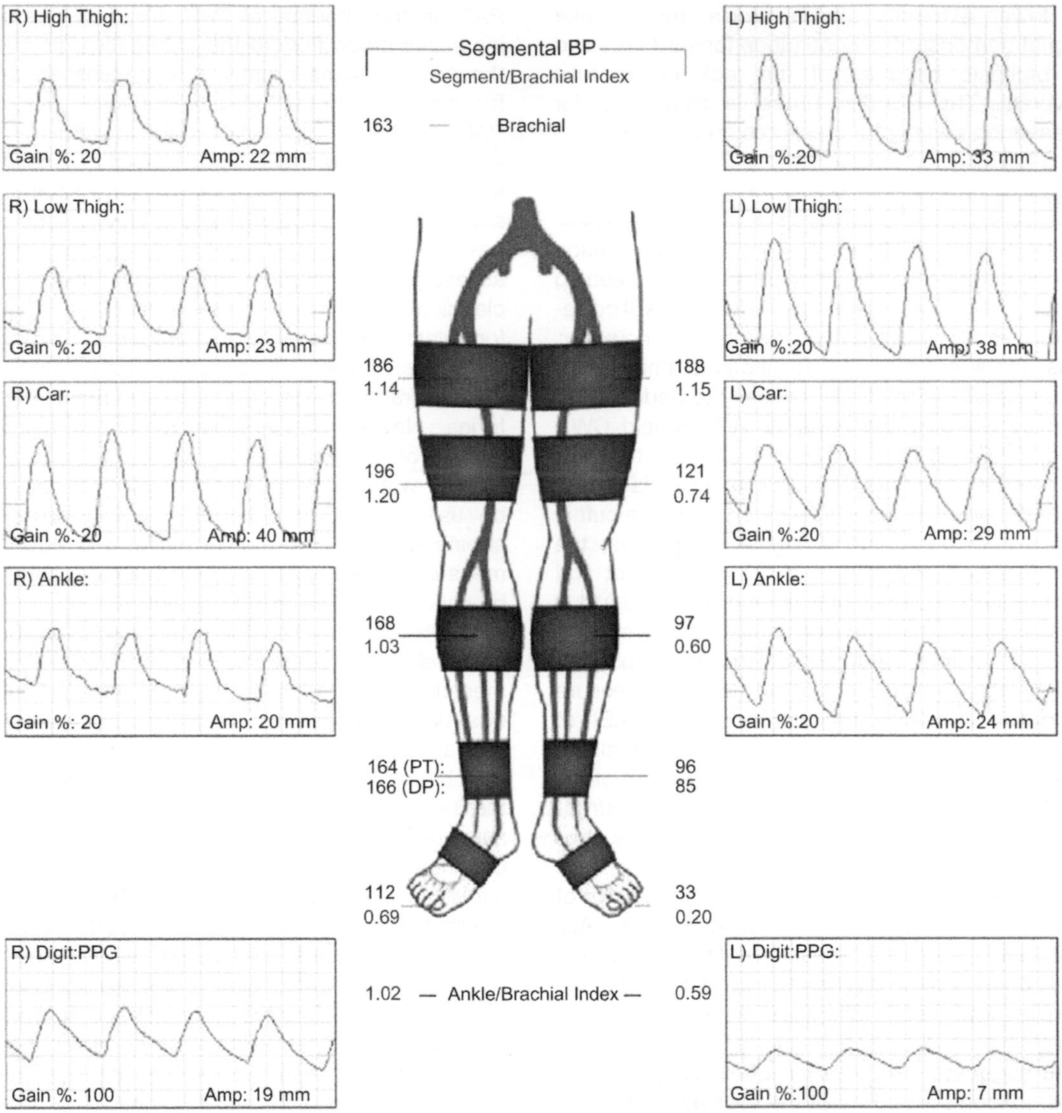


**Fig. 1.** Demonstration of segmental arterial pressures and pulse volume recording (PVR) of the lower extremities. The ABI is normal on the right (ABI = 1.02) and demonstrates moderate disease on the left (ABI = 0.59). Both the segmental pressure measurements and PVR waveforms suggest obstruction at the level of the left femoral and popliteal arteries. Amp, amplitude; BP, blood pressure; DP, dorsalis pedis; PT, posterior tibial.

instrument. The pulse volume recording (PVR) is a form of APG. A blood pressure cuff is placed on the lower extremity and inflated to a baseline pressure of approximately 65 mm Hg. Placement of the cuffs is similar to those used for segmental pressures, and the cuff is attached to the plethysmograph. The lower extremity pulsatile flow causes small changes in limb volume, which are recorded as arterial contours and provide indirect qualitative information about the arterial blood flow and correspond to direct arterial pressure waveform recording at that level. The normal PVR tracing has a sharp upstroke (anacrotic slope), a distinct pulse peak, and a rapid decline (catacrotic slope), which bows toward the baseline. With increasing arterial obstruction, the PVR tracing becomes progressively flattened and prolonged.[14] The PVR only allows for qualitative interpretation of the waveform. The PVR is useful in predicting the outcome in critical limb ischemia and risk of amputation as well as in monitoring limb perfusion after revascularization. A severely flattened PVR tracing at the ankles suggests a limited opportunity for wound healing. In patients with noncompressible vessels, the PVR tracing is more reliable than segmental pressure or the ABI. Therefore, PVRs are often combined with segmental pressure measurement, particularly in patients with noncompressible vessels (see **Fig. 1**).[30] PVR waveforms may be abnormal in patients with low cardiac output or influenced by technologist inexperience with cuff placement.

## *Duplex Ultrasonography*

Duplex ultrasonography combines B-mode imaging and pulsed wave Doppler imaging. Duplex ultrasonography is an accurate, cost-effective, noninvasive method to localize stenosis and differentiate stenosis from occlusion. This technique does not require any intravenous contrast administration or radiation. Gray-scale or B-mode imaging creates a 2-dimensional (D) image of the arterial wall and lumen, which allows the operator to identify morphologic changes in the arterial wall, including atherosclerotic plaque and other abnormalities, such as aneurysms or cystic adventitial disease, that may be the source of ischemic symptoms. Pulsed wave Doppler imaging, which may be augmented by the use of color flow Doppler, allows an estimation of the degree of stenosis based on the blood flow velocity. In the peripheral arteries, a peak systolic velocity greater than 200 cm/s or a systolic velocity ratio greater than 2.5 across the stenosis correlates with an obstruction of more than 50% (**Fig. 2**). Using the combined modalities of B-mode imaging and pulsed wave Doppler, duplex ultrasonography allows for the assessment of the degree of stenosis as well as the character and length of stenosis in the peripheral arteries.[31–33] Duplex ultrasonography is also used to diagnose renal artery stenosis, mesenteric occlusive disease, carotid disease, and aortic and/or aneurysmal disease. Duplex ultrasonography is frequently used in surveillance programs after endovascular therapy or surgical revascularization. Recurrent leg symptoms or significant decrease in ABI of more than 0.15 detects a failing bypass graft in only 50% of cases, which underscores the importance of routine surveillance. Serial monitoring to assess for recurrent stenosis or preocclusive lesions allows for repeat intervention before the primary repair fails.[34]

Although duplex ultrasonography provides excellent anatomic and physiologic information, some of the imaging studies are quite time-consuming. Accuracy is operator dependent, and studies should be performed by an experienced vascular technologist. Obesity and overlying bowel gas can interfere with the visualization of the aorta and renal, mesenteric, and iliac arteries. Severe calcification, overlying skin disorders, or edema of the lower extremities can also interfere with the imaging of the tibial arteries. Ultrasound cannot penetrate bony structures; therefore, the proximal intrathoracic vessels, such as the aortic arch, supra-aortic trunk, and distal cervical and intracranial carotid arteries, are not amendable to ultrasound imaging.[14]

Although not yet approved by the Food and Drug Administration (FDA), the newly developed ultrasound contrast agents show promise in the imaging of lower extremities and renal arteries as well as for endograft surveillance.[35–39] Several other imaging advances stand to change the current ultrasound imaging technology. Three-dimensional ultrasound imaging and ultrasonic computed tomography for precisely determining the location, extent, and configuration of vascular disease are under development.[40,41]

## *Magnetic Resonance Angiography*

Magnetic resonance angiography (MRA) provides excellent-quality images of the aorta and the peripheral vasculature, including identification of small runoff vessels in the foot. In many centers, MRA meets or exceeds the quality of traditional catheter-based angiography and has replaced angiography as the procedure of choice for planning intervention or surgical therapy.[42,43] Gadolinium-enhanced 3D MRA affords the opportunity to acquire angiographic-like images.[44–47] Compared with conventional digital subtraction angiography (DSA), contrast-enhanced 3D MRA has a sensitivity and specificity of more than 90% and 97%, respectively, for detecting hemodynamically significant lower extremity disease.[3,34] Magnetic resonance imaging (MRI) also provides excellent soft tissue imaging, vessel wall information, and qualitative aspects of plaque, including lipid-rich plaque, intraplaque hemorrhage, and so forth. Combining MRI and MRA allows simultaneous visualization of muscular and tendinous structures and can help determine the cause of popliteal artery entrapment.

Some of the limitations of MRA include claustrophobia and inability to perform the technique in patients with pacemakers and intracranial arterial aneurysm clips.[48] Increased venous contamination used to be a problem in patients with critical limb ischemia or diabetic foot ulcers owing to rapid arterial-venous transit.[49] However, this problem has been largely circumvented by the use of venous cuffs and judicious use of timing techniques. Although use of gadolinium-based contrast does not have strong propensity to cause contrast nephropathy compared with iodinated contrast agents used for computed tomographic angiography (CTA) and catheter-based angiography, the recent FDA warnings regarding nephrogenic systemic fibrosis after gadolinium administration

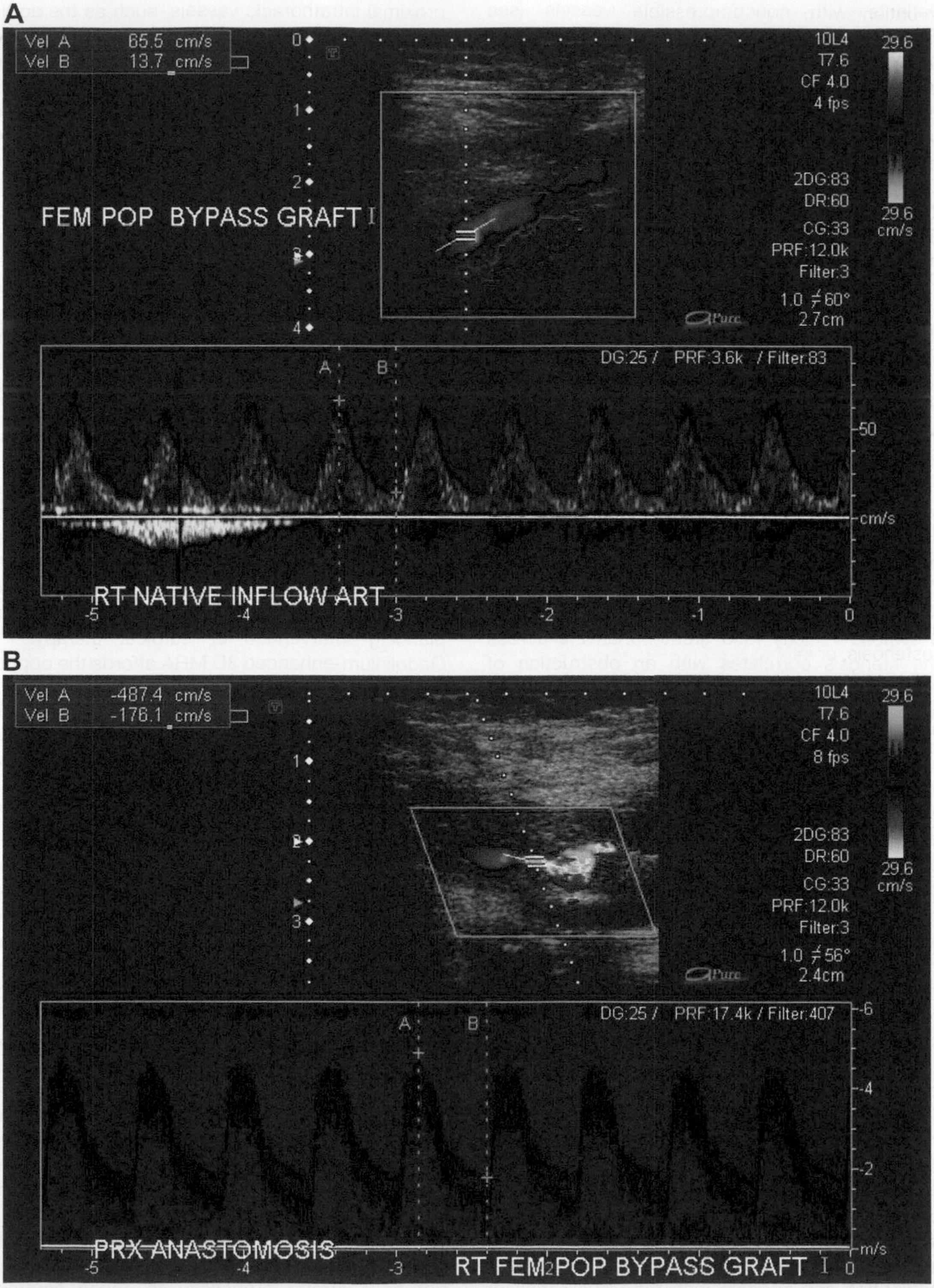


**Fig. 2.** Duplex ultrasonographic image of the proximal anastomosis of a femoropopliteal bypass graft. (*A*) Inflow from the native common femoral artery with biphasic arterial Doppler signals. At the anastomosis (*B*), a velocity shift is noted. Systolic velocity ratio is (487 cm/s:66 cm/s) 7.4, which is consistent with severe stenosis.

in patients with severe renal insufficiency (glomerular filtration rate <30–35 mL/min) have limited the use of contrast-enhanced MRA in this patient population.[14,50] Noncontrast MRA discussed in this issue by Mihai and colleagues can be particularly advantageous in the setting of advanced chronic kidney disease or in patients on dialysis.

## *CTA*

Current multidetector CTA scanners can generate high-resolution arterial images at an isotropic voxel resolution of 500 μ, which allows superb delineation of small vessels in the foot.[51] The volumetric acquisition of axial images and software-based reformatting allows the practitioner to visualize the anatomy from multiple angles and in multiple planes after a single acquisition. Postprocessing software can be used to create 3D reconstructions; multiplanar reconstruction in coronal, sagittal, and axial images; as well maximum-intensity projection images. Unlike DSA, CTA provides improved visualization of the arterial wall and surrounding soft tissues as well as other adjacent anatomic structures. Arterial calcification, plaque ulceration, intravascular thrombus, stent fracture, in-stent restenosis, or intimal hyperplasia, which may influence endovascular or surgical procedures, can also be assessed by CTA. This technique is less invasive, with fewer complications than conventional angiography.[34,52,53]

CTA has a sensitivity and specificity of greater than 95% for identifying greater than 50% stenoses or occlusion in the peripheral vessels.[54,55] Most surgeons have acquired considerable experience with both preoperative planning and postoperative surveillance for endovascular aneurysm repair using CTA.[14] Limitations of CTA are exposure to radiation as well as administration of intravenous contrast and risk of contrast nephropathy. For a typical CTA, visualization of the vasculature is obtained using 100 to 150 mL of iodinated contrast. Once again, timing of the contrast bolus is the key to providing adequate visualization of the vasculature. Extensive vascular calcification can obscure the lumen and overestimate the degree of stenosis. CTA techniques are covered in more detail in a subsequent article by Walls and colleagues.

## *DSA and Intravascular Ultrasonography*

In many centers, duplex ultrasonography, CTA, and MRA have replaced traditional catheter-based imaging in the initial evaluation of PAD. However, traditional DSA still plays a vital role in the management of patients with PAD. One major advantage of DSA is the ability to selectively evaluate individual vessels; obtain physiologic measurements, such as pressure gradients across stenotic lesions; investigate the vessel wall using intravascular ultrasound (IVUS); and perform a therapeutic intervention in the same setting.[56,57] Advances in IVUS technology, such as 3D reconstruction, virtual histology, and color flow, can provide information regarding plaque characterization and may influence intervention strategy.[40,58] Intravascular optical coherence tomography is a developing technology that has proved useful in coronary imaging and intervention. Although not well studied, this technology may have a role in monitoring disease progression and outcomes of therapeutic intervention in PAD.[59–61]

Limitations of this technique include exposure to ionizing radiation, use of iodinated contrast agents, and risk of complications from vascular access and catheterization. Carbon dioxide ($CO_2$) can be used as a nonnephrotoxic contrast agent in the evaluation of PAD below the diaphragm. Injection of compressed $CO_2$ results in displacement of blood, creating negative contrast within the target vessel. $CO_2$ is rapidly absorbed in the blood and therefore limits the evaluation of tibial vessels. Faster frame acquisition rates and specialized injection equipment are necessary for $CO_2$ angiography. Therefore, this technique may not be applicable to all imaging centers.[62,63]

## *Positron Emission Tomography*

Positron emission tomography (PET) is a nuclear medicine functional imaging modality that analyzes nutrient flow and uptake into perfused tissues, including the brain, lungs, and heart. Recent studies have demonstrated the utility of fludeoxyglucose F 18 and water labeled with oxygen O 15 in evaluating skeletal muscle tissue and quantifying regional muscle blood flow in patients with lower extremity PAD.[64–66] PET has not been studied as a diagnostic modality. However, the role of PET in monitoring changes for disease severity over time and after therapeutic interventions has been examined. Further investigation is needed to establish the utility and cost-effectiveness of PET imaging in relation to other imaging modalities for diagnosing PAD.

## *Other Imaging Technologies*

Hyperspectral imaging is a noninvasive technology that relies on scanning spectroscopy based on local chemical composition and can create a 2D anatomic oxygenation map of imaged tissue. Although still in the early stages of development, hyperspectral imaging may prove useful in following the outcomes of intervention, managing medical therapies for PAD, as well as assessing wound healing.[59,67,68] Molecular imaging of plaques by administering traceable molecules, such as magnetic nanoparticles and radionuclides, into the body and subsequently imaging them could potentially identify high-risk plaques. Being in early developmental phase, the infrastructure, duration of procedure, and costs are present limitations of molecular imaging. Nevertheless, this technique may prove potentially useful and cost effective in select patients.[40,69]

## SUMMARY

Most patients with PAD are symptomatic. Symptomatic patients may present with typical or atypical symptoms. Both symptomatic and asymptomatic patients are at an increased risk of MI, stroke, and cardiovascular and all-cause mortalities. Furthermore, progression of PAD results in a decreased quality of life for the affected individual. Patients with known risk factors for PAD should be actively screened with appropriate physical examination and diagnostic testing. Timely referral to a vascular specialist is also warranted. There are numerous modalities available to clinicians to evaluate patients with suspected PAD. All the different imaging techniques play a role in the evaluation, management, and follow-up of patients with PAD. **Fig. 3** outlines one clinical approach in patients with suspected PAD. Clinically, the first step involves a thorough history taking and physical examination, including obtaining an ABI or TBI in patients with noncompressible vessels. Patients with an abnormal ABI can be further evaluated with PVRs and segmental pressure measurements to determine the location of disease within the lower extremities. In addition, patients with normal ABIs and high suspicion of PAD should be evaluated with exercise testing to unmask hemodynamically significant disease.

Once a diagnosis of PAD is established, appropriate treatment can be instituted, which includes aggressive risk factor modification, medical therapy, and, if indicated, invasive intervention. CTA or MRA studies are usually sought as preprocedural planning for either surgical or percutaneous intervention. DSA, however, may allow for

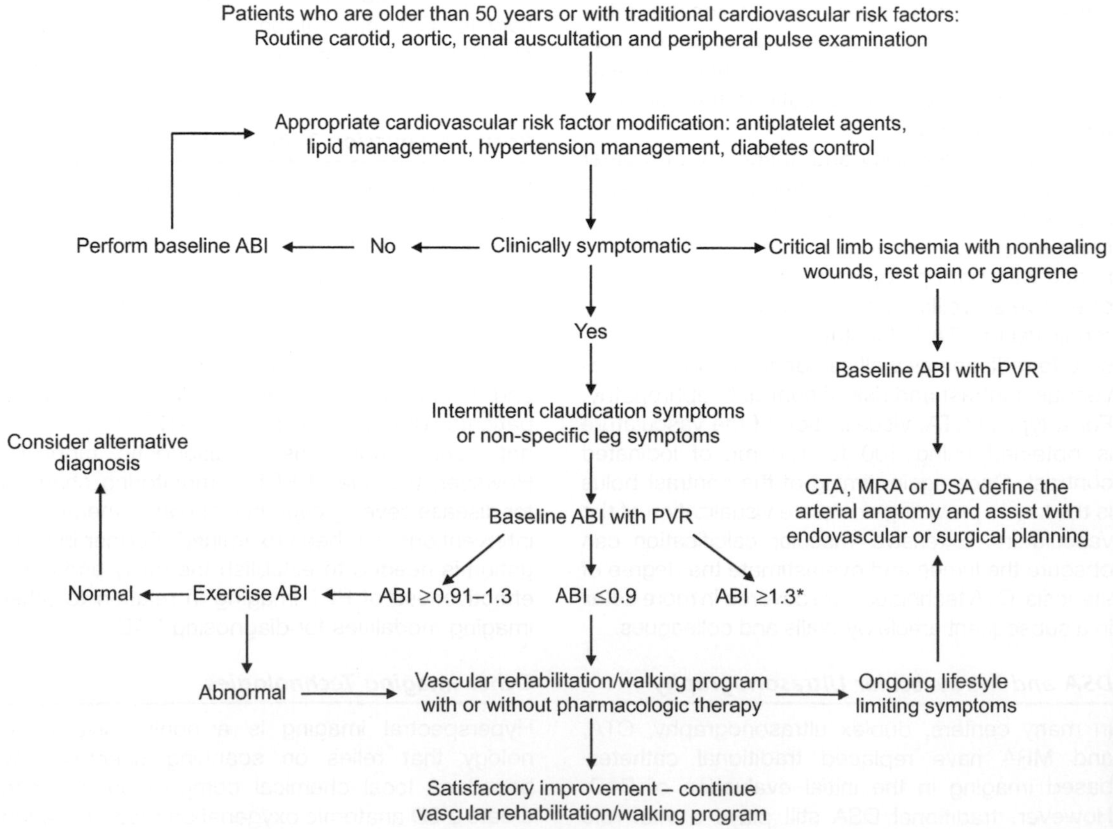


**Fig. 3.** The evaluation of a patient with suspect lower extremity atherosclerotic PAD. * If ABI is greater than 1.3, use TBI and PVR waveforms to determine the presence of vascular disease and follow the appropriate algorithm for ABI of 0.9 or less or of 0.91 to 1.3 or more.

imaging and intervention in a single setting. Once surgical or percutaneous intervention is performed, patients should be placed in surveillance programs, typically using duplex ultrasonography, to identify potential problems and help manage restenosis or impending occlusion. Adoption of recently developed performance measures and national guidelines for the diagnosis and treatment of PAD in clinical practice should improve both the overall care provided to patients with this systemic disease process and outcomes.

## REFERENCES


1. Norgren L, Hiatt WR, Dormandy JA, et al. Inter-Society Consensus for the Management of Peripheral Arterial Disease (TASC II). Eur J Vasc Endovasc Surg 2007;33(Suppl 1):S1–75.
2. Hirsch AT, Haskal ZJ, Hertzer NR, et al. ACC/AHA 2005 Practice Guidelines for the management of patients with peripheral arterial disease (lower extremity, renal, mesenteric, and abdominal aortic): a collaborative report from the American Association for Vascular Surgery/Society for Vascular Surgery, Society for Cardiovascular Angiography and Interventions, Society for Vascular Medicine and Biology, Society of Interventional Radiology, and the ACC/AHA Task Force on Practice Guidelines (Writing Committee to Develop Guidelines for the Management of Patients With Peripheral Arterial Disease): endorsed by the American Association of Cardiovascular and Pulmonary Rehabilitation; National Heart, Lung, and Blood Institute; Society for Vascular Nursing; TransAtlantic Inter-Society Consensus; and Vascular Disease Foundation. Circulation 2006; 113(11):e463–654.
3. Olin JW, Sealove BA. Peripheral artery disease: current insight into the disease and its diagnosis and management. Mayo Clin Proc 2010;85(7):678–92.
4. Hiatt WR. Medical treatment of peripheral arterial disease and claudication. N Engl J Med 2001; 344(21):1608–21.
5. Hirsch AT, Criqui MH, Treat-Jacobson D, et al. Peripheral arterial disease detection, awareness, and treatment in primary care. JAMA 2001; 286(11):1317–24.
6. Criqui MH, Fronek A, Barrett-Connor E, et al. The prevalence of peripheral arterial disease in a defined population. Circulation 1985;71(3):510–5.
7. McDermott MM, Guralnik JM, Ferrucci L, et al. Asymptomatic peripheral arterial disease is associated with more adverse lower extremity characteristics than intermittent claudication. Circulation 2008; 117(19):2484–91.
8. McDermott MM, Greenland P, Guralnik JM, et al. Depressive symptoms and lower extremity functioning in men and women with peripheral arterial disease. J Gen Intern Med 2003;18(6):461–7.
9. Regensteiner JG, Hiatt WR, Coll JR, et al. The impact of peripheral arterial disease on health-related quality of life in the Peripheral Arterial Disease Awareness, Risk, and Treatment: New Resources for Survival (PARTNERS) Program. Vasc Med 2008;13(1):15–24.
10. Resnick HE, Lindsay RS, McDermott MM, et al. Relationship of high and low ankle brachial index to all-cause and cardiovascular disease mortality: the Strong Heart Study. Circulation 2004;109(6):733–9.
11. Criqui MH, Langer RD, Fronek A, et al. Mortality over a period of 10 years in patients with peripheral arterial disease. N Engl J Med 1992;326(6):381–6.
12. Fowkes FG, Murray GD, Butcher I, et al. Ankle brachial index combined with Framingham Risk Score to predict cardiovascular events and mortality: a meta-analysis. JAMA 2008;300(2):197–208.
13. Bundo M, Munoz L, Perez C, et al. Asymptomatic peripheral arterial disease in type 2 diabetes patients: a 10-year follow-up study of the utility of the ankle brachial index as a prognostic marker of cardiovascular disease. Ann Vasc Surg 2010;24(8): 985–93.
14. Rasmussen TE, Clouse WD, Tonnessen BH. Handbook of patient care in vascular diseases. 5th edition. Philadelphia: Lippincott Williams & Wilkins; 2008.
15. Leng GC, Fowkes FG. The Edinburgh Claudication Questionnaire: an improved version of the WHO/Rose Questionnaire for use in epidemiological surveys. J Clin Epidemiol 1992;45(10):1101–9.
16. Rose G, McCartney P, Reid DD. Self-administration of a questionnaire on chest pain and intermittent claudication. Br J Prev Soc Med 1977;31(1):42–8.
17. Pickett CA, Jackson JL, Hemann BA, et al. Carotid bruits as a prognostic indicator of cardiovascular death and myocardial infarction: a meta-analysis. Lancet 2008;371(9624):1587–94.
18. Carter SA. Indirect systolic pressures and pulse waves in arterial occlusive diseases of the lower extremities. Circulation 1968;37(4):624–37.
19. Carter SA. Clinical measurement of systolic pressures in limbs with arterial occlusive disease. JAMA 1969;207(10):1869–74.
20. Newman AB, Tyrrell KS, Kuller LH. Mortality over four years in SHEP participants with a low ankle-arm index. J Am Geriatr Soc 1997;45(12):1472–8.
21. Vogt MT, Cauley JA, Newman AB, et al. Decreased ankle/arm blood pressure index and mortality in elderly women. JAMA 1993;270(4):465–9.
22. McKenna M, Wolfson S, Kuller L. The ratio of ankle and arm arterial pressure as an independent predictor of mortality. Atherosclerosis 1991;87(2–3): 119–28.
23. Newman AB, Shemanski L, Manolio TA, et al. Ankle-arm index as a predictor of cardiovascular disease

and mortality in the Cardiovascular Health Study. The Cardiovascular Health Study Group. Arterioscler Thromb Vasc Biol 1999;19(3):538–45.
24. Criqui MH, Coughlin SS, Fronek A. Noninvasively diagnosed peripheral arterial disease as a predictor of mortality: results from a prospective study. Circulation 1985;72(4):768–73.
25. Newman AB, Siscovick DS, Manolio TA, et al. Ankle-arm index as a marker of atherosclerosis in the Cardiovascular Health Study. Cardiovascular Heart Study (CHS) Collaborative Research Group. Circulation 1993;88(3):837–45.
26. Zheng ZJ, Sharrett AR, Chambless LE, et al. Associations of ankle-brachial index with clinical coronary heart disease, stroke and preclinical carotid and popliteal atherosclerosis: the Atherosclerosis Risk in Communities (ARIC) Study. Atherosclerosis 1997;131(1):115–25.
27. Kasapis C, Gurm HS. Current approach to the diagnosis and treatment of femoral-popliteal arterial disease. A systematic review. Curr Cardiol Rev 2009;5(4):296–311.
28. McPhail IR, Spittell PC, Weston SA, et al. Intermittent claudication: an objective office-based assessment. J Am Coll Cardiol 2001;37(5):1381–5.
29. Gornik HL, Garcia B, Wolski K, et al. Validation of a method for determination of the ankle-brachial index in the seated position. J Vasc Surg 2008; 48(5):1204–10.
30. Rutherford RB, Lowenstein DH, Klein MF. Combining segmental systolic pressures and plethysmography to diagnose arterial occlusive disease of the legs. Am J Surg 1979;138(2):211–8.
31. Kohler TR, Nance DR, Cramer MM, et al. Duplex scanning for diagnosis of aortoiliac and femoropopliteal disease: a prospective study. Circulation 1987;76(5):1074–80.
32. Moneta GL, Yeager RA, Antonovic R, et al. Accuracy of lower extremity arterial duplex mapping. J Vasc Surg 1992;15(2):275–83 [discussion: 283–4].
33. Whelan JF, Barry MH, Moir JD. Color flow Doppler ultrasonography: comparison with peripheral arteriography for the investigation of peripheral vascular disease. J Clin Ultrasound 1992;20(6):369–74.
34. Olin JW, Kaufman JA, Bluemke DA, et al. Atherosclerotic Vascular Disease Conference: Writing Group IV: imaging. Circulation 2004;109(21):2626–33.
35. Correas JM, Claudon M, Tranquart F, et al. The kidney: imaging with microbubble contrast agents. Ultrasound Q 2006;22(1):53–66.
36. Eiberg JP, Hansen MA, Jensen F, et al. Ultrasound contrast-agent improves imaging of lower limb occlusive disease. Eur J Vasc Endovasc Surg 2003;25(1):23–8.
37. Mirza TA, Karthikesalingam A, Jackson D, et al. Duplex ultrasound and contrast-enhanced ultrasound versus computed tomography for the detection of endoleak after EVAR: systematic review and bivariate meta-analysis. Eur J Vasc Endovasc Surg 2010;39(4):418–28.
38. Helck A, Hoffmann RT, Sommer WH, et al. Diagnosis, therapy monitoring and follow up of renal artery pseudoaneurysm with contrast-enhanced ultrasound in three cases. Clin Hemorheol Microcirc 2010;46(2–3):127–37.
39. Fischer T, Dieckhofer J, Muhler M, et al. The use of contrast-enhanced US in renal transplant: first results and potential clinical benefit. Eur Radiol 2005;15(Suppl 5):E109–16.
40. Tang GL, Chin J, Kibbe MR. Advances in diagnostic imaging for peripheral arterial disease. Expert Rev Cardiovasc Ther 2010;8(10):1447–55.
41. Janvier MA, Destrempes F, Soulez G, et al. Validation of a new 3D-US imaging robotic system to detect and quantify lower limb arterial stenoses. Conf Proc IEEE Eng Med Biol Soc 2007;2007:339–42.
42. Grist TM. MRA of the abdominal aorta and lower extremities. J Magn Reson Imaging 2000;11(1):32–43.
43. Menke J, Larsen J. Meta-analysis: accuracy of contrast-enhanced magnetic resonance angiography for assessing steno-occlusions in peripheral arterial disease. Ann Intern Med 2010;153(5):325–34.
44. Prince MR, Meaney JF. Expanding role of MR angiography in clinical practice. Eur Radiol 2006; 16(Suppl 2):B3–8.
45. Ersoy H, Zhang H, Prince MR. Peripheral MR angiography. J Cardiovasc Magn Reson 2006;8(3):517–28.
46. Prince MR. Peripheral vascular MR angiography: the time has come. Radiology 1998;206(3):592–3.
47. Prince MR, Narasimham DL, Stanley JC, et al. Breath-hold gadolinium-enhanced MR angiography of the abdominal aorta and its major branches. Radiology 1995;197(3):785–92.
48. Leiner T. Magnetic resonance angiography of abdominal and lower extremity vasculature. Top Magn Reson Imaging 2005;16(1):21–66.
49. Dinter DJ, Neff KW, Visciani G, et al. Peripheral bolus-chase MR angiography: analysis of risk factors for nondiagnostic image quality of the calf vessels—a combined retrospective and prospective study. AJR Am J Roentgenol 2009;193(1):234–40.
50. Leiner T, Kessels AG, Nelemans PJ, et al. Peripheral arterial disease: comparison of color duplex US and contrast-enhanced MR angiography for diagnosis. Radiology 2005;235(2):699–708.
51. Fleischmann D, Hallett RL, Rubin GD. CT angiography of peripheral arterial disease. J Vasc Interv Radiol 2006;17(1):3–26.
52. Rubin GD, Shiau MC, Leung AN, et al. Aorta and iliac arteries: single versus multiple detector-row helical CT angiography. Radiology 2000;215(3): 670–6.
53. Rubin GD, Schmidt AJ, Logan LJ, et al. Multi-detector row CT angiography of lower extremity

arterial inflow and runoff: initial experience. Radiology 2001;221(1):146–58.

54. Sun Z. Diagnostic accuracy of multislice CT angiography in peripheral arterial disease. J Vasc Interv Radiol 2006;17(12):1915–21.
55. Menke J. Diagnostic accuracy of multidetector CT in acute mesenteric ischemia: systematic review and meta-analysis. Radiology 2010;256(1):93–101.
56. Tutein Nolthenius RP, van den Berg JC, Moll FL. The value of intraoperative intravascular ultrasound for determining stent graft size (excluding abdominal aortic aneurysm) with a modular system. Ann Vasc Surg 2000;14(4):311–7.
57. van Essen JA, Gussenhoven EJ, van der Lugt A, et al. Accurate assessment of abdominal aortic aneurysm with intravascular ultrasound scanning: validation with computed tomographic angiography. J Vasc Surg 1999;29(4):631–8.
58. Kohno H, Sueda S. Rupture of a peripheral popliteal artery plaque documented by intravascular ultrasound: a case report. Catheter Cardiovasc Interv 2009;74(7):1102–6.
59. Farooq MU, Khasnis A, Majid A, et al. The role of optical coherence tomography in vascular medicine. Vasc Med 2009;14(1):63–71.
60. Meissner OA, Rieber J, Babaryka G, et al. Intravascular optical coherence tomography: comparison with histopathology in atherosclerotic peripheral artery specimens. J Vasc Interv Radiol 2006;17(2 Pt 1):343–9.
61. Karnabatidis D, Katsanos K, Paraskevopoulos I, et al. Frequency-domain intravascular optical coherence tomography of the femoropopliteal artery. Cardiovasc Intervent Radiol December 30 2010. [Epub ahead of print].
62. Chao A, Major K, Kumar SR, et al. Carbon dioxide digital subtraction angiography-assisted endovascular aortic aneurysm repair in the azotemic patient. J Vasc Surg 2007;45(3):451–8 [discussion: 458–60].
63. Perry JT, Statler JD. Advances in vascular imaging. Surg Clin North Am 2007;87(5):975–93, vii.
64. El-Haddad G, Zhuang H, Gupta N, et al. Evolving role of positron emission tomography in the management of patients with inflammatory and other benign disorders. Semin Nucl Med 2004;34(4):313–29.
65. Rudd JH, Myers KS, Bansilal S, et al. Atherosclerosis inflammation imaging with 18F-FDG PET: carotid, iliac, and femoral uptake reproducibility, quantification methods, and recommendations. J Nucl Med 2008;49(6):871–8.
66. Sinusas AJ. Imaging of angiogenesis. J Nucl Cardiol 2004;11(5):617–33.
67. Nouvong A, Hoogwerf B, Mohler E, et al. Evaluation of diabetic foot ulcer healing with hyperspectral imaging of oxyhemoglobin and deoxyhemoglobin. Diabetes Care 2009;32(11):2056–61.
68. Khaodhiar L, Dinh T, Schomacker KT, et al. The use of medical hyperspectral technology to evaluate microcirculatory changes in diabetic foot ulcers and to predict clinical outcomes. Diabetes Care 2007;30(4):903–10.
69. Jaffer FA, Libby P, Weissleder R. Molecular and cellular imaging of atherosclerosis: emerging applications. J Am Coll Cardiol 2006;47(7):1328–38.

# Advances in CT Angiography for Peripheral Arterial Disease

Michael C. Walls, MD[a],
Paaladinesh Thavendiranathan, MD, FRCPC[a],
Sanjay Rajagopalan, MD[b,*]

**KEYWORDS**
- CT Angiography • Peripheral arterial disease
- Vascular imaging • Computed tomography

Multidetector CT scan (MDCT) has clearly revolutionized the diagnosis of peripheral arterial disease (PAD). Adequate imaging of the peripheral vascular system during a single acquisition and a single injection of contrast medium became feasible with the introduction of a 4-slice system with 0.5 second gantry rotation (collimation 4 × 2.5 mm) in 1998.[1] The introduction of 16-slice CT allowed acquisition of large anatomic volumes with isotropic submillimeter spatial resolution. Two approaches were introduced by different vendors in 2004. The "volume concept" pursued by GE (GE Medical Systems, Milwaukee, WI, USA), Philips (Philips Healthcare, The Netherlands), and Toshiba (Toshiba Medical Systems, Tochigi-ken, Japan) aimed at a further increase in volume coverage speed by using larger arrays of detectors without changing the physical parameters of the scanner. The "resolution concept" pursued by Siemens (Siemens Medical Solutions, Forchheim, Germany) used a lower number of physical detector rows (eg, 32) in combination with double z-sampling, a technique enabled by a periodic motion of the focal spot in the z-direction, to simultaneously acquire overlapping slices with the goal of pitch-independent increase of longitudinal resolution and reduction of spiral artifacts.[2–4] The most recent generation of CT scan systems further increase the number of detector arrays (eg, 320), which allows further increases in volume coverage and acquisition of large volumes rapidly.[5] Although clearly advantageous in coronary imaging, these have provided advantages in vascular imaging, including arterial phase imaging and diagnosis of vascular disorders such as dissection. Furthermore, the introduction of dual-source scanners has allowed the possibility of tissue characterization in CT scans.[6,7] This article briefly discusses the basic principles of MDCT and provides an overview of its application in vascular diseases.

## TECHNOLOGICAL CONSIDERATIONS

### *Major Components of a CT Scanner*

The major components of a CT scanner are an x-ray tube and generator, a collimator, and photon detectors.[4,8] These components are mounted on a rotating gantry. The x-ray tube produces the x-rays necessary for imaging. The predetector collimator helps shape the x-ray beams that emanate from the x-ray tube in order to cut out unnecessary radiation. The detectors consist of multiple rows of detector elements (>900 elements per row in the

The authors have nothing to disclose.
[a] Division of Cardiovascular Medicine, Department of Internal Medicine, The Ohio State University, 473 West 12th Avenue, Suite 200 DHLRI, Columbus, OH 43210, USA
[b] Division of Cardiology, The Ohio State University, 200 Davis Heart and Lung Research, 473 West 12th Avenue, Columbus, OH 43210, USA
* Corresponding author.
*E-mail address:* Sanjay.Rajagopalan@osumc.edu

Cardiol Clin 29 (2011) 331–340
doi:10.1016/j.ccl.2011.04.001

current scanners), which receive x-ray photons that have traversed through the patient, with the postdetector collimators preventing back-scatter. The newer scanners have as many as 320 detector rows. With the increase in detector rows the width of each detector ("detector collimation") has decreased from 2.5 mm in 4-slice systems to 0.5 mm in the 320-slice systems. The most important benefit of increasing the detector rows is the increased coverage per gantry rotation (a 320 row detector CT scan with a detector width of 0.5 mm will have coverage in the z-axis of 160 mm). Decreased detector width improves spatial resolution in the z-axis, whereas increased coverage shortens scan time. Each detector element consists of a radiation-sensitive solid state material (such as cadmium tungstate, gadolinium-oxide, or gadolinium oxysulfide with suitable dopings), which converts the absorbed x-rays into visible light.[2] The light is then detected by a silicone photodiode. The resulting electrical current is amplified and converted into a digital signal. The gantry rotation time determines the temporal resolution of the images with older scanners having a rotation time of 0.75 seconds, whereas the more contemporary scanners have a rotation time of 0.33 seconds. The temporal resolution of a single source scanner is slightly higher than half the time it takes for the gantry to rotate 360 degrees as it is possible to generate the entire data set with a little more than 180 degrees of rotation. Thus, a 0.33 second gantry rotation will effectively provide a temporal resolution of 0.17 seconds.

### *CT Scan Attenuation Data for Image Reconstruction*

CT scan measures the local x-ray attenuation coefficients of the tissue volume elements, or voxels, in an axial slice of the patient's anatomy. The attenuation coefficients are translated into the gray-scale values (CT scan value) of the corresponding picture elements (pixels) in the displayed two-dimensional image of the slice. The numeric value $I_{ij}$ assigned to a pixel (i,j) corresponds to the average x-ray attenuation $\mu(x_i,y_j)$ within its associated voxel $(x_i,y_j)$, after normalization to the attenuation properties of water. Pixel values are stored as integers, in the range −1024 Hounsfield units (HU) to 3071 HU, corresponding to 4096 different values. In general, lung and fat have negative CT scan values, while bone has large CT scan values up to 2000 HU. Administration of iodine contrast agent increases the CT scan value with contrast-filled vessels typically having CT scan values in the range 200 HU to 600 HU. In most cases, they can be easily differentiated from the surrounding tissue that does not exceed a CT scan value of 100 HU with the exception of bone. The gantry rotates around the patient collecting attenuation data from different angles. The attenuation coefficient also varies depending on the energy of the photons (measured in kiloelectron volt [keV]) that pass through them. The measured intensity of photons at the CT scan detector can be expressed using a formula (below) describing the relationship between the photon flux coming through the x-ray tube and that detected at the detector elements.

$$I = I_o e^{-\mu}$$

*I* is the intensity measured at the detector, $I_o$ is the photon flux from the x-ray tube measured in mA, and *e* is the exponent, and $\mu$ is the attenuation coefficient.

Therefore as the attenuation of the tissue increases, the fraction of photons that are detected at the detector element decreases. Photon energy (keV) and photon flux (mA) are variables that are set by the user. $I_0$ or tube current expressed as mA may be defined as the number of photons emanating from the focal spot. Thus, a high $I_0$ improves image quality but also increases radiation dose. Often an effective tube current ($I_{eff}$ or effective mA) is given by the equation below.

$$I_{eff} = I_{tube} \cdot T$$

*T* is the illumination time.

Tube voltage [keV] determines the energy of the x-ray beam or the hardness of the x-ray. A high keV results in a smaller fraction of the x-ray beam being absorbed (reduced attenuation) but will result in improvements in contrast. Some manufacturers, such as Siemens, have introduced an "effective" mA-concept for spiral or helical scanning, which includes the factor 1/pitch (*p*) into the mA; see definition below.

$$(\text{mAs})_{eff} = \text{mA} \times t_{rot} \times 1/p = \text{mAs} \times 1/p$$

### *Scanning Modes*

The two scanning modes used in CT angiography (CTA) are the axial mode and the spiral or helical mode. The major differences between these modes include (1) table movement during image acquisition, (2) assignment of data to each channel, and (3) need for interpolation for data reconstruction. Each mode has its benefits; however, the mode used for vascular CTA is the spiral or helical mode. For coronary CTA there has been a shift toward using axial mode due to its benefit in significantly reducing radiation exposure. During spiral scanning there is continuous table movement and the tube is on the whole time; however, the tube current can be made to fluctuate (current modulation). Because the table is moving during the acquisition, the detector channels are not dedicated to a slice of the patient and, hence, it receives data from multiple contiguous slices of the patient. An interpolation algorithm would be necessary to reconstruct "virtual" axial slices with some loss in image quality.[9] Spiral imaging is fast and can provide infinite reconstruction of data; however, this is at the cost of higher radiation.

### *Beam Pitch*

Pitch is an expression of the relationship between the table distance moved per gantry rotation and the coverage of the scanner. Pitch = [table feed per gantry rotation (mm)/coverage (mm)]. If the pitch is 1, then there are no gaps between the data set; however, if the pitch is greater than 1, gaps are present and, if the pitch is less than 1, there is overlap in the data acquisition. The pitch for ECG-gated cardiac scanning the pitch is 0.2 to 0.3. For most vascular CT scans, the pitch ranges between 0.5 and 1.2.[3,8]

### *Radiation Dose Reduction Techniques Relevant in Peripheral CTA*

Radiation exposure of the patient by CT scan and the resulting potential radiation hazard has recently gained considerable attention both in the public and in the scientific literature. There are several ways to lower the dose that can be used alone or together. Using EKG-gated tube current modulation is not relevant as peripheral CTA is typically done without EKG gating.

#### *Reduction of tube current*

Lowering the mA settings according to the patient's body habitus can lead to decreases in radiation dose.

#### *Reduction of tube voltage*

Clinical studies have demonstrated a potential for dose reduction of about 30% to 50% when using 80 kV instead of 120 kV for performing CTA. One study recommended 100 kV as the standard mode for aortoiliac CTA and reports dose savings of 30% without loss of diagnostic information, so this is one potential approach.[10] Another study evaluated use of 80 kV and reduced contrast dose in PAD and reported no differences in visual quality but a 30% reduction in radiation dose and contrast dose.[11]

#### *Anatomic tube current modulation*

The tube output is modulated based on the tissue attenuation characteristics of the localizer scan. This allows reduction of dose by 15% to 35% without degrading image quality, depending on the body region. A more sophisticated variation of anatomic tube current modulation varies the tube output according to the patient geometry and in the longitudinal direction to maintain adequate dose when moving to different body regions, for instance from thorax to abdomen (automatic exposure control). Automatic adaptation of the tube current to patient size prevents both over-irradiation and under-irradiation, which considerably simplifies the clinical workflow for the technician and eliminates the need for look-up tables of patient weight and size for adjusting the mA settings.

## APPROACH TO LOWER-EXTREMITY IMAGING

### *General Acquisition Protocol for Lower-Extremity Arterial CTA*

Low-osmolar nonionic contrast agents are most commonly used for CTA applications.[12] Patients' renal function should be assessed before administration of contrast and decisions regarding prophylactic medication use should be made if necessary. The selection of the specific acquisition parameters of imaging depends on the employed scanner model, the patient's body habitus, and the clinical question. The voltage is typically set at 120 kV, although 100 kV or even 80 kV provides acceptable images with significantly reduced radiation and can be employed in most individuals with PAD who are not obese.[10,11] Tube current is usually 200 to 300 mA and can be adjusted upward if the patient is very large. Breath-holding is required only for the chest and abdomen CTA acquisitions to reduce motion artifact. Although current generation scanners offer improved spatial resolution, their increased coverage and rotation speeds pose the risk of "out-running" the bolus of contrast in CTA applications. Accordingly, adjustments in both the pitch and the gantry rotation speed must be made to achieve a table translation speed of no more than 30 to 32 mm/s for CTA applications. In a 64-slice scanner, this usually is achieved by a reduction in $t_{rot}$ to 0.5 seconds and a decrease in pitch to less than or equal to 0.8. Patients are placed in a supine position on the scanner table in a feet-first orientation. The typical field-of-view (FOV) should extend from the diaphragm to the toes with an average scan length of 110 to 130 cm. The scanning protocol begins with a scout image of the entire FOV followed by a test bolus or bolus triggering acquisition. When an automated bolus detection algorithm is used, the region of interest is set up in the aorta immediately below the level of the diaphragm. A repetitive monitor acquisition (120 kV, 10 mA, 1-second interscan delay) is started 10 seconds after contrast injection begins. The actual peripheral CTA acquisition is then started when the contrast enhancement reaches a prespecified level (typically set between 150–200 HU). Breath-holding may be necessary for the more proximal abdominal station, but not for the distal stations. A second late acquisition of the calf vessels can be prescribed in the event of inadequate pedal opacification during the arterial phase. For most CTA applications, 100 to 140 mL of contrast (with an iodine concentration between 350–370 mg/mL) is administered at a rate of 4 mL/s followed by a saline flush.[13] Recently a fixed-time strategy has been recommended and may provide a better strategy to image peripheral arterial disease (**Table 1**).[14] In this strategy the pitch is varied to accomplish a fixed scan time of 40 seconds in all patients. A biphasic injection protocol is used that provides for sustained opacification of the arterial system. This approach standardizes PAD-imaging protocols and consistently provides for good quality scans.

### *Image Reconstruction at the Scanner Console*

Various image reconstruction filters are offered by each manufacturer and are referred to as "sharp" or "soft" filters. Sharper reconstruction filters will provide more details but also more noise and are best for assessment of stents and areas of calcifications.[15] Softer reconstruction filters provide less image detail but less noise. Soft-to-medium filters are used for most CTA applications. Slice width and slice increment used for image reconstruction at the scanner console depends on the anatomy being assessed and scanner capabilities. Reconstruction thickness for vascular imaging can be performed at the same width (thin) or several times the detector width (thick) to reduce noise (thinner slices are associated with higher image noise compared with thicker slices and take a longer time to review). A slice increment of approximately 50% of the slice thickness is typically used.

### *Image Postprocessing*

Multiple postprocessing techniques can be used and include (1) multiplanar reformats (MPR), (2) maximal intensity projections (MIP), (3) curved planer reformats (CPR), (4) volume rendering (VR), and (5) shaded surface display (SSD).[16] For CTA, the evaluation of the data set begins with review of the axial images to assess gross anatomy and scan quality.[17] This is followed by use of a MIP format in traditional projections as well as in oblique projections. Care must be taken viewing MIP images when calcium is present, as it can overestimate the severity of stenotic lesions and severely affect diagnostic quality.[18] For detailed evaluation, especially when calcium and stents are present, the raw MPR images should be reviewed. Each of these reconstruction methods has its pitfalls and it is important to assess an abnormality identified in a systematic manner, in multiple different planes, using different techniques, and different phases of the cardiac cycle if available.

## CLINICAL APPLICATION IN LOWER-EXTREMITY ARTERIAL DISEASE

### *Peripheral Arterial Disease*

Atherosclerotic disease is the most common indication for CTA evaluation of the peripheral arterial system (**Fig. 1**). The goal of CTA in PAD is to determine the length, number, severity, and location of stenoses. In conjunction with the patient's

**Table 1**
**Recommended injection protocol for PAD imaging**

| Suggested Injection Protocol | |
|---|---|
| Contrast Agent | Low-osmolar nonionic 350–370 mg/mL |
| Site of Bolus Detection | Aorta, below diaphragm |
| Scan Time | Fixed at 40 s |
| Injection Duration | 35 s |
| Pitch | Variable and adjusted to scan time of 40 s |
| Delay | Bolus trigger to occur on reaching threshold of 150–200 HU |
| Weight-based Biphasic Injection Rate | <55 kg: 20 mL (4 mL/s) + 96 mL (3.2 mL/s)<br>56–65 kg: 23 mL (4.5 mL/s) + 108 mL (3.6 mL/s)<br>66–85 kg: 25 mL (5.0 mL/s) + 120 mL (4.0 mL/s)<br>86–95 kg: 28 mL (5.5 mL/s) + 132 mL (4.4 mL/s)<br>>95 kg: 30 mL (6.0 mL/s) + 144 mL (4.8 mL/s) |

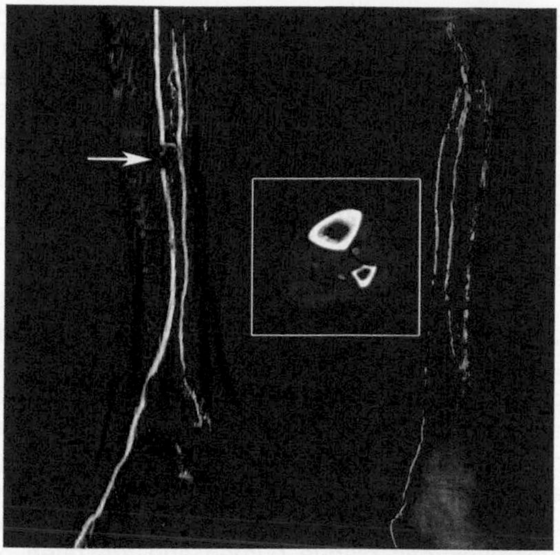

Fig. 1. Distal lower-extremity atherosclerotic disease. Three-dimensional, CTA volume-rendered image shows a segmental occlusion of the anterior tibial artery (*arrow*) with small bridging collateral arteries (*left panel*) and severe, three-vessel atherosclerotic disease of the leg (*right panel*). Axial CTA image (inset) shows calcification within the walls of the anterior tibial, posterior tibial, and peroneal arteries with poor luminal visualization. (*Adapted from* Cohen E, et al. CT angiography of the lower extremity circulation with protocols. In: Mukherjee D, Rajagopalan S, editors. CT and MR angiography of the peripheral circulation. Hampshire [United Kingdom]: Informa UK Ltd; 2007. p. 143; with permission.)

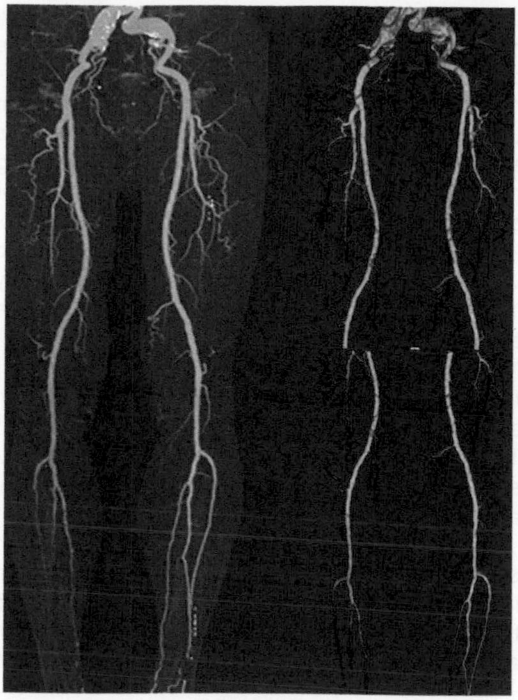

Fig. 2. Abdominal CTA with runoff. Maximal intensity projection (*left panel*) and three-dimensional, CTA volume-rendered images (*right panel*) showing bilateral common iliac aneurysms with distal runoff disease of the right, lower extremity. (*Adapted from* Cohen E, et al. CT angiography of the lower extremity circulation with protocols. In: Mukherjee D, Rajagopalan S, editors. CT and MR angiography of the peripheral circulation. Hampshire [United Kingdom]: Informa UK Ltd; 2007. p. 140; with permission.)

manifestations, activity status and goals, findings on CTA may help determine choice of therapy (conservative, interventional, or surgical). Data from a CTA can help plan the access route as well as the equipment that will be necessary for endovascular repair.[19] CTA is equally useful for surgical planning as it can define proximal and distal anastomotic sites, concomitant disease processes (eg, aneurysm, dissection), and sizing of prostheses or stents. Atherosclerotic disease affecting the inflow vessels (**Fig. 2**) can often be treated by catheter-based therapy with good results and little morbidity. Often the success of therapy, whether surgical or endovascular, depends on the extent of disease in the vessels distal to the area of disease and/or the presence of diabetes. CTA is also commonly the modality of choice in the setting of acute lower-extremity ischemia. A meta-analysis of CTA in PAD, published in 2007, using mostly four-slice systems reported a pooled sensitivity and specificity for detecting a stenosis of greater than 50% or segment of 92% (95% CI of 89%–95%) and 93% (95% CI of 91%–95%), respectively. The diagnostic performance of CTA in the infrapopliteal tract was lower but not significantly different from that in the aortoiliac and femoropopliteal levels.[20] CTA findings clearly influence treatment decisions correctly in the vast majority of cases and are a definitive part of the imaging approach, especially when the decision to intervene percutaneously or surgically must be made.[21,22] At least one study has compared the comparative effectiveness of various imaging approaches in PAD. The outcome measures included the clinical utility, functional patient outcomes, quality of life, and actual diagnostic and therapeutic costs related to the initial imaging test during 6 months of follow-up. Significantly higher confidence and less additional imaging were found for magnetic resonance angiography and CTA compared with duplex sonography at lower costs.[23]

## *Buerger Disease and Vasculitis*

Buerger disease typically affects the small-to-medium–sized arteries of the extremities. It manifests angiographically with a "corkscrew" appearance to the distal arteries (this is, however, not specific for this disorder) and, clinically, the patient can present with claudication (predominantly foot or calf claudication) with or without ulcerations of the digits.[24] Buerger disease is strongly associated with smoking and a smoking cessation program has been shown to halt or dramatically slow the progression of the disease.

Takayasu arteritis generally affects the aorta and visceral vessels. The disease predominantly involves the media and it is rare for the disease to extend to the iliac vessels and the lower extremities. It affects young female patients and manifests as wall-thickening of the aorta with associated narrowing, stenosis, and occlusions.[25] The extent of contrast enhancement of the thickened wall has been correlated with the degree of acute inflammation.

Giant cell arteritis presents in older patients and classically affects medium-sized vessels. It can involve the great vessels off the arch as well as the lower-extremity vessels.[26] It can present in a fashion similar to Takayasu arteritis but the patient's age and the pattern of the diseased vessels will help differentiate it.

Polyarteritis nodosa typically presents with nonspecific vascular symptoms and is strongly associated with hepatitis B infection. When vascular involvement is present it is usually restricted to the visceral vessels but, clinically, the patient can present with microvascular PAD and bilateral symmetric gangrene.

Drug-induced vasculitis is often seen in the patient engaged in recreational drug use as well as patients on clinically indicated therapy. The drugs most often associated with vasculitis are amphetamine derivatives and cocaine. Vasculitis can also be a side effect of some drugs including ephedrine and l-dopa. These patients usually present with vascular stenosis without significant atherosclerotic plaque burden and are often of a younger age. The small-to-medium–sized vessels are typically affected. CTA is particularly useful in this patient group as it allows for accurate assessment of vessel wall thickness and inflammation.

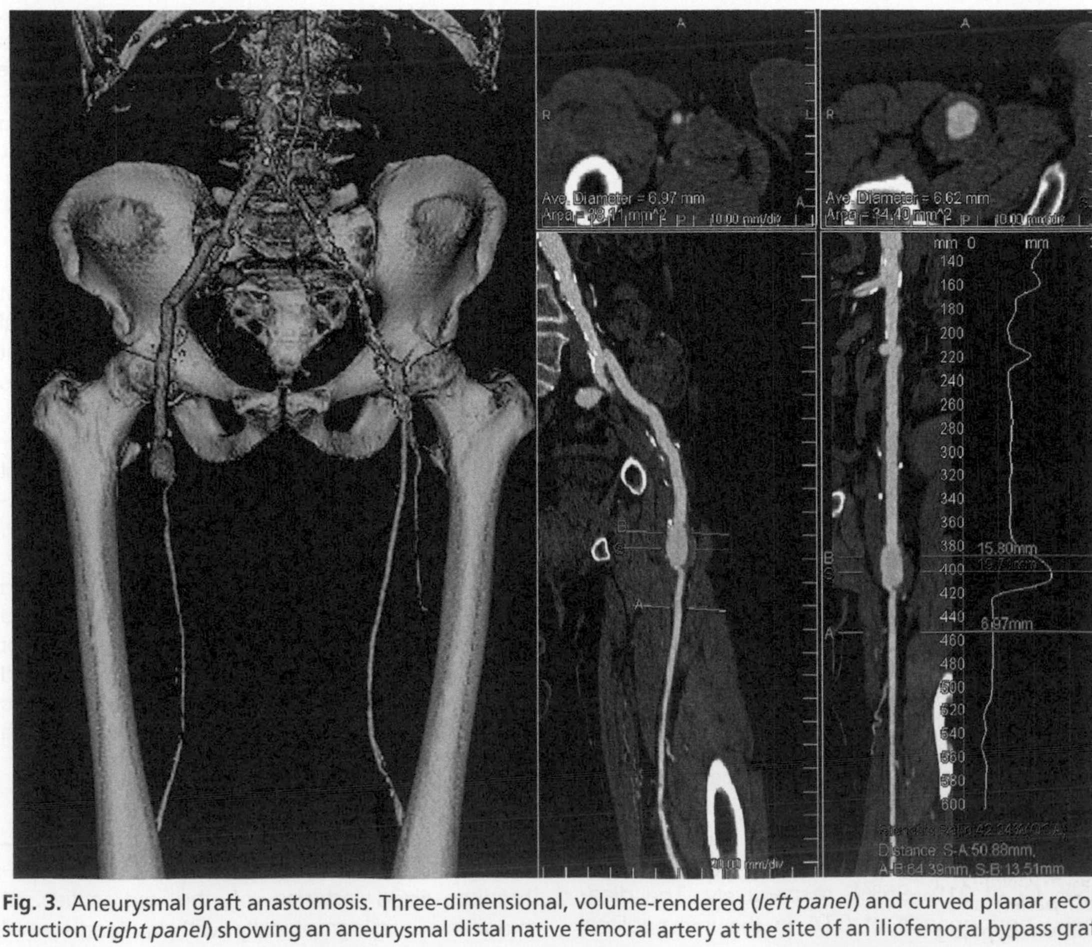


**Fig. 3.** Aneurysmal graft anastomosis. Three-dimensional, volume-rendered (*left panel*) and curved planar reconstruction (*right panel*) showing an aneurysmal distal native femoral artery at the site of an iliofemoral bypass graft.

## *Aneurysms*

CTA is very useful in the assessment of aneurysm location, number, size, and complication (eg, thrombosis, rupture, distal embolization). Aneurysms of the abdominal aorta and lower-extremity vasculature are a frequent complication of atherosclerotic, inflammatory disease, and disorders of collagen metabolism.[27] The most frequent site of extra-aortic aneurysms is in the popliteal region, but they can also involve other vascular territories and are frequently bilateral. Therapy is usually indicated if the aneurysm exceeds 2 cm and/or there is mural thrombus. As the popliteal region is difficult to dissect without significant damage to adjacent structures, the usual course of therapy is to bypass the affected region, usually with a saphenous vein graft. Preventive measures may also be pursued if the vessels distal to the aneurysm are diseased and thereby increase the risk of eventual thrombosis.

## *Stent and Endovascular Graft Evaluation*

CTA may be used for evaluation of in-stent restenosis particularly in proximal vessels such as the iliac and femoral arteries (**Figs. 3** and **4**). This may require reconstruction with alternate kernels and adjustment of window-levels. There is only limited data comparing the performance of CT versus other modalities for the evaluation of peripheral stents.[15] However, there is emerging data for other circulatory beds similar or even smaller compared with lower-extremity vessels. For instance, in a recent prospective study involving assessment of renal in-stent restenosis in 86 patients (95 stents), CT had a negative predictive value of 100%.[28] One case of nonsignificant in-stent restenosis seen at selective x-ray angiography was interpreted as significant by using CT angiography, giving a specificity of 99% and a positive predictive value of 90%. In 4 of 78 patients without in-stent restenosis (ISR) seen at selective catheter renal artery (RA) angiography, CT RA angiography showed no significant ISR, giving a specificity of 95% and a positive predictive value of 56%. In the coronary circulation, sensitivity and specificity using 64-slice systems exceed 90%.[29] However, in practice, these rates may be considerably lower owing to significant publication bias in these reports.

CTA can be used to evaluate patients with aortoiliac, aortofemoral, or axillofemoral bypass grafts who present again with extremity symptoms and have abnormal noninvasive, nonangiographic

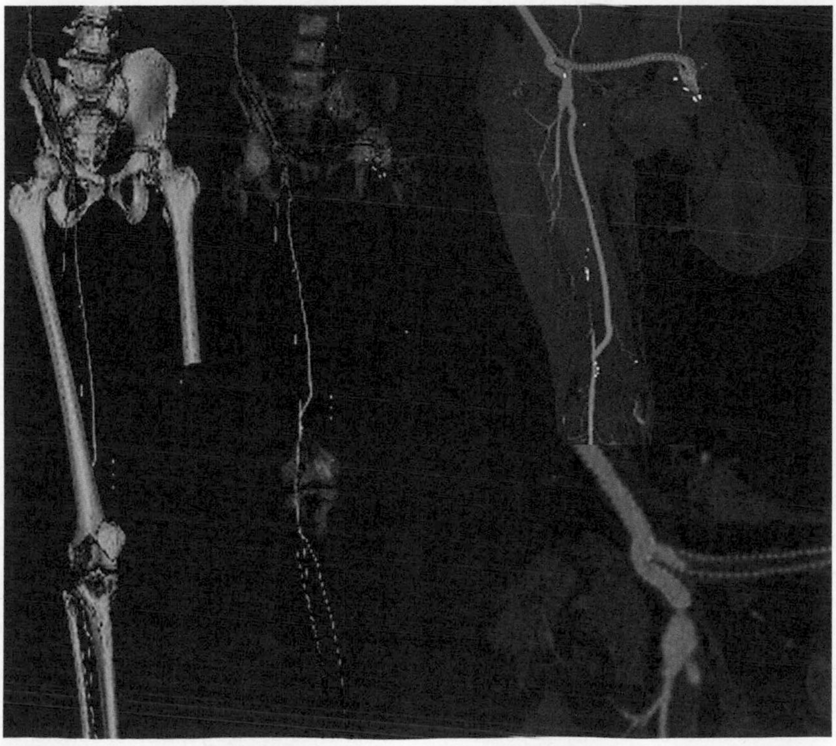

**Fig. 4.** Axillary graft with thrombosed fem-fem bypass graft. Three-dimensional, volume-rendered images (*left panel*) and curved planar images (*right panel*) showing a patent axillary-femoral bypass and occluded fem-fem bypass grafts.

imaging test results.[25] Surveillance of grafts is important and is primarily performed by sonographic evaluation. Nevertheless, recent studies suggest that CTA may be superior to duplex ultrasound evaluation.[30] The regular use of duplex ultrasound for screening is still the recommended approach. However, if symptoms progress or if there is concern regarding disease in other areas, CTA may be an ideal approach; but attention must be paid to the radiation dose especially cumulatively and the use of contrast agents. Assessment of the graft should include careful evaluation of the proximal anastomotic area to exclude stenosis or aneurysm, the body of the graft, and the touch-down site of the graft.

## *Other Indications*

A variety of other conditions may represent less common indications for the use of a peripheral CTA, including persistent sciatic artery (**Fig. 5**), popliteal entrapment (**Fig. 6**), and cystic medial adventitial disease.[31] For instance, arteriovenous malformations and fistulas may be well delineated by acquiring images during the arterial and venous phase. CTA imaging may also significantly contribute to the characterization of congenital abnormalities with direct or indirect involvement of the peripheral vessels.

## *Artifacts and Pitfalls*

There are several artifacts that can been seen with CT imaging that one should be aware of to avoid erroneous interpretation. Artifacts could include those that are related to the patient, procedure, or reconstruction. Three of the most common artifacts include motion artifact, beam hardening, and partial-volume effects. Motion artifacts can occur due to body motion during scanning or inability to hold breath. Beam-hardening artifacts occur due to the passage of photons through structures such as pacemaker leads, metal clips, or calcium

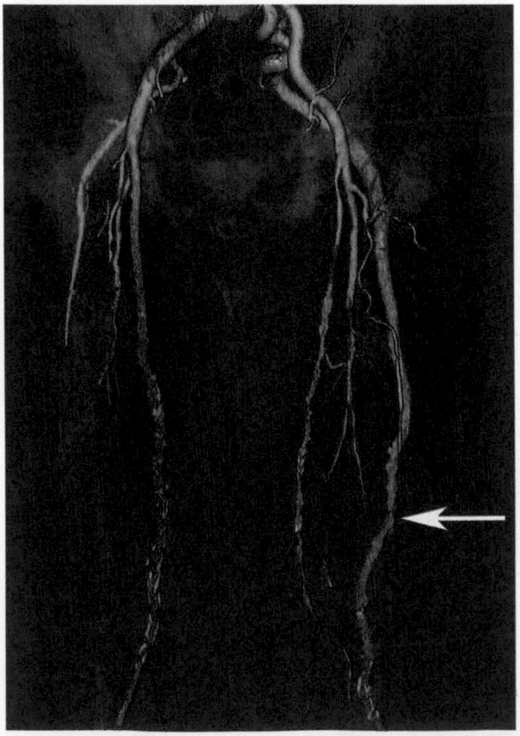

**Fig. 5.** Persistent sciatic artery. Three-dimensional, CTA volume-rendered image shows occlusion of the distal left superficial femoral artery. The left popliteal artery is supplied by a persistent left sciatic artery fed by the internal iliac artery (*arrow*). (*Adapted from* Cohen E, et al. CT angiography of the lower extremity circulation with protocols. In: Mukherjee D, Rajagopalan S, editors. CT and MR angiography of the peripheral circulation. Hampshire [United Kingdom]: Informa UK Ltd; 2007. p. 143; with permission.)

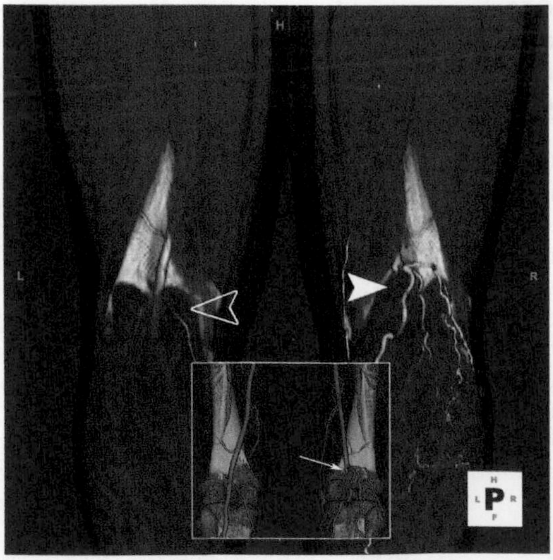

**Fig. 6.** Popliteal artery entrapment. Three-dimensional, CTA volume-rendered image (posteroanterior view) of a young patient with right calf pain on exertion. The medial head of the right gastrocnemius muscle demonstrates an abnormal origin lateral to the popliteal artery (*closed arrowhead*). Inset image shows complete occlusion of the right popliteal artery (*arrow*) with multiple superficial collateral arteries originating just proximal to this level. The normal origin of the medial head of the left gastrocnemius medial to the popliteal artery (*open arrowhead*) is shown for comparison. (*Adapted from* Cohen E, Doshi A, Lookstein R. CT angiography of the lower extremity circulation with protocols. In: Mukherjee D, Rajagopalan S, editors. CT and MR angiography of the peripheral circulation. Hampshire [United Kingdom]: Informa UK Ltd; 2007. p. 143; with permission.)

resulting in lower-energy photons being filtered out. Consequently, dark areas are created next to these structures that can affect assessment of lumen patency. Partial-volume effects occur when parts of the voxel representing a structure has other structures with different attenuation properties resulting in averaging of the CT values for that voxel; therefore, the image appears distorted. The most frequent pitfall encountered during the interpretation of CTA images is represented by the difficulty in the evaluation of vascular segments affected by moderate-to-severe calcification or occupied by a stent. The selection of the adequate windowing set (~1500 window width) may help in reducing the unavoidable blooming effect produced by structures with high signal attenuation. Cross-sectional MPR images of the vessel of interest are very helpful in visualizing, at least in part, the underlying lumen in presence of intense calcification or stent. Other interpretation pitfalls such as pseudostenosis or pseudo-occlusions may potentially be generated by inadequate image postprocessing (eg, partial or total vessel removal during MIP-image editing and inaccurate centerline definition in CPR images).

## SUMMARY

CT scan technology has continued to evolve and its application for the diagnosis of PAD has gained significant momentum. There are multiple publications of clinical studies documenting its accuracy when compared with other modalities. The high spatial resolution and rapid throughput of CTA has enabled its widespread acceptance into evaluation of patients with PAD. CTA is now routinely used in clinical practice and rivals magnetic resonance angiography for evaluation of vascular disease.

## REFERENCES

1. Ligon BL. Biography: history of developments in imaging techniques: Egas Moniz and angiography. Semin Pediatr Infect Dis 2003;14:173.
2. Flohr T, Ohnesorge B. Fundamentals of multislice CT scanning and its application to the periphery. In: Mukherjee D, Rajagopalan S, editors. CT and MR angiography of the peripheral circulation: practical approach with clinical protocols. 1st edition. London (United Kingdom): Informa UK Ltd; 2007. p. 1.
3. Flohr T, Stierstorfer K, Raupach R, et al. Performance evaluation of a 64-slice CT system with z-flying focal spot. Rofo 2004;176:1803.
4. Flohr TG, Schaller S, Stierstorfer K, et al. Multidetector row CT systems and image-reconstruction techniques. Radiology 2005;235:756.
5. Flohr TG, Klotz E, Allmendinger T, et al. Pushing the envelope: new computed tomography techniques for cardiothoracic imaging. J Thorac Imaging 2010;25:100.
6. Boroto K, Remy-Jardin M, Flohr T, et al. Thoracic applications of dual-source CT technology. Eur J Radiol 2008;68:375.
7. Petersilka M, Bruder H, Krauss B, et al. Technical principles of dual source CT. Eur J Radiol 2008; 68:362.
8. Mukherjee D, Rajagopalan S. In: Ct and MR angiography of the peripheral circulation: practical approach with clinical protocols. 1st edition. London (United Kingdom): Informa UK Ltd; 2007. p. 3213.
9. Prokop M. Multislice CT: technical principles and future trends. Eur Radiol 2003;13(Suppl 5):M3.
10. Wintersperger B, Jakobs T, Herzog P, et al. Aorto-iliac multidetector-row CT angiography with low kV settings: improved vessel enhancement and simultaneous reduction of radiation dose. Eur Radiol 2005;15:334.
11. Utsunomiya D, Oda S, Funama Y, et al. Comparison of standard- and low-tube voltage MDCT angiography in patients with peripheral arterial disease. Eur Radiol 2010;20:2758.
12. Mukherjee D, Rajagopalan S. X ray contrast agents and contrast timing considerations. In: Mukherjee D, Rajagopalan S, editors. CT and MR angiography of the peripheral circulation: practical approach with clinical protocols. 1st edition. London (United Kingdom): Informa UK Ltd; 2007. p. 53–62.
13. Cohen Ei, Doshi A, Lookstein RA. CT angiography of the lower extremity circulation with protocols. In: Mukherjee D, Rajagopalan S, editors. CT and MR angiography of the peripheral circulation: practical approach with clinical protocols. 1st edition. London (United Kingdom): Informa UK Ltd; 2007. p. 133–46.
14. Fleischmann D. CT angiography: injection and acquisition technique. Radiol Clin North Am 2010; 48:237.
15. Blum MB, Schmook M, Schernthaner R, et al. Quantification and detectability of in-stent stenosis with CT angiography and MR angiography in arterial stents in vitro. AJR Am J Roentgenol 2007;189:1238.
16. Jang JJ. Image postprocessing in CT. In: Mukherjee D, Rajagopalan S, editors. CT and MR angiography of the peripheral circulation: practical approach with clinical protocols. 1st edition. London (United Kingdom): Informa UK Ltd; 2007. p. 43–52.
17. Ota H, Takase K, Igarashi K, et al. MDCT compared with digital subtraction angiography for assessment of lower extremity arterial occlusive disease: importance of reviewing cross-sectional images. AJR Am J Roentgenol 2004;182:201.
18. Ouwendijk R, Kock MC, van Dijk LC, et al. Vessel wall calcifications at multi-detector row CT angiography in patients with peripheral arterial disease: effect

on clinical utility and clinical predictors. Radiology 2006;241:603.
19. Fleischmann D, Lammer J. Peripheral CT angiography for interventional treatment planning. Eur Radiol 2006;16(Suppl 7):M58.
20. Heijenbrok-Kal MH, Kock MC, Hunink MG. Lower extremity arterial disease: multidetector CT angiography meta-analysis. Radiology 2007;245:433.
21. Dellegrottaglie S, Sanz J, Macaluso F, et al. Technology Insight: magnetic resonance angiography for the evaluation of patients with peripheral artery disease. Nat Clin Pract Cardiovasc Med 2007; 4:677.
22. Schernthaner R, Fleischmann D, Lomoschitz F, et al. Effect of MDCT angiographic findings on the management of intermittent claudication. AJR Am J Roentgenol 2007;189:1215.
23. Ouwendijk R, de Vries M, Stijnen T, et al. Multicenter randomized controlled trial of the costs and effects of noninvasive diagnostic imaging in patients with peripheral arterial disease: the DIPAD trial. AJR Am J Roentgenol 2008;190:1349.
24. Piazza G, Creager MA. Thromboangiitis obliterans. Circulation 2010;121:1858–61.
25. Foley WD, Stonely T. CT angiography of the lower extremities. Radiol Clin North Am 2010;48:367.
26. Tato F, Hoffmann U. Giant cell arteritis: a systemic vascular disease. Vasc Med 2008;13:127.
27. Mattar SG, Kumar AG, Lumsden AB. Vascular complications in Ehlers-Danlos syndrome. Am Surg 1994;60:827.
28. Steinwender C, Schutzenberger W, Fellner F, et al. 64-Detector CT angiography in renal artery stent evaluation: prospective comparison with selective catheter angiography. Radiology 2009;252:299.
29. Sun Z, Almutairi AM. Diagnostic accuracy of 64 multislice CT angiography in the assessment of coronary in-stent restenosis: a meta-analysis. Eur J Radiol 2009;73:266.
30. Willmann JK, Mayer D, Banyai M, et al. Evaluation of peripheral arterial bypass grafts with multi-detector row CT angiography: comparison with duplex US and digital subtraction angiography. Radiology 2003;229:465.
31. Deutsch AL, Hyde J, Miller SM, et al. Cystic adventitial degeneration of the popliteal artery: CT demonstration and directed percutaneous therapy. AJR Am J Roentgenol 1985;145:117.

# Noncontrast MRA for the Diagnosis of Vascular Diseases

Georgeta Mihai, PhD[a,*], Orlando P. Simonetti, PhD[a,b], Paaladinesh Thavendiranathan, MD, FRCPC[a]

**KEYWORDS**

• Angiography • Noncontrast • Vascular imaging
• Magnetic resonance imaging

Magnetic resonance angiography (MRA) has become the modality of choice for noninvasive imaging of diverse vascular beds. MRA techniques can be divided into 2 main categories: contrast agent–enhanced and noncontrast angiographic approaches. Both techniques have benefited from recent improvements in MR hardware, software, and rapid acquisition methodologies such as parallel imaging. Until recently, noncontrast techniques have played mostly a back-up role when contrast-enhanced sequences were suboptimal owing to artifacts or poor timing of contrast injection. However, the association between the usage of gadolinium (Gd) contrast and nephrogenic systemic fibrosis (NSF) disease in individuals with intrinsic renal dysfunction has rekindled interest in noncontrast angiography techniques.

The purpose of this article is to summarize and briefly describe noncontrast MRA techniques that are useful in the clinical context. Noncontrast techniques are divided, as they usually are, based on the appearance of the imaged vascular lumen into bright-blood and black-blood angiographic techniques. A section of the article is dedicated to summarize NSF description, and another section discusses application of noncontrast MRA approaches in carotid, thoracic/abdominal, renal, and peripheral vascular territories.

## BRIGHT-BLOOD NONCONTRAST MRA

### *Time-of-Flight Angiography*

The most commonly used noncontrast angiographic technique, time-of-flight (TOF), has been available for at least 2 decades.[1,2] It produces magnitude images that display increased vessel signal intensity, as it takes advantage of the through-plane blood flow. TOF acquisition, which mostly uses spoiled gradient-echo T1-weighted pulse sequences, relies on the differences in radiofrequency (RF) exposure between stationary tissue of a slab (imaging slab) and the blood that moves into the slab from the surrounding tissue. The imaging slab experiences RF excitation pulses meant to null its signal, while the inflowing blood brings fully magnetized protons into the image slice. As it carries unsaturated protons into the imaging slab, the flowing blood shows brighter signal compared with nulled/saturated stationary tissue. This hyperintense blood signal effect depends on the transverse relaxation time (T1), velocity, and direction of the moving blood. The repetition time (TR) in TOF is generally chosen to balance acquisition time and flow enhancement, as a shorter TR will not give enough time for the fresh spins to enter the imaging slab. The placement of a presaturation pulse on an adjacent slab superior or inferior to the imaging slab can be

The authors have nothing to disclose.
[a] Division of Cardiovascular Medicine, Department of Internal Medicine, The Ohio State University, 473 West 12th Avenue, Suite 200 DHLRI, Columbus, OH 43210, USA
[b] Department of Radiology, The Ohio State University, 410 West 10th Avenue, 527 Doan Hall, Columbus, OH 43210, USA
* Corresponding author.
*E-mail address:* georgeta.mihai@osumc.edu

Cardiol Clin 29 (2011) 341–350
doi:10.1016/j.ccl.2011.04.006
0733-8651/11/$ – see front matter 

used to selectively suppress signals from either veins or arteries, allowing the respective generation of MR arteriograms (MRA) or MR venograms (MRV). The choice of 2-dimensional (2D) sequential slices or 3-dimensional (3D) volume for imaging is dictated by how quickly the blood becomes saturated because of repeatedly experiencing the RF excitation pulses as it flows through the imaging slab. Although it may be desirable to cover the imaging volume with a single slab of 3D thin slices with increased signal-to-noise ratio (SNR) compared with a 2D acquisition, long vessels are difficult to visualize simultaneously in a 3D-TOF volume. This is due to an overall decrease in vessel SNR as a result of blood saturation that results in progressively attenuated blood signal from the entrance point to the exit slice. However, in clinical practice, multiple overlapping thin-slab acquisition (MOTSA),[3] a hybrid of 2D-TOF and 3D-TOF is used particularly in vascular beds with rapid flow (such as intracranial vessels) where the issue of saturation of blood flow in multiple slices can be compensated owing to the rapid flow. MOTSA has some of the advantages of both types of acquisitions (coverage, higher SNR, thin slices), as it covers the imaging volume with multiple, thin slabs that are acquired sequentially and are fused to form a 3D volume. Some of the limitations of TOF angiography in addition to blood saturation effects that may mimic pathology are related to susceptibility to artifacts from pulsatile flow, tortuous vessels not in the plane of imaging, and vessel movement (may be corrected by cardiac triggering), as well as from breathing, swallowing, and any other bulk patient motion.

## *Phase-Contrast Angiography*

A less infrequently used noncontrast angiographic technique, phase-contrast (PC) angiography,[4–6] relies on the phase change that occurs in moving spins such as the ones in the blood. This phase change is dependent on the application of a bipolar gradient (one gradient with positive polarity followed by same-strength second gradient with a negative polarity, separated by a time delay $\Delta T$). When a bipolar gradient is applied, stationary protons do not gain a net phase (assuming homogeneous magnetic field), but for protons moving perpendicular to the plane of imaging, the effect of the first gradient field is not perfectly counteracted by the second gradient field, resulting in a phase offset. The degree of phase shift is proportional to the velocity of the spins within the excited volume and the time $\Delta T$ between the positive and negative lobes of the bipolar gradients. To correct for magnetic field inhomogeneities, in a second similar acquisition of the imaged tissue, the polarity of the bipolar gradient is reversed, and moving spins of the blood are encoded with negative phase, while the stationary spins exhibit no phase change. Subtracting the second excitation from the first cancels the magnetization owing to stationary spins, but enhances the magnetization generated by the moving blood. Because of the phase change's direct relationship to the velocity, PC imaging allows for flow quantification. Proper choice of imaging parameters and knowledge of expected spin velocities are necessary to avoid phase wrap, as phase can take only values between $+180^\circ$ and $-180^\circ$. Although some of the strengths of PC angiography are that it offers flow quantification, has an excellent background suppression, and is highly sensitive to turbulent and slow flow,[7] having to repeat the acquisition twice makes (especially 3D-PC) PC angiography a time-consuming technique.

## *Balanced Steady State-Free Precession Angiography*

Balanced steady-state free precession (b-SSFP) is a gradient record echo (GRE)-based sequence, for which the excitation train consists of an initial $\alpha/2$ pulse followed at a time equal to TR by a train of alternating $\pm\alpha$ excitation pulses separated by TR/2 time.[8] The TR of the applied alternating pulse is much shorter than longitudinal recovery-T1 time, hence maintaining residual transverse magnetization between excitations. The image contrast in b-SSFP angiography is mainly determined by the ratio of intrinsic transversal relaxation time (T2)/T1 differences between blood and surrounding tissue; however, depending on the choice of slice thickness and orientation, the observed image contrast could be actually a mixture of T2/T1 ratio of b-SSFP contrast and signal-enhancing inflow effect. As a result, b-SSFP angiography shows high SNR images with very bright blood, especially when fat is suppressed by additional excitation pulses. Higher SNR of this sequence makes it well suited for 3D angiography in conjunction with parallel imaging,[9] electrocardiogram (ECG)-triggered,[10] and navigator-gated free-breathing techniques.[7,11,12] Both arteries and veins are bright on b-SSFP acquisition and, as such, additional preparation modules are required to selectively enhance arteries or veins depending on the clinical application and indication. b-SSFP angiographic sequences are sensitive to flow and are vulnerable to susceptibility artifacts owing to field inhomogeneity, tissue interface, metallic implants, and stents.[8] In addition, free-breathing 3D b-SSFP could take a relatively long time to acquire.

### *ECG-Gated 3D Partial-Fourier Fast Spin-Echo Angiography*

This newer, clinically promising noncontrast angiography technique is based on an ECG-gated spin-echo sequence.[13,14] Improvements in magnetic resonance imaging (MRI) hardware and software that led to single-shot partial-Fourier fast spin-echo sequence (FSE) has made this noncontrast angiography method clinically feasible.[15–17] This technique uses a 3D partial-FSE sequence (usually with fat suppression preparation) triggered for systolic and diastolic acquisition. It uses different trigger time delays to acquire images during systole and diastole, with a TR of 2 to 3 cardiac cycles or R-R intervals. The exact triggering times for a structure of interest are generated by getting 1 or 2 ECG-gated, single-shot 2D partial-Fourier FSE scans to obtain images at different delay times. Because of the faster arterial flow during systole, the blood arterial signal is nulled (black blood); the opposite happens during diastole when arterial blood shows hyperintense signal in T2-weighted images. For both systolic and diastolic acquisitions, venous blood is bright because of its slow flow compared with the arterial flow. A bright arteriogram is obtained by subtracting the systolic from diastolic images or a black-blood image may be obtained by just looking at the systolic acquired images.

Although promising, this technique is dependent on exact timing of the 2 separate systolic and diastolic acquisitions. This may be problematic in patients with arrhythmias, motion, or other time-varying artifacts that may compromise image quality.

### *Arterial Spin-Labeling Angiography*

Arterial spin-labeling (ASL) imaging frequently used for blood perfusion measurements is capable of generating angiographic images using spin tagging upstream of the arteries of interest. Most recently, this method was implemented using fast imaging methods such as b-SSFP and partial-Fourier FSE methods.[18,19] The tagging of the spins outside the imaging plane is followed by a delay time that allows blood to travel to the imaging slab before images are acquired. The same time delay could be used to insert preparation modules to selectively suppressed unwanted signal from the imaging plane. For perfect background suppression, an ASL angiogram usually requires 2 separate acquisitions, one in which spins in a slab upstream of imaging volume are tagged (usually by an inversion pulse) and one with no tagging. After subtracting the 2 sets of images, a bright-blood angiogram with no background signal could be obtained. By combining ASL with tagged and untagged b-SSFP and/or partial-Fourier FSE readout, the advantages of the latter methods are enhanced, by either minimizing the flow sensitivity (with b-SSFP) or improving the vascular signal by cardiac triggering for diastolic imaging (with partial-Fourier FSE).[7] Some of the limitations of ASL angiography are related to susceptibility to motion between the tagged and untagged acquisition, and the failure of the sequence to perform in vascular regions with slow flow that may lose the tagging effect.

## BLACK-BLOOD NONCONTRAST MRA

Black-blood imaging techniques are commonly used to asses vessel wall pathologies, such as atherosclerosis, aneurysms, intramural hematoma, aortic dissections, and vasculitides. Most black-blood sequences are fast SE sequences with preparation modules for blood-signal suppression. These techniques allow for depiction of lumen and vascular wall, and are able to deliver all contrast types (T1, T2, and PD) but need efficient suppression of flowing blood. The latter is accomplished either by inflow–outflow saturation bands (IOSB; flowing blood experiences an extra 90° RF pulse outside the imaging slice),[20] double inversion recovery (DIR),[21–23] or variants.[24,25] However, these methods are time consuming and they do not allow for coverage of large vascular territories in a reasonable scanning time; as such, they are mostly used for research. Lately 3D b-SSFP angiographic sequences with preparation modules to null the blood signal were specifically developed for either carotid artery[26] or thoracic aorta[27] wall depiction. Recently, an efficient 3D-FSE method with variable flip angle (Sampling Perfection with Application of optimized Contrasts using different flip angle Evolution [SPACE]) has been developed and has shown promise for clinical implementation as a dark-blood angiographic method[28–30] and even as a whole-body noncontrast angiography approach (WB-DBMRA).[12,31]

### *3D-Variable Flip-Angle FSE Angiography (SPACE)*

This technique is based on a 3D-FSE method originally developed for brain imaging.[32,33] SPACE uses variable refocusing flip angles to allow for longer echo train duration, as well as nonselective refocusing pulse to minimize echo spacing. The latter significantly improve time efficiency of SPACE over conventional 3D FSE sequences. Additionally, flowing blood is dephased and blood signal is suppressed without the need for DIR preparation pulses, hence permitting the use of thick 3D slabs and efficient coverage of large vascular territories. Two mechanisms are responsible for blood suppression (dark blood) in SPACE. First, strong spoiler gradient pulses are applied in the frequency-encoding direction before and after radiofrequency refocusing pulses to suppress unwanted stimulated echoes. Additionally, the spoiler gradients dephase moving spins when a long echo-time (TE) is used. Second, the variable flip angle refocusing pulses generate numerous stimulated echoes that refocus for stationary tissues but cause destructive interference during long echo-time collection for the flowing blood. The latter is more effective for blood flowing in the readout (frequency-encoded) direction; this is the main reason coronal or sagittal acquisitions are necessary and facilitate efficient vascular coverage.[31] To acquire large slabs of vascular structures, such as the thoracic aorta, ECG-gating to systole and free-breathing respiratory navigator gating is used. As such, the 3D volumetric acquisition can take up to 15 to 20 minutes at 1.5 T to acquire high-resolution, isotropic images with 1.0-$mm^3$ to 1.8-$mm^3$ resolution[31] necessary to quantify and characterize arterial wall composition in atherosclerotic disease. Other than for vessel wall pathology, SPACE can be used when significant stent susceptibility artifact precludes the use of GRE sequences, as it allows imaging outside of the stent without any signal loss.[34] As a flow-dependent method, SPACE is susceptible to show unsuppressed blood that could mask wall visualization when blood flow is turbulent, moving slow or not parallel to the frequency encode direction.[31] In patients with arrhythmias, the usage of both ECG gating and navigator-gated free breathing may prolong acquisition time excessively.

## NSF AND GADOLINIUM USE FOR MRA

The latest efforts to develop and use nonenhanced MR angiographic techniques were mostly influenced by the association between NSF and Gd-based contrast-enhanced agents seen almost exclusively in patients with end-stage renal disease (ESRD), advanced chronic kidney disease, or acute renal failure (ARF) with severe reductions in glomerular filtration rate (GFR).[35,36] NSF is a rare, but extremely debilitating, largely untreatable acquired systemic disease characterized by induration, thickening, and tightening of the skin. Pathologically there are thickened collagen bundles, mucin deposition, and proliferation of fibroblasts and elastin fibers. The increased retention of Gd contrast in the body owing to renal failure may result in free, more toxic Gd, as well as bioactivation of chelated Gd that initiates pathologic processes associated with NSF.[37] Gd is highly toxic in the free unchelated form in contrast to the chelated form, which is rapidly excreted by the kidneys. Several factors have been reported to contribute to the development of NSF, including the type of Gd chelate; the total dose administered and factors including renal failure; inflammatory state (lupus, recent major vascular surgery, recent thrombosis); and comorbidities of renal failure, including acidosis, elevated phosphate levels, and high-dose erythropoietin therapy as well as the patient's own susceptibility.[37,38] The type of chelate (linear vs macrocyclic) may influence stability of preparation and the release of free unchelated Gd. Although the overwhelming majority of cases have been reported in patients on dialysis, a GFR less than 30 mL per minute is a contraindication for administration of Gd-based contrast. These facts have led to widespread screening of MRI patients for renal dysfunction and using caution in administering Gd-based contrast agents in such situations unless the benefits obviate the risks. Changes in patient screening approaches, using weight-based guidelines and avoidance in the previously mentioned situations have resulted in a virtual disappearance of NSF.[38,39]

## APPLICATIONS OF NONCONTRAST MRA

The selection of specific noncontrast angiographic techniques for each vascular region reflects the performance of the sequence in this location and specifically its ability to overcome challenges intrinsic to each vessel bed.

### *Carotid Angiography*

Angiography of carotid artery can delineate carotid bifurcation disease and aortic arch branch vessel stenosis/occlusion, and can help differentiate atherosclerotic disease, fibromuscular dysplasia, carotid and vertebral artery dissection, vascular neoplasms, and carotid artery aneurysms. Carotid arteries are medium-sized vessels with moderately high flow and a supero-inferior orientation that makes them ideal for 3D TOF angiography. In a very cooperative, still patient, with dedicated neck coils to improve the SNR and parallel imaging to speed up scan time, a high-resolution, axial multislab TOF acquisition can be generated in less than 5 minutes. Localized PC imaging can be performed to assess hemodynamic significance of stenosis or flow direction using in-plane acquisitions as well as to quantify the severity by using through-plane acquisitions. Black-blood imaging, using variable flip angle 3D TSE

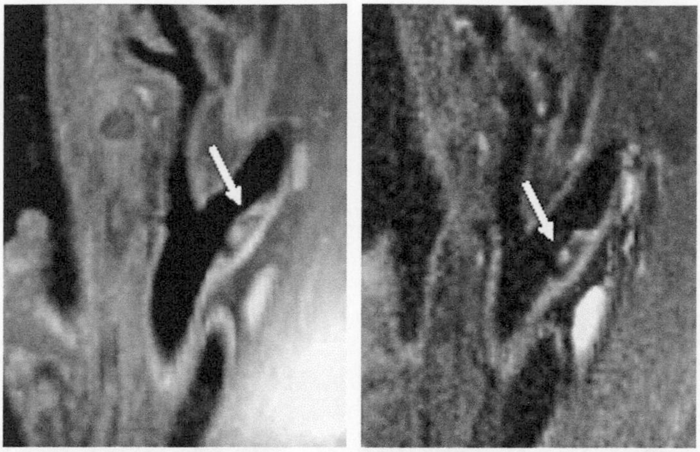

**Fig. 1.** Sagittal maximum projection reconstruction (MPR) reformats of T1-weighted (*left*) and T2-weighted 3D SPACE (*right*) data sets acquired at 3 T field strength (MAGNETOM Avanto, Siemens, Erlangen) of a subject with atherosclerotic carotid disease. White arrows point to the atherosclerotic lesion located approximately at the carotid bifurcation. Observe the varied composition of the lesion showing different contrasts in T1-weighted and T2-weighted images (image resolution: $0.7 \times 0.7 \times 0.7$ mm$^3$).

sequence allows for high-resolution ($\leq$0.8 mm$^3$) luminal and vascular wall interrogation of carotid arteries in only a few minutes.[30,31] Vessel wall morphometry, plaque localization, and characterization is possible using the aforementioned SPACE sequence with different contrasts (**Fig. 1**). Alternative plaque characterization can be provided using localized 2D-FSE approaches.

## *Thoracic Angiography*

Noncontrast MRA is capable of accurately assessing any congenital or acquired disease of the thoracic aorta and as such is perhaps the widest application for these techniques. The most used sequence for noncontrast assessment of thoracic aorta assessment is SSFP, followed more recently by the ECG-gated 3D partial-Fourier FSE sequences with different preparation modules to null the fat and enhance the blood signal. Single-shot SSFP images in the axial plane could be obtained in the transversal direction for quick luminal assessment. ECG-gated "segmented" SSFP cine sequences[10] can be used to depict functional abnormalities of the entire thoracic aorta throughout the cardiac cycle in a single "candy cane" plane (**Fig. 2**). This may be useful in patients with aortic dissection for the evaluation of the dynamic behavior of the intimal flap or the pulsatility of the true or false lumens, when the aorta is not tortuous. For a comprehensive assessment of the entire thoracic aorta, a 3D MRA b-SSFP with free-breathing respiratory navigator and ECG triggered to diastolic acquisition can be obtained in less than 10 minutes, with image quality and diagnostic accuracy as high as the contrast-enhanced MRA.[12,40] Dark-blood 3D imaging for quantification and depiction of the arterial wall could also be obtained using variable flip-angle SPACE acquisition with free-breathing navigator and ECG gated to systolic acquisition (**Fig. 3**). PC imaging is useful in specific cases to assess

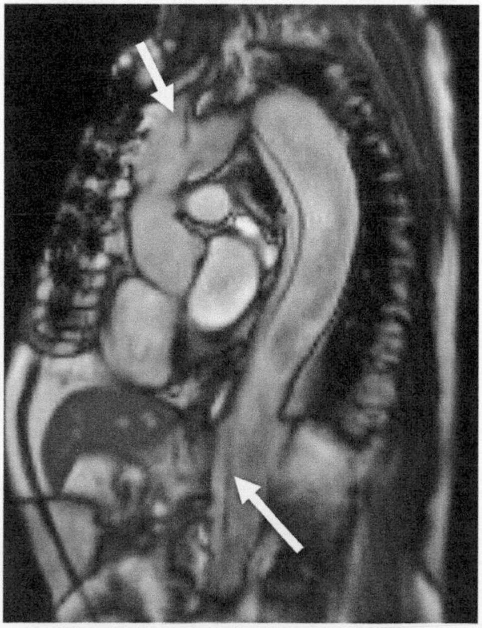

**Fig. 2.** Balanced SSFP image acquired at 1.5 T (MAGNETOM Avanto) in a "candy cane" view of a patient with Type A dissection with previous repair of the proximal ascending aorta. There is ongoing dissection starting just distal to the graft and extending well into the abdominal aorta (*white arrows*).

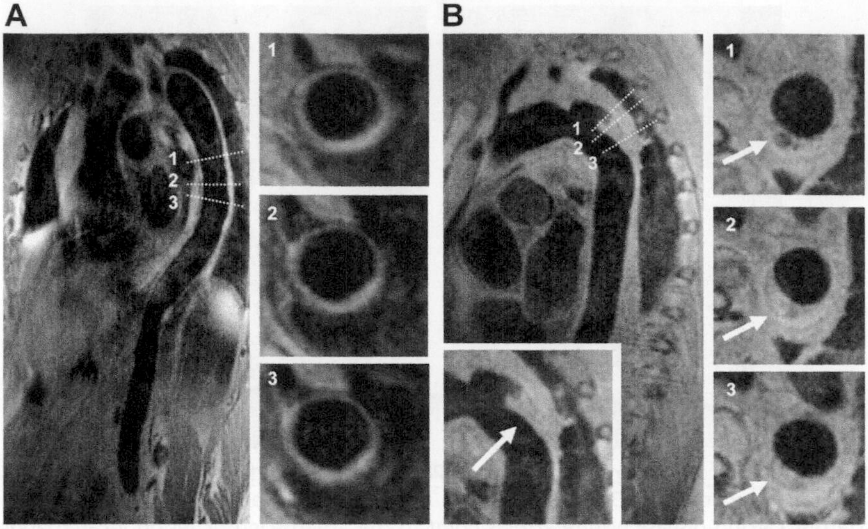


**Fig. 3.** Sagittal and axial MPR reformats of T1-weighted 3D SPACE acquisitions of thoracic aorta (TR = R-R interval, TE = 25 ms, parallel imaging factor 2, acquired image resolution = $1.2 \times 1.2 \times 1.2$ mm$^3$) obtained at 1.5 T (MAGNETOM Avanto). (*A*) Diffuse atherosclerosis disease shows thickening of the thoracic arterial wall more visible in axial images. (*B*) Aortic ulcer with intramural hematoma (*white arrow* in the magnified cropped segment of diseased aorta) visible in the axial reformatted images. The white dotted lines delineate the exact position on the sagittal view where the axial cuts were generated.

for turbulence and to quantify blood flow, as well as to determine the presence and direction of flow (eg, in a communication between the true and false lumen through an intimal tear in cases of dissection or to assess flow turbulence at the site of coarctation) (**Fig. 4**). Similar noncontrast angiographic approaches can be implemented in the diagnosis of abdominal aorta diseases.

## *Renal Angiography*

Patients evaluated for renal diseases usually have contraindications to Gd usage, and, as such, noncontrast MR angiography is a necessary approach in the assessment of renal artery stenosis, aneurysms, and dissection, as well as the evaluation of transplanted renal arteries. The development of noncontrast MRA techniques had to take into

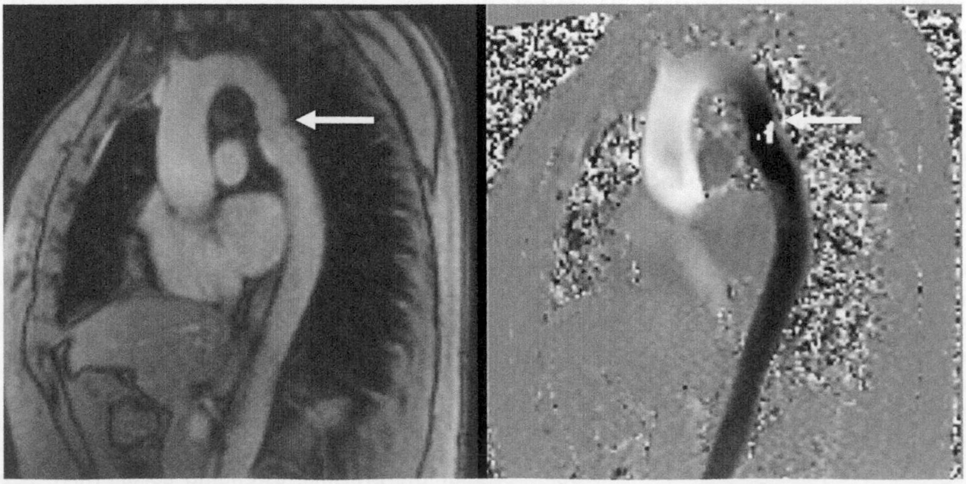

**Fig. 4.** Phase-contrast imaging with illustration of magnitude image (*left*) and phase image (*right*) illustrating a mild juxta-ductal coarctation with flow acceleration seen in the phase image (aliasing).

consideration some of the main challenges of imaging renal arteries, such as small size, different orientation of renal artery branches, and motion with breathing. Currently, 3D b-SSFP sequences with different modifications, such as ASL,[18] navigator or respiratory gating, ECG gating,[17] and venous and background suppression with saturation bands or slab selective inversion pre-pulses (**Fig. 5**), have been proven to have high specificity and sensitivity for stenosis detection when compared directly with contrast-enhanced MRA.[17,41] The functional assessment of stenosis can be evaluated using PC angiography[42,43] with good results. Further refinements in the noncontrast techniques will likely increase the sensitivity and specificity for diagnosis of renal artery diseases.

## *Lower-Extremity Angiography*

Lower-extremity angiography is perhaps the most challenging application for noncontrast MRA techniques, as they call for extensive anatomic coverage (from renal arteries to the toes) at high resolution (<1 mm) and these 2 attributes mandate specific modifications in sequences. Owing to the flow dependence with cardiac cycle, the noncontrast angiographic approaches have to be ECG triggered (systolic phase) to allow acquisition of usable images. Although TOF angiography of lower peripheral vasculature has failed to attain the diagnosis performance of contrast-enhanced MRA,[44] the PC angiographic technique has been showing high specificity and sensitivity for

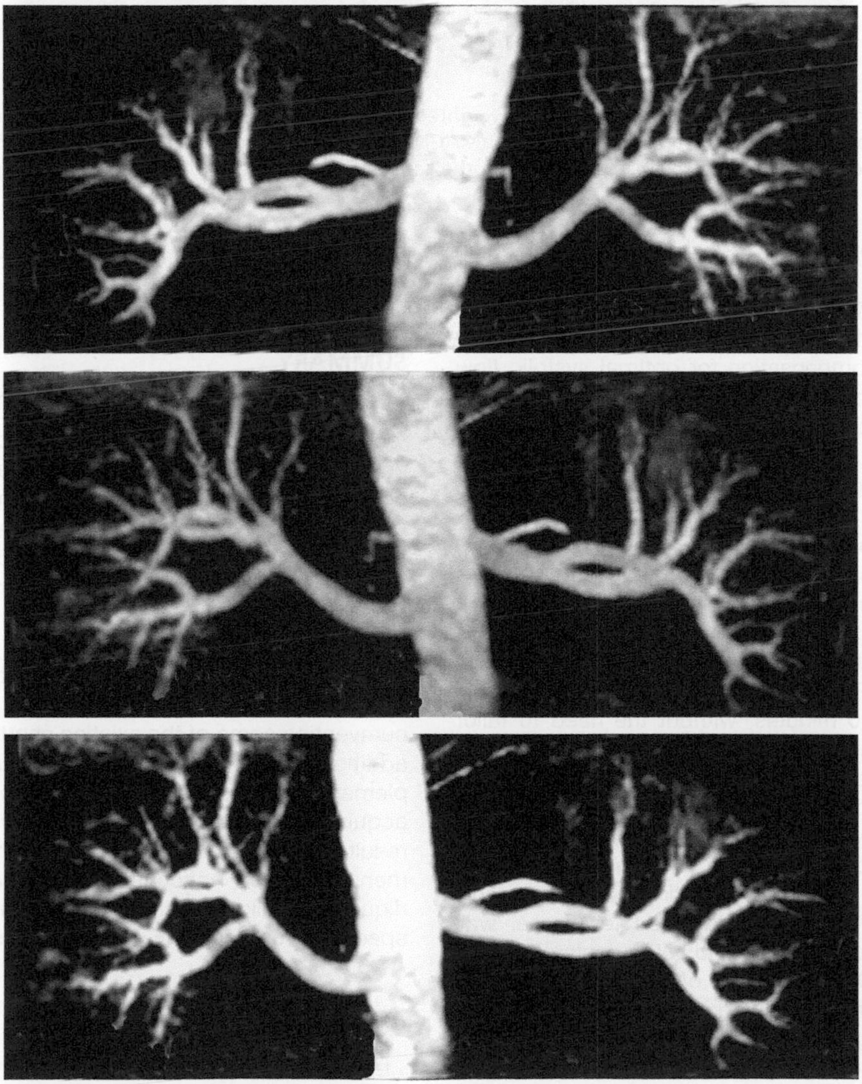

**Fig. 5.** Nonenhanced renal angiography in a healthy subject obtained at 3 T (Trim Trio, Siemens, Erlangen) using a respiratory navigated 3D b-SSFP with selective inversion slab (to null background tissue and venous blood). Frontal and slightly left and right lateral *maximum intensity projections (MIPs)* are shown.

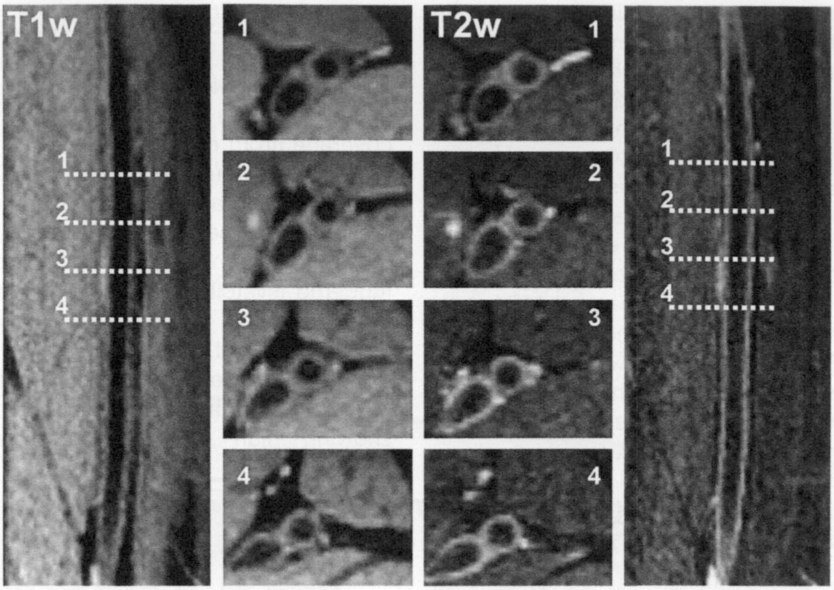


**Fig. 6.** Coronal and axial MPR reformats of a T1-weighted (*left*) and T2-weighted 3D SPACE (*right*) acquisition of a normal superficial femoral artery obtained at 3 T (MAGNETOM Avanto) (image resolution: 0.8 × 0.8 × 0.8 mm$^3$). White dotted lines delineate the exact position on the sagittal view where the axial cuts were generated.

stenosis depiction,[45,46] despite the relatively high acquisition time (up to 30 minutes) for the entire peripheral vascular bed. Lately, ECG-gated 3D partial-Fourier FSE sequence with flow spoiling and flow compensation for optimal systolic flow void was applied for noncontrast peripheral angiography with good results.[7,16] The main drawback of the latest approach as well as b-SSFP in peripheral imaging resides in the necessity for perfect timing of the triggered acquisition. Quiescent-interval, single-shot b-SSFP method[47] was able to address this issue by implementing slice-selective saturation followed by a quiescent interval for maximum flow enhancement. This method showed excellent agreement with contrast MRA to assess peripheral vasculature in less than 10 minutes, without the need to tailor the technique for individual patients. This technique is the strongest runner up for the noncontrast peripheral angiography challenge. In angiography of the upper limbs, b-SSFP with ASL proved to be useful for imaging the small vessels of the hand and fingers.[15] The dark-blood approaches mostly used for vessel wall depiction of normal and atherosclerotic wall include 3D-SPACE T1 of iliac and femoral arteries[28] or T2-weighted[29] images of the femoral arteries (**Fig. 6**). The high-resolution acquisitions necessary to depict vessel wall of the vasculature below the pedal arteries prevents SPACE from being applied for lower leg and foot angiography, as the imaging time would be extremely long and motion artifacts would most likely affect the image quality.

## SUMMARY

Although challenging, noncontrast angiographic techniques are available to be applied when NSF risk outweighs the benefit of Gd-contrast MR angiography. Nevertheless, the application of noncontrast angiographic methods in different vascular beds has to balance the imaging requirements of each vessel bed with the specific strengths and pitfalls of the noncontrast method. Imaging at a higher magnetic field may provide incremental benefits (SNR, higher resolution, and/or shorter imaging time), and may provide future utility in circumventing some of the existing shortcomings. In addition, further higher-order parallel imaging implementation has the potential to speed up the acquisition of noncontrast angiography that may result in fewer motion artifacts. Further refinements in these noncontrast angiographic techniques will likely increase the sensitivity and specificity for diagnosis of vascular diseases.

## REFERENCES

1. Laub GA. Time-of-flight method of MR angiography. Magn Reson Imaging Clin N Am 1995;3(3):391–8.
2. Kaufman JA, McCarter D, Geller SC, et al. Two-dimensional time-of-flight MR angiography of the

lower extremities: artifacts and pitfalls. AJR Am J Roentgenol 1998;171(1):129–35.
3. Parker DL, Yuan C, Blatter DD. MR angiography by multiple thin slab 3D acquisition. Magn Reson Med 1991;17(2):434–51.
4. Moran PR. A flow velocity zeugmatographic interlace for NMR imaging in humans. Magn Reson Imaging 1982;1(4):197–203.
5. Bryant DJ, Payne JA, Firmin DN, et al. Measurement of flow with NMR imaging using a gradient pulse and phase difference technique. J Comput Assist Tomogr 1984;8(4):588–93.
6. Moran PR, Moran RA, Karstaedt N. Verification and evaluation of internal flow and motion. True magnetic resonance imaging by the phase gradient modulation method. Radiology 1985;154(2):433–41.
7. Miyazaki M, Lee VS. Nonenhanced MR angiography. Radiology 2008;248(1):20–43.
8. Scheffler K, Lehnhardt S. Principles and applications of balanced SSFP techniques. Eur Radiol 2003;13(11):2409–18.
9. Niendorf T, Hardy CJ, Giaquinto RO, et al. Toward single breath-hold whole-heart coverage coronary MRA using highly accelerated parallel imaging with a 32-channel MR system. Magn Reson Med 2006;56(1):167–76.
10. Carr JC, Simonetti O, Bundy J, et al. Cine MR angiography of the heart with segmented true fast imaging with steady-state precession. Radiology 2001;219(3):828–34.
11. Katoh M, Spuentrup E, Stuber M, et al. Free-breathing renal magnetic resonance angiography with steady-state free-precession and slab-selective spin inversion combined with radial k-space sampling and water-selective excitation. Magn Reson Med 2005;53(5):1228–33.
12. Krishnam MS, Tomasian A, Malik S, et al. Image quality and diagnostic accuracy of unenhanced SSFP MR angiography compared with conventional contrast-enhanced MR angiography for the assessment of thoracic aortic diseases. Eur Radiol 2010;20(6):1311–20.
13. Wedeen VJ, Meuli RA, Edelman RR, et al. Projective imaging of pulsatile flow with magnetic resonance. Science 1985;230(4728):946–8.
14. Meuli RA, Wedeen VJ, Geller SC, et al. MR gated subtraction angiography: evaluation of lower extremities. Radiology 1986;159(2):411–8.
15. Miyazaki M, Sugiura S, Tateishi F, et al. Non-contrast-enhanced MR angiography using 3D ECG-synchronized half-Fourier fast spin echo. J Magn Reson Imaging 2000;12(5):776–83.
16. Miyazaki M, Takai H, Sugiura S, et al. Peripheral MR angiography: separation of arteries from veins with flow-spoiled gradient pulses in electrocardiography-triggered three-dimensional half-Fourier fast spin-echo imaging. Radiology 2003;227(3):890–6.
17. Mohrs OK, Petersen SE, Schulze T, et al. High-resolution 3D unenhanced ECG-gated respiratory-navigated MR angiography of the renal arteries: comparison with contrast-enhanced MR angiography. AJR Am J Roentgenol 2010;195(6):1423–8.
18. Spuentrup E, Manning WJ, Bornert P, et al. Renal arteries: navigator-gated balanced fast field-echo projection MR angiography with aortic spin labeling: initial experience. Radiology 2002;225(2):589–96.
19. Katoh M, Stuber M, Buecker A, et al. Spin-labeling coronary MR angiography with steady-state free precession and radial k-space sampling: initial results in healthy volunteers. Radiology 2005;236(3):1047–52.
20. Felmlee JP, Ehman RL. Spatial presaturation: a method for suppressing flow artifacts and improving depiction of vascular anatomy in MR imaging. Radiology 1987;164(2):559–64.
21. Edelman RR, Chien D, Kim D. Fast selective black blood MR imaging. Radiology 1991;181(3):655–60.
22. Parker DL, Goodrich KC, Masiker M, et al. Improved efficiency in double-inversion fast spin-echo imaging. Magn Reson Med 2002;47(5):1017–21.
23. Song HK, Wright AC, Wolf RL, et al. Multislice double inversion pulse sequence for efficient black-blood MRI. Magn Reson Med 2002;47(3):616–20.
24. Yarnykh VL, Yuan C. Simultaneous outer volume and blood suppression by quadruple inversion-recovery. Magn Reson Med 2006;55(5):1083–92.
25. Sampath S, Raval AN, Lederman RJ, et al. High-resolution 3D arteriography of chronic total peripheral occlusions using a T1-W turbo spin-echo sequence with inner-volume imaging. Magn Reson Med 2007;57(1):40–9.
26. Koktzoglou I, Chung YC, Carroll TJ, et al. Three-dimensional black-blood MR imaging of carotid arteries with segmented steady-state free precession: initial experience. Radiology 2007;243(1):220–8.
27. Koktzoglou I, Kirpalani A, Carroll TJ, et al. Dark-blood MRI of the thoracic aorta with 3D diffusion-prepared steady-state free precession: initial clinical evaluation. AJR Am J Roentgenol 2007;189(4):966–72.
28. Mihai G, Chung YC, Kariisa M, et al. Initial feasibility of a multi-station high resolution 3D dark blood angiography protocol for the assessment of peripheral arterial disease. J Magn Reson Imaging 2009;30(4):785–93.
29. Zhang Z, Fan Z, Carroll TJ, et al. Three-dimensional T2-weighted MRI of the human femoral arterial vessel wall at 3.0 Tesla. Invest Radiol 2009;44(9):619–26.
30. Fan Z, Zhang Z, Chung YC, et al. Carotid arterial wall MRI at 3T using 3D variable-flip-angle turbo

spin-echo (TSE) with flow-sensitive dephasing (FSD). J Magn Reson Imaging 2010;31(3):645–54.
31. Mihai G, Chung YC, Merchant A, et al. T1-weighted-SPACE dark blood whole body magnetic resonance angiography (DB-WBMRA): initial experience. J Magn Reson Imaging 2010;31(2):502–9.
32. Mugler JP 3rd, Bao S, Mulkern RV, et al. Optimized single-slab three-dimensional spin-echo MR imaging of the brain. Radiology 2000;216(3):891–9.
33. Park J, Mugler JP 3rd, Horger W, et al. Optimized T1-weighted contrast for single-slab 3D turbo spin-echo imaging with long echo trains: application to whole-brain imaging. Magn Reson Med 2007; 58(5):982–92.
34. Winner MW III, Raman SV, Simonetti OP, et al. Post-interventional three-dimensional dark blood MRI in the adult with congenital heart disease. Int J Cardiol 2011. [Epub ahead of print].
35. Marckmann P, Skov L, Rossen K, et al. Nephrogenic systemic fibrosis: suspected causative role of gadodiamide used for contrast-enhanced magnetic resonance imaging. J Am Soc Nephrol 2006;17(9):2359–62.
36. Grobner T. Gadolinium—a specific trigger for the development of nephrogenic fibrosing dermopathy and nephrogenic systemic fibrosis? Nephrol Dial 2006;21(4):1104–8.
37. Newton BB, Jimenez SA. Mechanism of NSF: new evidence challenging the prevailing theory. J Magn Reson Imaging 2009;30(6):1277–83.
38. Prince MR, Zhang HL, Roditi GH, et al. Risk factors for NSF: a literature review. J Magn Reson Imaging 2009;30(6):1298–308.
39. Martin DR, Krishnamoorthy SK, Kalb B, et al. Decreased incidence of NSF in patients on dialysis after changing gadolinium contrast-enhanced MRI protocols. J Magn Reson Imaging 2010;31(2):440–6.
40. Amano Y, Takahama K, Kumita S. Non-contrast-enhanced MR angiography of the thoracic aorta using cardiac and navigator-gated magnetization-prepared three-dimensional steady-state free precession. J Magn Reson Imaging 2008;27(3): 504–9.
41. Glockner JF, Takahashi N, Kawashima A, et al. Non-contrast renal artery MRA using an inflow inversion recovery steady state free precession technique (Inhance): comparison with 3D contrast-enhanced MRA. J Magn Reson Imaging 2010;31(6):1411–8.
42. Meyers SP, Talagala SL, Totterman S, et al. Evaluation of the renal arteries in kidney donors: value of three-dimensional phase-contrast MR angiography with maximum-intensity-projection or surface rendering. AJR Am J Roentgenol 1995;164(1):117–21.
43. de Haan MW, Kouwenhoven M, Thelissen RP, et al. Renovascular disease in patients with hypertension: detection with systolic and diastolic gating in three-dimensional, phase-contrast MR angiography. Radiology 1996;198(2):449–56.
44. Hahn WY, Hecht EM, Friedman B, et al. Distal lower extremity imaging: prospective comparison of 2-dimensional time of flight, 3-dimensional time-resolved contrast-enhanced magnetic resonance angiography, and 3-dimensional bolus chase contrast-enhanced magnetic resonance angiography. J Comput Assist Tomogr 2007;31(1):29–36.
45. Steffens JC, Link J, Muller-Hulsbeck S, et al. Cardiac-gated two-dimensional phase-contrast MR angiography of lower extremity occlusive disease. AJR Am J Roentgenol 1997;169(3):749–54.
46. Reimer P, Boos M. Phase-contrast MR angiography of peripheral arteries: technique and clinical application. Eur Radiol 1999;9(1):122–7.
47. Edelman RR, Sheehan JJ, Dunkle E, et al. Quiescent-interval single-shot unenhanced magnetic resonance angiography of peripheral vascular disease: technical considerations and clinical feasibility. Magn Reson Med 2010;63(4):951–8.

# Advances in Percutaneous Therapy for Upper Extremity Arterial Disease

Quinn Capers IV, MD[a,*], John Phillips, MD[b]

**KEYWORDS**

- Subclavian artery • Stent • Angioplasty • Innominate
- Intervention

Upper extremity arterial occlusive disease is an important manifestation of peripheral atherosclerosis. As with all patients with peripheral atherosclerosis, the leading cause of death in patients with upper extremity atherosclerosis is ischemic cardiac and cerebrovascular disease. Thus, when treating these patients, attention needs to be paid to cardiovascular risk reduction, such as encouraging physical activity, avoiding tobacco abuse, and complying with a regimen of medications proven to reduce the risk of cardiovascular events. Although diseases and disorders other than atherosclerosis can cause upper extremity arterial obstructions, such as arteritis (Takayasu and giant cell arteritis), thoracic outlet obstruction, fibromuscular disease, radiation-induced injury, traumatic (crutch) injury, and so forth, atherosclerosis is by far the most common cause.[1] Arterial stenosis/occlusion of the upper extremities can be classified into large-vessel and small-vessel diseases. This article focuses on the catheter-based management of obstructive disease confined to the large vessels of the upper extremities.

## RISK FACTORS AND PATHOPHYSIOLOGY

The risk factors that are associated with atherosclerosis in other vascular beds increase the risk of developing atherosclerosis in the upper extremity arteries (diabetes, hyperlipidemia, hypertension, advanced age, and tobacco abuse). Tobacco abuse is particularly prevalent in patients with upper extremity atherosclerotic disease and seems to be a stronger risk factor than the others. Atherosclerosis develops slowly for several decades before a critical narrowing is evident and arterial flow is impaired. This slow progression allows collateralization to develop, maintaining blood flow to the arms and hands. This and the rather robust collateralization response in the upper extremity are possible reasons why upper extremity arterial disease is frequently asymptomatic. Embolization of the upper extremities, either from proximal arteries or from the heart, can cause acute symptoms. Similar to carotid atherosclerotic disease, plaque rupture and disruption can occur, leading to macroembolization of plaque components with thrombus or microembolization of platelet aggregates. Thus, unilateral vasospastic symptoms or embolic phenomena should trigger a work-up for proximal sources of embolization.

## DIAGNOSIS OF UPPER EXTREMITY ARTERIAL OCCLUSIVE DISEASE

### *History*

Most cases of upper extremity arterial stenoses are asymptomatic. They are often diagnosed

The authors have nothing to disclose.

[a] Peripheral Vascular Interventions, Division of Cardiovascular Medicine, The Ohio State University Medical Center, The Ohio State University College of Medicine, 473 West 12th Avenue, Suite 200, Columbus, OH 43210, USA
[b] Division of Cardiovascular Medicine, The Ohio State University Medical Center, The Ohio State University College of Medicine, 473 West 12th Avenue, Suite 200, Columbus, OH 43210, USA
* Corresponding author.
*E-mail address:* Quinn.capers@osumc.edu

Cardiol Clin 29 (2011) 351–361
doi:10.1016/j.ccl.2011.04.007

incidentally when a discrepancy in arm blood pressures is detected. However, some patients do present with symptoms. The brachiocephalic or innominate artery supplies blood to the entire right side of the brain via the right carotid and right vertebral arteries, and to the right arm via the right subclavian artery. If the innominate artery is the affected, the symptoms can be right arm or hand ischemia, cerebrovascular ischemia, or a combination of both. Arm claudication can be mild to severe but is seldom crippling. Arm fatigue and aching with exertion is the classic story, yet it can be described as numbness or heaviness. These symptoms are often self-diagnosed or misdiagnosed as arthritis or as secondary to a pinched nerve or other neuromusculoskeletal disorders. Digital embolization can result in discoloration, pain, and even digital loss. Some patients complain of the affected arm being cooler in temperature than the other, although this is often only realized in retrospect after successful arterial intervention. Posterior circulation ischemia manifests as dizziness and is generally postural, or at least worse when standing. Vertebrobasilar transient ischemic attacks manifest as sudden loss of consciousness or drop attacks and can be quite dramatic. Because the basilar artery is formed by the union of both vertebral arteries, a single patent vertebral artery should be sufficient to perfuse the posterior brain. Therefore, posterior circulation ischemic symptoms typically occur in the presence of bilateral vertebral artery stenosis, and usually a combination of lesions are found on angiography in such individuals, such as an occluded subclavian artery with a severely stenosed contralateral vertebral artery, bilateral vertebral artery stenoses, or bilateral critical subclavian artery stenoses. In cases where both the arms and the brain are affected, the stenosis is located in the proximal or ostial innominate, whereas symptoms confined to the right arm occur if the stenosis is located beyond the bifurcation of the innominate artery and into the right subclavian artery. Severe stenosis of the left subclavian artery is more common than in the right subclavian artery. Symptoms related to severe left subclavian artery stenosis range from arm claudication to digital ischemia in the case of embolization, to vertebrobasilar ischemia if the right vertebral artery flow is also compromised. Because the left internal mammary artery (LIMA) is commonly used in coronary artery bypass surgeries as a conduit to bypass the left anterior descending coronary artery, proximal left subclavian artery stenosis puts the postbypass surgery patient at risk for myocardial ischemia of the anterior portion of the left ventricle and may result in angina pectoris. Axillary artery stenosis is unusual and is discovered less frequently than subclavian artery stenosis. When symptoms occur, patients usually complain of arm claudication, numbness, or that the affected arm feels cold. The most common cause of brachial artery stenosis or occlusion is iatrogenic injury from brachial artery catheterization, usually during cardiac catheterization procedures. Patients presenting with these symptoms should have complete evaluation (**Fig. 1**), starting with a detailed cardiovascular history and physical examination.

The combination of retrograde vertebral flow and neurologic symptoms in response to upper extremity exertion has been labeled subclavian steal syndrome (SSS). In this disorder, blood flows from the unaffected subclavian artery and vertebral artery branch to the basilar artery, where it is shunted down the contralateral vertebral artery to ameliorate blood flow to the diseased subclavian artery beyond a tight proximal stenosis. This is mostly encountered in the context of contralateral carotid or posterior circulation disease or hypoplastic posterior communicating arteries (a common anomaly) causing inadequate blood flow to the ipsilateral vertebral artery and resulting in posterior circulation ischemia. The Joint Study of Extracranial Arterial Occlusion found that 80% of patients with SSS had concomitant lesions in the contralateral carotid or vertebral circulation.[2] The existence of this clinical entity has, however, been questioned, because there can be imprecise correlation between the presence of these symptoms and the existence of stenosis.

### *Physical Examination*

The diagnosis of upper extremity arterial disease relies heavily on the physical examination and is confirmed by appropriate testing. The examination starts with bilateral brachial artery blood pressure determinations. Frequently, the only sign that upper extremity arterial disease is present is a discrepancy in blood pressure readings in the arms. Up to 15 mm Hg can be expected; a difference greater than this should alert the clinician to the possible presence of an arterial stenosis. Once bilateral arm blood pressures are measured, the clinician should palpate all pulses of the upper extremities, comparing the amplitude and contour of each pulse with its corresponding artery on the other arm. Radial, ulnar, brachial, axillary, and carotid pulses should all be palpated, and the stethoscope should be placed over the carotid and subclavian areas to listen for bruits. The fingers and hands should be inspected for hemorrhages, discoloration, pallor, and differences in temperature.

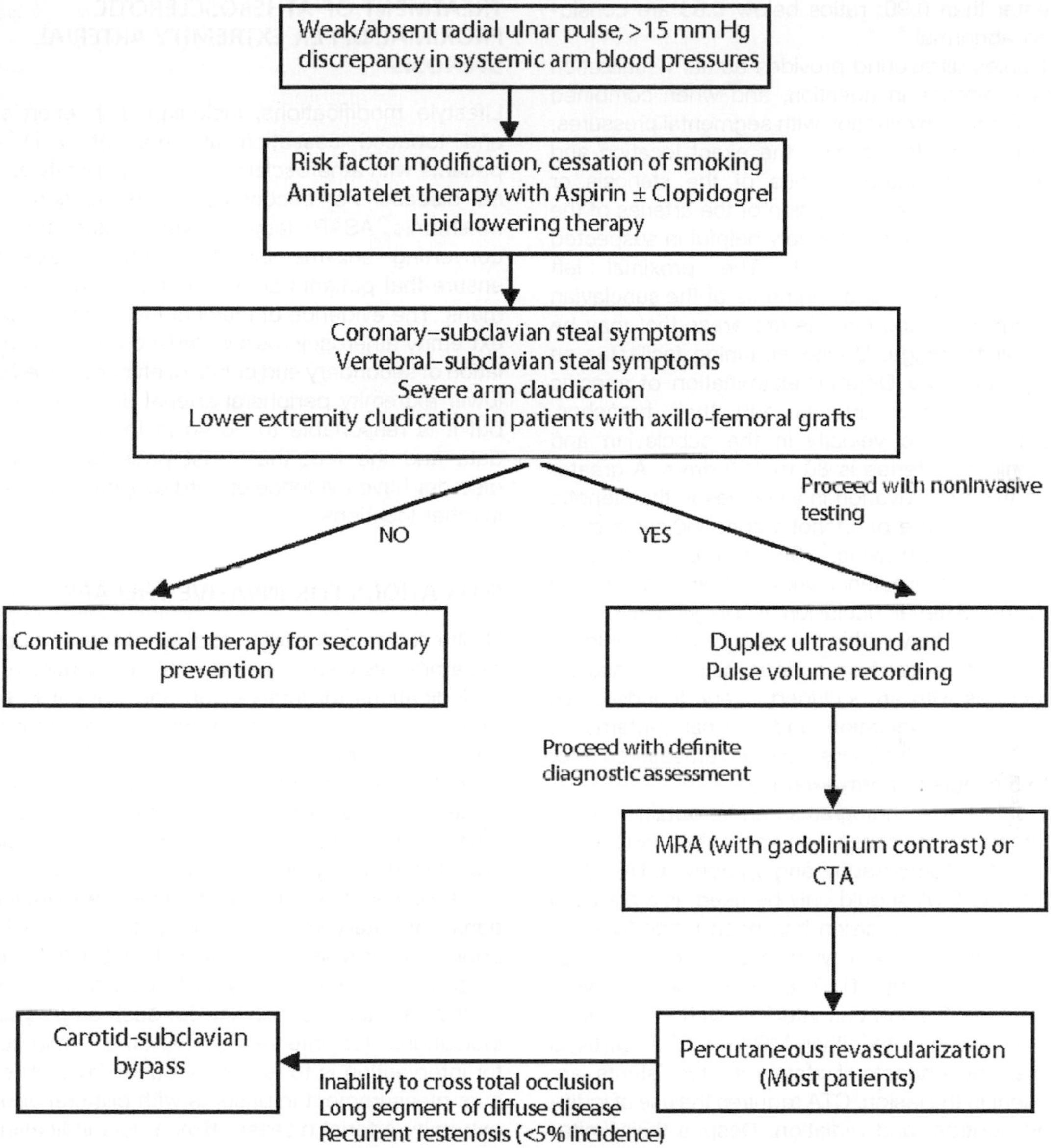


**Fig. 1.** A simplified approach to the patient with suspected subclavian/innominate artery stenosis.

### *Noninvasive Testing*

The simplest noninvasive test to screen for upper extremity large artery disease is bilateral brachial artery blood pressure determination with a sphygmomanometer. If the difference is greater than 15 mm Hg, this indicates a significant stenosis in the upper extremity proximal to the site of measurement. A full upper extremity arterial Doppler study includes segmental pressures, whereby a series of cuffs are placed on the arm and the Doppler probe is used to detect systolic blood pressures at each level. Simultaneous Doppler or pulse volume recordings are also obtained. This technique is useful for locating the affected segment. Normally the pulse contours in the upper extremity arteries are triphasic or biphasic. The normal pressure differential between adjacent levels of the same limb or compared with the same level of the contralateral limb is less than 7 mm Hg. A significant pressure drop (more than 10 mm Hg) or an index below 0.80 indicates disease at that level. The brachial/brachial, forearm/forearm, wrist/wrist, wrist/brachial (same arm) or forearm/brachial indices (same arm) ratio is normally greater than 0.90; ratios below 0.85 are considered abnormal.[3]

Duplex ultrasound provides actual visualization of the arteries in question, and when combined with Doppler evaluation with segmental pressures, can be used to visualize the exact location and morphologic characteristics of the stenosis or occlusion. Duplex evaluation of the arteries of the upper extremity is extremely helpful in suspected large-vessel involvement. The proximal left subclavian artery and segments of the subclavian system under the clavicle are areas that may be difficult to image. Duplex scanning facilitates an image directed Doppler examination of specific upper extremity arteries and their branches. Normal systolic velocity in the subclavian and innominate arteries is 80 to 120 cm/s. A greater than twofold elevation in velocities in the stenotic zone versus the prestenotic zone indicates more than 50% narrowing.[1] Spectral characteristics that suggest turbulence are very helpful adjunctive findings. Arterial occlusion is diagnosed by the absence of flow within the artery; care should be taken not to confuse various solid nonvascular structures with an occluded artery. In individuals with arm claudication and normal patterns at baseline, Doppler flow should be remeasured after 3 to 5 minutes of arm exercise.

Noninvasive angiograms can be obtained using magnetic resonance angiography (MRA) or computed tomography angiography (CTA). Both MRA and CTA should only be used as a planning modality if the decision has been made to intervene in the lesion or when arch lesions are suspected (see **Fig. 1**). The presence of severe lesion calcification can interfere with visualization of the lesion with either MRA or CTA; MRA is limited by artifacts if stainless steel stents are present in the lesion. CTA requires the use of iodinated contrast and radiation. Despite their limitations, both tests can yield high-quality road maps of the vasculature, and the three-dimensional perspective that these modalities give make them superior to invasive contrast angiograms for preinterventional planning.

### *Invasive Angiography*

For the interventionalist, the contrast angiogram remains the gold standard, especially when combined with an intervention. Digital subtraction angiography is superior to standard, nonsubtracted angiography in terms of visualization of small branches and collateral vessels, as surrounding bone and soft tissue structures can be filtered or subtracted out, leaving only the high-quality silhouette of the lumen.

## TREATMENT OF ATHEROSCLEROTIC PROXIMAL UPPER EXTREMITY ARTERIAL STENOSIS

Lifestyle modifications, including diet, exercise, and tobacco cessation are mandatory in all patients with atherosclerotic upper extremity arterial disease. For secondary risk prevention, the mnemonic ASAP (aspirin, statin, angiotensin-converting enzyme inhibitor, Plavix) helps to ensure that patients are on optimal medical regimens. The evidence of medical therapy for upper extremity atherosclerosis is derived from extrapolation of secondary end points of efficacy based on lower extremity peripheral arterial disease (PAD), but it is reasonable to do so in the absence of data and the fact that most patients with this disorder have evidence of cardiovascular disease in other locations.[1]

## INDICATIONS FOR INVASIVE THERAPY

Unlike lower extremity vascular disease, upper extremity disease is usually asymptomatic, and so indications for intervention only appear in the rare cases of severe symptoms or when a target organ is compromised by the diminished blood flow. Severe arm claudication, upper extremity ischemia secondary to embolization, including digital embolization, and symptoms of vertebrobasilar insufficiency in the presence of bilateral compromise of vertebral artery flow are all indications for intervention. Proximal left subclavian artery stenosis in a patient with a LIMA to left anterior descending artery (LAD) coronary bypass graft or a patient scheduled for such surgery are indications for intervention. Another indication for intervention is to restore accurate blood pressure measurement in patients with bilateral upper extremity arterial disease. **Box 1** lists indications for intervention on upper extremity arterial stenoses.

**Box 1**
**Indications for intervening on upper extremity arterial stenoses**

- Severe arm claudication
- Ischemia secondary to embolization
- Vertebrobasilar insufficiency
- Proximal left subclavian artery stenosis in the presence of LIMA to LAD coronary bypass graft
- Bilateral severe upper extremity arterial stenoses interfering with accurate blood pressure measurement

## SURGICAL MANAGEMENT

Surgery for subclavian artery stenosis was first described by Crawford and colleagues[4] in 1958 with additional surgical procedures to treat upper extremity occlusive disease introduced in the 1960s and 1970s. These include bypass graft placement, endarterectomy, and extra-anatomic reconstructions, such as carotid to subclavian bypass using synthetic grafts. Long-term patency after surgery approaches 90%; however, a high rate of complications has severely dampened enthusiasm for the surgical management of upper extremity arterial disease. Mortality after surgical reconstruction ranges from 19% in older series of major intrathoracic procedures to 0% to 2% in modern series using less invasive, extrathoracic procedures.[5] Stroke rates for surgical revascularization in some series have been as high as 14%.[6] In contrast, multiple series have documented stroke and death rates of 0% after percutaneous intervention.[7] Although surgical revascularization still has a role, it is mainly a secondary option in the case of failed percutaneous therapy or incessant restenosis after percutaneous stenting.

## PERCUTANEOUS THERAPY FOR UPPER EXTREMITY ARTERIAL DISEASE

### *Choice of Access Site*

Planning for a percutaneous approach to an upper extremity intervention involves thoughtful consideration of an access site. The brachial artery has the highest complication rate but sometimes is a good option in the case of a complete occlusion of the subclavian artery or innominate. This is especially true when there is an ostial occlusion that is flush with the aorta, or the nub of the occlusion is so shallow that obtaining a stable guide catheter position from which to cross the occlusion is very difficult from the femoral approach. **Fig. 2** illustrates a case of subclavian artery occlusion approached via simultaneous femoral and brachial access sites. Care must be taken during the case and when obtaining hemostasis afterwards to minimize the risk of brachial artery injury, thrombosis, and occlusion. **Box 2** lists approaches to minimizing brachial artery injury and subsequent occlusion when using the brachial artery as an access site. The femoral artery has been the most commonly used access site for all catheterization laboratory and angiography suite procedures, and remains so. It usually provides excellent backup for a long sheath or guide catheter placed into the ostial or proximal left subclavian artery, because the path is relatively straight. Because the innominate tends to be on the proximal portion of the arch, a guide catheter or sheath from the femoral artery must tend toward the left to engage the ostium. This feat is much easier with a preformed, shaped, guide catheter such as a multipurpose or JR4 guide catheter than with a standard straight sheath. The radial artery is an excellent option for accessing the upper extremity vasculature and performing interventions. The radial artery has the lowest complication rate of all the access sites and is geographically close to the target vessels. The authors have used the transradial approach with great success when performing axillary artery interventions and mid to distal subclavian artery interventions. **Figs. 3** and **4** demonstrate axillary artery stenting cases approached from the ipsilateral radial artery. When the lesion is a total occlusion located at the ostium of the innominate or left subclavian, the radial approach is not ideal. The remote location does not allow for maximal backup or optimal opacification with contrast injections, although a longer catheter placed inside the radial artery sheath improves both of these limitations. The authors like the low complication rates and the superior patient comfort that is afforded by taking the transradial approach. Although sheath size limitations might seem to be a drawback, in actuality, most interventions these days with miniaturized equipment compatible with 0.014 to 0.018 thousandths of an inch guidewires, can be performed through 6Fr sheaths. The authors advise performing an intravascular ultrasound (IVUS) of the radial artery through a 6Fr sheath to determine that the radial artery is at least 3 mm in diameter before upsizing to an 8Fr sheath. It is sometimes very useful to have dual access sites; the femoral artery to opacify the target vessel from below and either the radial or brachial to opacify the lesion from above. This approach is also useful for identification of the true ostium, when placing a stent in the ostial innominate or subclavian via a brachial or radial artery approach. **Fig. 5** illustrate a case of severe disease of the ostium of the innominate, approached by both the femoral and brachial sites. Although it is desirable to have the edge of the stent protrude into the aorta a few millimeters (to ensure that the entire ostial lesion is covered), one can overshoot the ostium considerably if relying only on opacification from the brachial artery sheath or catheter. Contrast injections from a transfemoral catheter or sheath located at the ostium of the arch vessel is an excellent way to visualize the ostium when placing a stent from above. **Box 3** shows our algorithm for selecting an access site for upper extremity arterial intervention.

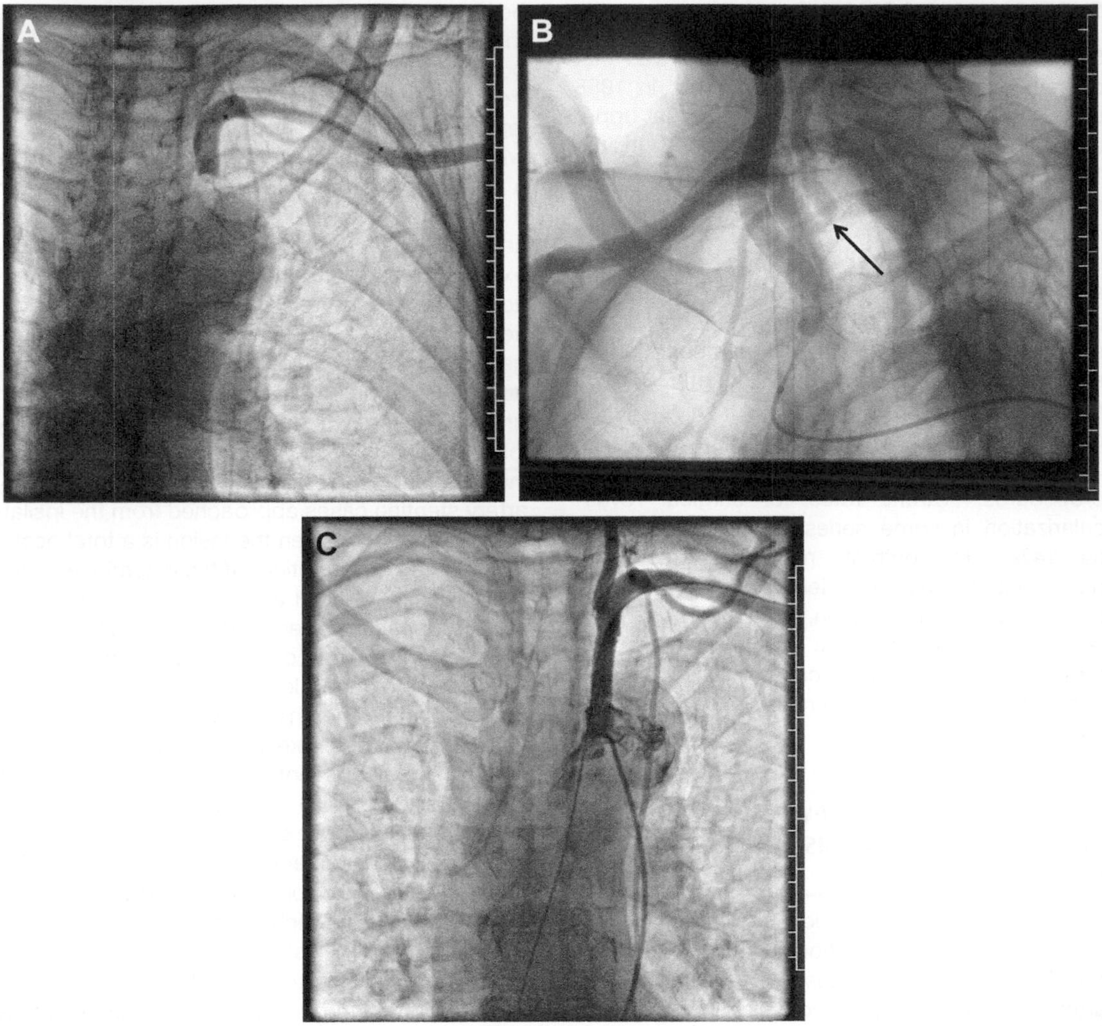


**Fig. 2.** Left subclavian occlusion with right vertebral artery stenosis. An 80-year-old white female smoker with known coronary artery disease had several episodes of frank syncope. A carotid duplex revealed mild carotid obstructions (<50%) and retrograde flow down the left vertebral artery. The left brachial systolic blood pressure was 70 mm Hg lower than the right. Left subclavian arteriography was performed via the left radial artery and confirmed a complete occlusion of the left subclavian artery proximal to the left vertebral artery (*A*). She was pretreated with clopidogrel and aspirin, and right femoral artery access was obtained. Aortography was performed, showing a right vertebral artery stenosis (*B, arrow*), with retrograde filling of the left vertebral artery. A weight-based bolus of bivalirudin followed by a continuous IV drip was started. From the radial artery sheath, a hydrophilic, 0.035-inch angled Glidewire (Terumo) was advanced slightly outside of a preloaded 0.035 Quick-Cross Support Catheter (Spectranetics) to perform blunt dissection and the lesion was crossed. The lesion was dilated followed by successful deployment of a 6 mm × 27 mm balloon-expandable, stainless steel stent. Zero residual stenosis was achieved (*C*), and there was no significant pressure gradient between the left subclavian artery and aorta at the conclusion of the procedure.

## *Periprocedural Pharmacotherapy*

Preprocedural planning includes deciding on the adjunctive antithrombotic agents to use. To optimize outcomes, platelets and thrombin activity must be optimally inhibited during the procedure. For antiplatelet therapy, pretreatment of all patients with aspirin (acetyl salicylic acid [ASA], 325 mg) and a thienopyridine (usually clopidogrel, 600 mg) is recommended. Postprocedure, all patients are treated with a minimum of 1 month of dual antiplatelet inhibition (ASA 81–325 mg/day and clopidogrel 75 mg/day) followed by lifelong ASA therapy. Many patients with coronary artery stents may require dual antiplatelet therapy for one full year or longer. Adjunctive platelet

**Box 2**
**Tips for minimizing brachial artery injury/occlusion when using the brachial artery as the access site for percutaneous interventions**

- Access the artery with micropuncture-sized needles
- Keep procedural activated clotting time more than 250 seconds
- Use the smallest diameter sheath possible
- When removing sheath:
  - Allow arterial site to bleed back 2 or 3 seconds to flush out thrombi
  - Hold brachial arteriotomy site to achieve hemostasis at the brachial arteriotomy site while allowing a faint radial pulse

glycoprotein IIb/IIIa antagonism using an agent such as eptifibatide is rarely indicated but may be used in situations where the patient has not received an adequate preload of oral antiplatelet agents. For antithrombin therapy, unfractionated heparin (a single intravenous [IV] bolus of 50–70 units/kg) or bivalirudin (weight-based bolus and drip, turned off at the end of the procedure) may be used.

## *Equipment Selection*

Equipment selection begins with selection of the guidewire that is used to cross the lesion. Traditional 0.035 inch guidewires are available as are miniaturized 0.014 inch guidewires based on coronary interventional equipment; 0.018 inch guidewires are an intermediate option. After guidewire selection, the balloons, stents, IVUS catheters, and other equipment are selected to be compatible with the size of the guidewire. The authors prefer 0.014-inch based systems and use them as our default systems as they are the smallest, and smaller profile balloons generally traverse severe lesions more easily. These systems also allow for smaller sheath sizes, which ultimately mean smaller punctures in the access site artery. The authors live by the adage that "When it comes to holes in arteries, the smaller the better." The larger 0.035-inch based systems are sometimes required, so it is necessary to be comfortable with both.

## *Percutaneous Transluminal Balloon Angioplasty*

Although few interventional procedures are stand-alone balloon angioplasty procedures, the balloon remains indispensable both in the predeployment

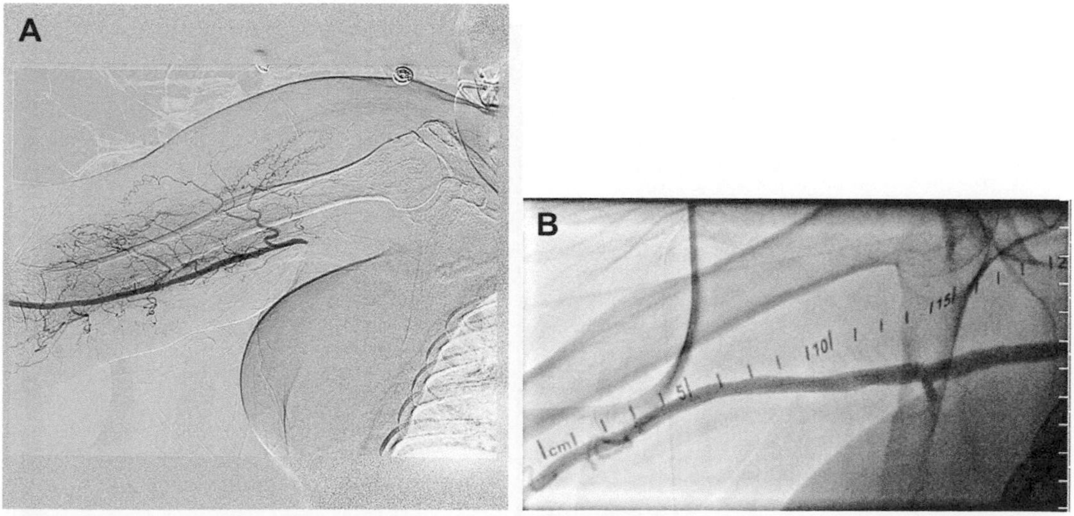


**Fig. 3.** Right axillary artery occlusion. A 64-year-old African American female smoker was noted to have a severely diminished right radial pulse and asymmetric upper extremity blood pressure readings on routine evaluation. After pretreatment with 600 mg of clopidogrel and 325 mg of aspirin, right radial arterial access was obtained. A bolus of 5000 units of unfractionated heparin was given in the radial artery sheath. Angiography revealed complete occlusion of the right axillary artery (*A*). A hydrophilic, 0.035-inch angled Glidewire (Terumo) was advanced slightly outside of a preloaded 0.035 Quick-Cross Support Catheter (Spectranetics) to perform blunt dissection, and the lesion was crossed. The catheter was then advanced distal into the ascending aorta, and the Glidewire was exchanged for a heavy 0.014-inch wire. Balloon angioplasty was performed, after which a 6 mm x 80 mm nitinol, self-expanding stent was successfully deployed, with zero residual stenosis (*B*) and normalization of the brachial index.

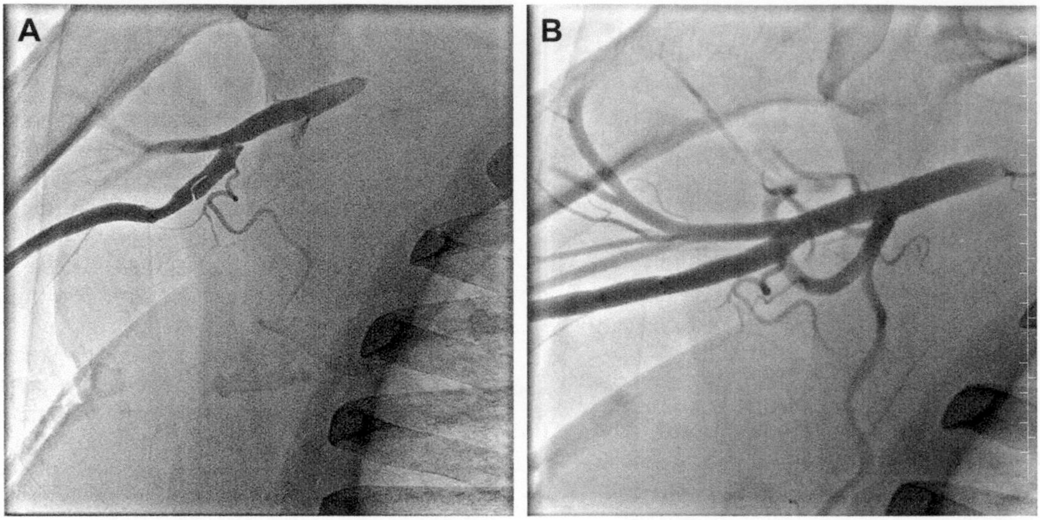


**Fig. 4.** Iatrogenic axillary artery dissection. A 60-year-old man with known coronary artery disease underwent a diagnostic left heart catheterization at an outside hospital. Right brachial arterial access was attempted and aborted because of difficulty in passing a wire through the axillary artery. At our institution femoral access was obtained, and a large dissection in the axillary artery was noted. (*A*) He was pretreated with aspirin and clopidogrel and right radial artery access was obtained, followed by a weight-based bolus and IV drip of bivalirudin. A 0.014-inch wire was advanced across the dissection and the vessel was stented using a 10 mm × 60 mm self-expanding, nitinol stent with excellent results (*B*). Cardiac catheterization and 2-vessel coronary artery stenting was then performed without incident.

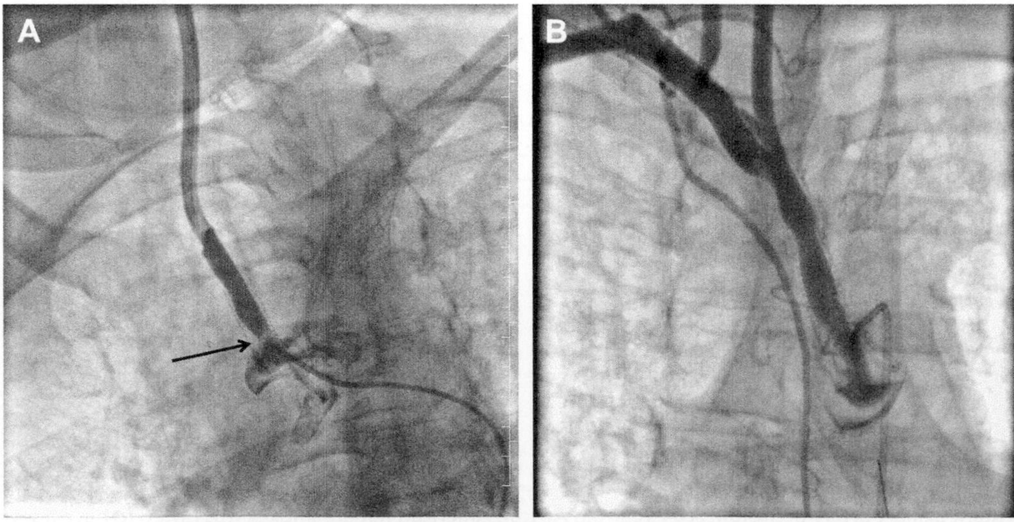


**Fig. 5.** Innominate artery in-stent restenosis. A 50-year-old woman with severe peripheral artery disease and prior stenting of the innominate artery presented with worsening chest pain, and the return of her previous right arm claudication. After right femoral arterial access was obtained, left heart catheterization and innominate artery angiography was performed. The angiography revealed high-grade in-stent restenosis of the innominate artery (*A, arrow*). Anticoagulation for the procedure included IV eptifibatide and weight-based, dose-adjusted, unfractionated heparin. Arterial access of the right brachial artery was then obtained and a 6Fr multipurpose guide catheter was advanced from the brachial artery sheath to the innominate. The lesion was crossed using 0.014-inch guidewire, and successive balloon inflations were performed. Minimal residual stenosis was noted at the conclusion of the procedure (*B*), and the translesion gradient was reduced from 90 mm Hg to 10 mm Hg.

**Box 3**
**Selecting an access site for upper extremity arterial intervention**

- Brachial artery
  - 100% occlusion of ostial innominate or subclavian
- Radial artery
  - Axillary artery occlusion or stenosis
  - Mid or distal subclavian artery
- Femoral artery
  - Proximal or mid subclavian artery
  - Stenosis in innominate artery
- Combined femoral and brachial/radial
  - Very proximal or ostial innominate or subclavian artery

and the postdeployment of stents. The balloon dilatation of the lesion tests the compliance of the lesion before it is traversed with a stent, allows for proper and accurate sizing of the stent, and is used to postdilate the stent to ensure adequate expansion and apposition against the arterial wall. For subclavian and innominate interventions, the balloon is typically undersized by 2 sizes for the first inflation (a 6-mm diameter artery is treated with a 4-mm balloon), which is done simply to test the compliance of the balloon and create a channel for the stent. There is no need to match the balloon and artery size if the ultimate goal is to place a stent; overaggressive balloon dilatation increases the risk of dissection, which can propagate quickly in the subclavian artery and jeopardize the vertebral and internal mammary arteries.

## *Percutaneous Stenting*

Percutaneous stenting of subclavian and innominate disease is the procedure of choice and involves both balloon-expandable and self-expanding stents. Balloon-expandable stents are typically indicated in procedures that require precise placement and for locations that are not compressible. They are made of stainless steel or cobalt chromium and have impressive radial strength, but are not elastic. When bent or pinched, they remain deformed. The ostium of the innominate or of the left subclavian artery is an ideal place for a stainless steel stent; its radial strength is an advantage at an aorto-ostial site where plaque tends to be difficult to compress and an abundance of fibrous tissue leads to recoil after balloon angioplasty. Self-expanding stents are made of an alloy of nickel and titanium. This nitinol material is elastic, and springs back to its original shape when exposed to compression and torsion, making it ideal for sites such as the axillary artery, the mid subclavian artery, and the cervical carotid artery. Hadjipetrou and colleagues[6] reported a 100% success rate in 18 patients undergoing aortic arch vessel stenosis who were treated with primary stent placement. There were no major complications. The follow-up at 17 months demonstrated no restenosis and all patients remained asymptomatic.

## *Thrombectomy/Fibrinolysis in Upper Extremity Arterial Disease*

Percutaneous thrombectomy/fibrinolysis is rarely needed in the upper extremity arteries, and when it is, it is usually secondary to thromboembolism from the heart. Artery-to-artery thromboembolism occurs when a complex plaque in the proximal portion of a large artery fractures or ruptures. Whatever the cause, acute limb ischemia from arterial thromboembolism represents a true emergency. A percutaneous approach usually involves attempts to remove the embolus via aspiration, using either a manual aspiration catheter or a mechanical aspiration thrombectomy system. The former is simply a hollow catheter with a syringe attached to the back end to generate suction. The most popular mechanical thrombectomy system uses a pump mechanism to create suction. With both types, the catheter is advanced over a wire to the embolus and several passes are made in which the catheter is repeatedly advanced distal and withdrawn proximal to the lesion. This can be done with or without adjunctive use of fibrinolytic drugs, and an attempt to improve the success rate of a catheter-based intervention by pretreatment with fibrinolytic agents seems reasonable. In the lower extremities, a well-defined protocol for fibrinolysis is usually performed with an overnight infusion of a fibrinolytic drug into a catheter wedged into the thrombotic lesion. In the upper extremity, thrombotic occlusions are less frequent and they tend to be more discrete than in the lower extremities. Thus, there is no universal well-defined protocol for fibrinolysis in this area, but several successful case series have been published.[8]

## COMPLICATIONS

Complications of upper extremity arterial interventions are familiar to the angiographer, as they are essentially the same complications that pose a risk to any percutaneous intervention. General complications of any angiographic and interventional procedure, such as radiographic dye allergy, contrast nephropathy, or radiation skin necrosis, can also accompany upper extremity arterial interventions.

### *Access Site Complications*

The most common complication is related to the access site and can include hemorrhage or thrombotic occlusion at the femoral, brachial, or radial artery. With normal collateral flow to the hand from the ulnar artery ensured by a normal Allen test, radial artery occlusion is usually a clinically silent event. Although some have had success with percutaneous therapies to treat access site occlusions, surgical thrombectomy may be required for occlusions of the brachial or femoral arteries. Access site complications related to bleeding can include large hematomas or sequelae such as arteriovenous fistulas or pseudoaneurysms. Therapies can range from expectant management to thrombin injection of pseudoaneurysms and surgical repair.

### *Target Vessel Complications*

Complications at the target vessel can include arterial dissection, rupture, or atherothromboembolism. Dissections need only be treated if they are occlusive or near occlusive and the authors do not treat small, hemodynamically insignificant dissections. Large dissections are usually effectively treated by implanting an additional stent. When this is not possible, prolonged balloon inflation sometimes helps to tack up the dissection. Small perforations can be effectively treated by placing covered stents, although these are large devices and may requiring upsizing the sheath to accommodate them. In the time necessary to do this, the patient can lose a large volume of blood. In such cases the authors recommend immediately inflating a balloon sized to the artery that can cover the perforation, and moving to a different access site to deploy the covered stent. If this strategy is unsuccessful, surgical repair may be required. Atherothromboembolism or thromboembolism downstream in the target vessel can be managed as described in the section on thrombectomy/fibrinolysis.

### *Other Major Complications*

Percutaneous interventions on aortic arch vessels carry the risk of embolic stroke secondary to atherothromboembolism or thromboembolism, the origin of which can be the subclavian, innominate or vertebral arteries, or the aorta. The embolus can also be composed wholly or mostly of platelet microaggregates. For this reason, pretreatment of patients with dual antiplatelet therapy, aspirin, and clopidogrel is recommended. If the procedure must be done before these patients can be pretreated, an intravenous platelet glycoprotein IIb/IIIa inhibitor, such as eptifibatide to achieve rapid platelet inhibition, may be used. Hadjipetrou and colleagues[6] documented a stroke rate of zero in a review of articles in which 108 patients were treated. Thus, the risk is clearly low but may not be zero in all patients. Careful technique, attention to adjunctive antithrombotic therapy, and careful patient selection will minimize the risk of stroke.

## SUMMARY

Upper extremity arteries are affected by occlusive diseases with diverse causes; atherosclerosis is by far the most common. Although mostly asymptomatic, very definite clinical consequences and symptoms can occur. Although the overriding principle in managing patients with upper extremity arterial occlusive disease should be cardiovascular risk reduction by noninvasive and pharmacologic means, when target organ ischemia produces symptoms or threatens the patient's well-being, revascularization is necessary. Given their minimally invasive nature and successful outcomes, percutaneous, catheter-based therapies are currently preferred to surgical approaches. The fact that expertise in these techniques resides in not one but several disciplines (vascular surgery, radiology, cardiology, vascular medicine) makes this an area ripe for multidisciplinary collaboration to the benefit of patients.

## REFERENCES

1. Mukherjee D, Rajagopalan S. Subclavian, innominate and axillary artery disease. In: Rajagopalan S, Dean SM, Mohler ER, et al, editors. Manual of vascular diseases. 2nd edition. Philadelphia: Lippincott Williams & Wilkins; 2011.
2. Fields WS, Lemak NA. Joint Study of extracranial arterial occlusion VII. Subclavian steal–a review of 168 cases. JAMA 1972;222(9):1139–43.
3. Coletti A, Rajagopalan S. Approach to the patient with upper extremity arterial disease. In: Rajagopalan S, Dean SM, Mohler ER, et al, editors. Manual of vascular diseases. 1st edition. Philadelphia: Lippincott Williams & Wilkins; 2005. p. 215–26.
4. Crawford ES, De Bakey ME, Morris GC Jr, et al. Surgical treatment of occlusion of the innominate, common carotid, and subclavian arteries: a 10 year experience. Surgery 1969;65(1):17–31.

5. Cina CS, Safar HA, Lagana A, et al. Subclavian carotid transposition and bypass grafting: consecutive cohort study and systematic review. J Vasc Surg 2002;35(3): 422–9.
6. Hadjipetrou P, Cox S, Piemonte T, et al. Percutaneous revascularization of atherosclerotic obstruction of aortic arch vessels. J Am Coll Cardiol 1999;33(5): 1238–45.
7. Stone PA, Srivastiva M, Campbell JE, et al. Diagnosis and treatment of subclavian artery occlusive disease. Expert Rev Cardiovasc Ther 2010;8(9): 1275–82.
8. Coulon M, Goffette P, Dondelinger RF. Local thrombolytic infusion in arterial ischemia of the upper limb: mid-term results. Cardiovasc Intervent Radiol 1994; 17(2):81–6.

# Medical Management of the Patient with Intermittent Claudication

Deepthi Vodnala, MD[a], Sanjay Rajagopalan, MD[b], Robert D. Brook, MD[c,*]

**KEYWORDS**

- Peripheral arterial disease • Atherosclerosis
- Cardiovascular risk factors • Vascular disease

Peripheral artery disease (PAD), an obstructive vascular disease of peripheral arteries, is most often caused by systemic atherosclerosis. Formal guidelines for management have been promulgated by many societies, including the Inter-Society Consensus for the Management of PAD (TASC II)[1] and the American Heart Association (AHA) in conjunction with the American College of Cardiology (ACC).[2] Additional articles of note that have affected therapeutic decisions include the AHA Conference Proceedings on Atherosclerotic Peripheral Vascular Disease Symposium II[3] and contemporary reviews on PAD.[4] Beyond summarizing these official recommendations, recent and important clinical updates with a potential to affect management are provided here. After briefly discussing the disease manifestation and overall approach to management, this review focuses on the medical treatment of PAD due to atherosclerosis.

## CLINICAL PRESENTATION AND EPIDEMIOLOGY OF PAD

Intermittent claudication (IC) is derived from Latin word "to limp" and derives at least in part from decreased perfusion to the relevant contracting muscles in the lower extremities during exertion. However, the relationship between blood flow limitations and symptoms is only moderate, and it has been suggested that intrinsic metabolic changes in the skeletal system could play a role in the pathophysiology of the disease.[1] The classic "Rose" symptoms of IC are a reproducible discomfort in a group of large leg muscles precipitated by activity that does not resolve with continued exertion and is rapidly abrogated (within 10 minutes) by rest.[1,3,4] The pain is typically reproducible with the same amount of exercise, and patients can frequently quantify the distance or the time of exercise that causes the pain. Symptoms are often limited to a group of muscles, which may vary depending on the extent and location of disease. For example, disease of aortoiliac arteries cause buttock and hip pain, common femoral artery PAD causes pain in thighs, superficial femoral artery disease causes pain in calf muscles, and disease of popliteal and peroneal-tibial arteries causes calf and foot pain. The pain of IC is produced in the group of muscles one segment below the level of disease. However, most often symptoms are contained to the calf, as calf muscles are metabolically very active and the superior femoral artery is commonly involved.[5] Nonetheless, recent studies have categorized patients who have rest pain and/or symptoms that are not classic as having atypical claudication.[6]

The authors have nothing to disclose. No applicable funding support.

[a] Michigan State University, East Lansing, MI, USA
[b] Section of Vascular Medicine, Division of Cardiovascular Medicine, Ohio State University, 460 West 12th Avenue Floor 3, Room 398, Biomedical Research Tower, Columbus, OH 43210-1252, USA
[c] Division of Cardiovascular Medicine, University of Michigan, 24 Frank Lloyd Wright Drive, PO Box 322, Ann Arbor, MI 48106, USA
* Corresponding author.
*E-mail address:* robdbrok@umich.edu

Cardiol Clin 29 (2011) 363–379
doi:10.1016/j.ccl.2011.04.003

Indeed, the majority of individuals with demonstrable PAD are asymptomatic (>40%) or have atypical leg pain symptoms (50%), whereas only 10% are estimated to present with classic IC as described.[1,4,7] Therefore, a high suspicion should be maintained in people with leg pain of any type and/or who are at risk for PAD, given the serious health risks and its role (alone or in conjunction with other disorders) in causing leg pain and impairing quality of life.

Of further note, the manifestations of PAD do not necessarily manifest by progressive deterioration. Patients presenting with critical limb ischemia (ie, pain at rest, tissue damage/loss or skin ulcers, leg systolic pressure <50 mm Hg, threatened limb loss) have often not complained of prior IC, and one-half to one-third of patients diagnosed with PAD by ankle brachial index (ABI; defined as the ratio of the blood pressure [BP] in the lower legs to the BP in the arms) testing report any symptomatology. The vast majority of patients with IC (≈70%) do not alter their symptoms with the progression of time. Worsening of symptoms occurs in 25% of cases over a 5-year period. The deterioration occurs most frequently during the first year after identification of PAD (7%–9%) compared with 2% to 3% per annum thereafter. Major amputation is relatively rare among patients with stable IC (1%–3% over 5 years).

## RISK FACTORS FOR PAD

Lower extremity PAD is common, with a prevalence rate in the United States of more than 8.5 million individuals.[8] The incidence increases with age, affecting up to 20% of patients older than 70 to 75 years. However, PAD is common with increasing age and is more prevalent among non-Hispanic Blacks (7.8%) than in Whites (4.4%).[9] Incidence and prevalence of asymptomatic and symptomatic PAD is more common in men than in women (relative risk of 0.7).[1] PAD also seems to occur more frequently in Hispanics (relative risk, 1.5) and African Americans (relative risk, 2.5).

The risk factors for developing IC due to atherosclerotic PAD are similar to coronary artery disease (CAD). These factors include smoking, male sex, increasing age, diabetes, and dyslipidemia (ie, elevated low-density lipoprotein cholesterol [LDL-C] and reduced high-density lipoprotein cholesterol [HDL-C]). However, the strongest age-independent risk factors are diabetes and tobacco smoking.[1,4] Given the commonality of risk factors and the systemic nature of atherosclerosis, it is not surprising that patients with PAD have a high prevalence of concurrent coronary artery and cerebrovascular disease.

Studies have shown that after multivariate adjustment for age, sex, and other risk factors, patients with PAD have a threefold higher risk of all-cause death and a sixfold higher risk of cardiovascular-related death. Patients with an ABI of less than 0.9 were found to have hazard ratios of 1.7 and 2.5 for all-cause and cardiovascular mortality, respectively, even without symptoms of IC.[1,4] In the REACH registry involving 55,814 patients, the majority of whom were on evidence-based risk-reduction therapy, the 1-year incidence of cardiovascular death, myocardial infarction (MI), stroke, and hospitalization was highest in patients with established PAD (21%) compared with 15% for CAD patients. The event rates increased with the number of symptomatic arterial disease locations, ranging from 5.3% for patients with risk factors only, to 13% for patients with 1, 21% for patients with 2, and 26% for patients with 3 arterial disease locations.

Patients with PAD are therefore at high risk for cardiovascular morbidity and mortality. The majority of patients with PAD die of MI or stroke.[10,11] As such, PAD is considered a "coronary heart disease (CHD) risk equivalent" by the National Cholesterol Education Program Adult Treatment Panel III.[12] Patients with PAD should be treated with risk factor optimization as aggressively as patients with diagnosed CHD, as discussed later. Unfortunately, the presence of PAD often masks CHD symptoms because of decreased exercise capacitance.[13] Patients with PAD have more incidence of CAD, die more often of cardiac causes, and perform poorly after coronary artery bypass graft surgery for significant CAD.[14,15]

## DIAGNOSIS OF PAD

Although diagnostic strategies are not the focus of this review and are covered in detail elsewhere,[1,3,4] a variety of other vascular and nonvascular diseases can cause lower extremity pain, or symptoms must be considered in the differential diagnosis before initiating treatment for PAD. It is also possible to have more than a single cause of leg pain.

In brief, nonatherosclerotic arterial causes of leg pain to consider include: thromboangiitis obliterans (Buerger disease), hypoplasia and acquired coarctation of the abdominal aorta ("mid-aortic syndrome"), vasculitis syndromes (eg, Takayasu vasculitis, giant cell arteritis, systemic lupus, small vessel disease), vascular trauma or irradiation injury, popliteal diseases (adventitial cystic disease, entrapment), fibromuscular dysplasia (external iliac artery), persistent sciatic artery (thrombosed), and iliac endofibrosis syndrome of the cyclist.

Nonvascular causes are also important drivers of lower extremity pain and can be concomitant with true PAD. Major causes include leg muscular cramps, nocturnal leg cramps or restless leg syndrome, radiculopathy (eg, sciatica), arthritis of any leg joint/hip/low back, Baker cyst, primary or secondary myopathy, venous claudication, compartment syndrome, peripheral large- or small-fiber neuropathy, erythromelalgia, and spinal stenosis. The latter disease often causes neurogenic "pseudoclaudication," and it is important to differentiate this from true PAD. Classic features that distinguish true arterial IC from pseudoclaudication include sharp and paresthetic nature of the discomfort, pain with variable walking distance, pain on standing alone, and relief with flexion of the spine (sitting or leaning forward).

A history and physical examination, along with initial diagnostic testing (eg, ABI, exercise ABI), will be helpful in determining the most pertinent cause of any leg symptoms. The traditional screening or first test to evaluate for PAD for patients with leg pain consistent with IC is to perform a resting ABI.[1,4] The ACC also recommends testing of all patients at risk for PAD with an ABI, including patients with exertion-related leg pain, those 50 to 69 years old with cardiovascular risk factors (particularly diabetes or smoking), people older than 70 years irrespective of risk factors, patients with an abnormal lower extremity pulse examination, and those with established or known cardiovascular, carotid, or renal artery atherosclerotic disease. Patients with a Framingham Risk Score between 10% and 20% may also benefit from an ABI test to help further discriminate cardiovascular risk. Those with an abnormal test are at higher risk and should be treated more aggressively.[2]

An ABI is an inexpensive and accurate diagnostic test for PAD. The test is 95% sensitive and almost 100% specific for PAD. A value of 0.9 to 1.3 is considered normal; a value less than 0.9 is abnormal and most often consistent with IC. An ABI between 0.7 and 0.89 is considered mild disease, 0.4 to 0.69 moderate disease, and less than 0.4 severe disease with a worse prognosis.[16] A value of high ABI, 1.3 to 1.4, is abnormal and indicates arterial calcification often due to underlying diabetes or renal disease, in which case a toe ABI value of less than 0.7 indicates PAD. Isolated or concomitant microvascular or small arteriole disease (as may occur with diabetes, Buerger disease, and atheroemboli) should not be overlooked and may cause more distal leg or isolated foot pain or IC, even with a normal or spuriously high ABI. A toe brachial index or imaging modality may be required to make the diagnosis.

Other diagnostic modalities include segmental arterial pressures analysis, Doppler waveform analysis, and a treadmill ABI if the symptoms are consistent with IC due to PAD but the resting ABI is normal or borderline. In the absence of severe immediate life-limiting ischemic symptoms (or perhaps very low ABI <0.4–0.5) or critical limb ischemia, follow-up studies to investigate the anatomy and confirm the degree of PAD are generally performed after the diagnosis has been made by an aforementioned test, treatment approaches have been given time to improve symptoms (typically 3–6 months), and a revascularization procedure is currently being considered. Such tests include duplex ultrasonography, computed tomographic angiography, magnetic resonance angiography, and/or conventional invasive angiography. Imaging tests can also be performed if the diagnosis remains in question, multiple causes of symptoms are suspected, screening tests are inconclusive and/or contradictory, or isolated small vascular disease is suspected.

## OVERALL MANAGEMENT OUTLINE

The overall treatment approach in the PAD patient focuses on (1) reducing cardiovascular events through risk factor optimization, (2) preventing progression of PAD and limb loss, and (3) improving symptoms and well-being through exercise regimen programs, pharmacotherapy, and surgical/endovascular interventions when required. The general management strategy is outlined in **Fig. 1**. IC cases due to PAD are categorized as mild, moderate, and severe based on symptoms and ABI, and therapy is guided accordingly.[2] Aggressive cardiovascular preventive strategies such as daily use of aspirin (or alternative antiplatelet regimens) should be considered, while complete smoking cessation is of critical importance. Cilostazol, proven to improve IC, should be considered for those with persistent life-limiting symptoms despite exercise and risk factor control (or perhaps concomitant with diagnosis and initiating exercise in selected patients). Endovascular and surgical approaches should be reserved for individuals who continue to have life-limiting IC, progression of PAD, and new critical limb ischemia, and/or who fail these initial approaches. Finally, patients with confirmed PAD may benefit from screening for underlying CAD (eg, pharmacologic stress testing if unable to adequately perform exercise stress modalities) and carotid atherosclerosis, because of the high probability of coexistent disease.[2]

To achieve treatment goals, patients with confirmed PAD should have testing for seated BP, a fasting CHD profile and glucose, as well as a hemoglobin $A_{1c}$ ($HbA_{1c}$) test. The measurement of a complete blood count (for hemoglobin and

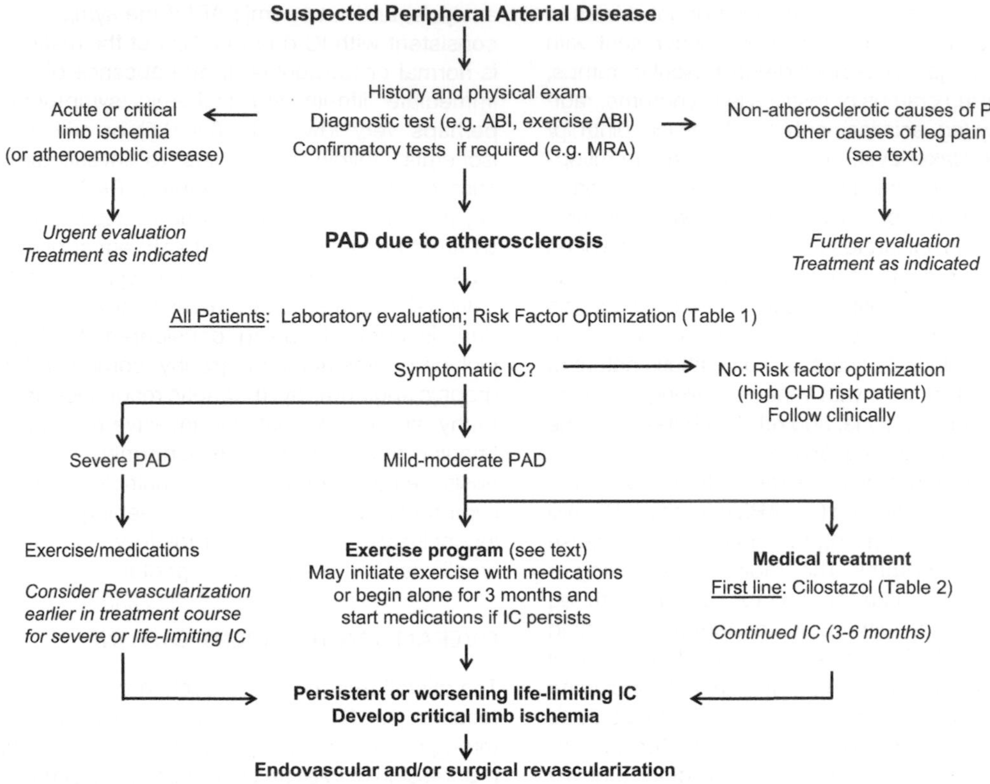


**Fig. 1.** Medical management algorithm for the treatment of patients with suspected intermittent claudication due to atherosclerotic peripheral vascular disease. ABI, ankle brachial index; CHD, coronary heart disease; MRA, magnetic resonance angiography.

platelet count), a basic chemistry panel (creatinine level), a urinalysis, and an electrocardiogram should be considered, particularly in patients who may undergo a revascularization. In some situations an evaluation for a hypercoagulable state and/or novel CHD risk factors associated with premature atherosclerosis may be considered.

## RISK FACTOR OPTIMIZATION

PAD is associated with a high prevalence of cardiovascular morbidity and mortality, and is thus considered a CHD risk equivalent by cholesterol guidelines.[12] Hence, all patients require aggressive management to optimize their traditional CHD risk factors. The overall recommended goals regarding the authors' review of the literature along with the formal TASC II guideline targets[1] are presented in **Table 1**. When present, for example if new trial evidence has become available since the TASC II publication, differences in recommendations are highlighted in the text sections.

### *Smoking Cessation*

Smoking is noted to be the most potent modifiable risk factor for the development of PAD,[17] and although no randomized controlled trials have seen the effect of smoking cessation in cardiovascular disease with PAD, observational studies have showed that the risk for MI, death, and amputation is less in patients who quit smoking.[18,19] Moreover, smoking cessation can improve overall exercise capacitance.[20,21] Although observational studies suggest a reduction in IC by smoking cessation, this remains incompletely proven among randomized trials.[22] However, this fact should not deter cessation efforts. Regardless of its effect on PAD, complete smoking cessation is a proven modality to substantially reduce CHD risk among all patients with or without atherosclerosis. Moreover, recent evidence corroborates its efficacy even among individuals taking modern-day aggressive medical therapy including high-dose statins.[23] The absolute risk reduction for cessation in terms of cardiovascular events (4.5%) is actually greater than intensive-dose versus moderate-dose statin therapy (1.7%–2.2%). Recently, the effectiveness of a smoking cessation program among patients with PAD in a randomized controlled trial was demonstrated.[24] Patients randomized to an intensive PAD-specific intervention for cessation were significantly more likely to be confirmed abstinent at 6 months than individuals undergoing standard practices. This clinical trial confirms the importance of multidisciplinary attempts to assure complete smoking cessation by providing specialized guidance to all patients with PAD who smoke.

It is recommended that every physician emphasize the importance of smoking cessation in patients with PAD. Pharmacologic interventions with nicotine replacement therapy such as transdermal nicotine patch, nicotine gum, nicotine spray, or nicotine inhalers have cessation rates of 15% to 30%.[25] Bupropion, an antidepressant, has approximately 25% efficacy in cessation. Varenicline, a partial nicotine agonist used to improve cravings and withdrawal symptoms, is the most effective agent for smoking cessation at this time.[26] There is no contraindication for its usage among patients with IC, even with stable CAD. Behavioral counseling should also be offered as a part of any comprehensive smoking cessation program.[2]

## *Diabetes Mellitus*

Diabetes mellitus is a strong risk factor for atherosclerosis of both systematic and coronary vasculature. Both PAD and diabetes pose an ominous presentation to patients as ischemic pain at rest and ulceration in a speedy manner. Patients with IC and diabetes have an amputation risk of 20% and 5-year mortality of 50%. Major factors contributing to amputation in diabetes patients include lack of outpatient diabetes education and neuropathic symptoms.[27] Falsely elevated ABI (1.3) is associated with calcified arteries of the lower extremities that are not compressible, most often due to diabetes. As per American Diabetes Association (ADA) recommendations, target $HbA_{1c}$ for patients with diabetes and PAD is 7% or lower, although this aggressive target has come under some criticism based on large trials such as the ACCORD trial (Action to COntrol Cardiovascular Risk in Diabetes).[28,29] Proper foot care including appropriate footwear with regular inspection, cleaning, and care of any foot ulcers should be addressed urgently.[2]

There are no clinical trials supporting the outcomes of antidiabetic therapy specifically in PAD. Strict glycemic control in type 1 and type 2 diabetics reduces the risk of microvascular complications such as neuropathy, retinopathy, and nephropathy. Intensive insulin therapy in both type 1 and type 2 diabetics had no significant effect on the risk for PAD.[30,31] Three large outcome studies have recently been completed comparing aggressive with more standard care for glucose lowering, though PAD outcomes were not specifically included.[32] None of the individual studies demonstrated an improvement in macrovascular events or overall mortality by achieving $HbA_{1c}$ values of less than 6.5% versus values ranging from 7.0% to 8.5%. Microvascular events, principally microalbuminuria, were reduced overall. A recent meta-analysis of 5 trials demonstrated the safety and possible benefit of reduction in CHD events by intensive glucose lowering.[33] However, the goal $HbA_{1c}$ was not evaluated and values less than 6.5% were not specifically investigated. Rather, it was shown that a 0.9% lower result produces a 15% reduction in CHD events. In light of these findings, we (the authors of this article) agree with the recent recommendation to achieve a target $HbA_{1c}$ of less than 7% as a reasonable goal[32] even among patients with PAD. We differ in our recommendations from those of the TASC II to try to achieve a target as close as possible to 6.0% (a lower goal) given the null findings of these clinical trials related to macrovascular event reduction. On an individual-level basis for certain patients, a lower goal of less than 6.5% could be considered to reduce microvascular events. We continue to recommend metformin as the first-line medication therapy as promoted by TASC II and ADA guidelines.[34]

## *Hypertension*

Hypertension is a strong cardiovascular risk factor, and contributes similarly to peripheral vascular disease. Antihypertensive agents should be given to lower BP at least to less than 140/90 mm Hg in all patients with PAD. The TASC II guidelines agree with the JNC VII recommendations for a more aggressive goal BP of lower than 130/80 mm Hg among diabetics and those with chronic kidney disease (CKD).[35] However, two major clinical trials have been published since these guidelines that substantively affect target BP levels as well as the initial antihypertensive agent to recommend. In the ACCORD study, a more aggressive approach (systolic BP ~119 mm Hg) did not reduce the primary composite cardiovascular end point compared with usual care (systolic BP ~134 mm Hg).[36] Although the secondary end point of stroke was reduced, the risks for serious side effects in the aggressive treatment limb were more numerous and therefore more than offset this benefit. There was no reduction in CHD-related events or the primary composite outcome in the more aggressively treated patients.[37] In addition, the primary results of the AASK study, though supporting the use of angiotensin-converting enzyme inhibitors (ACEIs)

**Table 1**
**Risk factor management and goals for PAD**

| Risk Factors | Goals Advocated | Therapies to Consider | Review of Efficacy[a] | Existing TASC II Guidelines |
|---|---|---|---|---|
| Smoking | Complete cessation | Counseling ± medications as required | +++ | Same as our recommendations |
| Diabetes mellitus | $HbA_{1c}$ of 7% to reduce microvascular disease and possibly CHD events<br>Lower goals (ie, <6.5% for select individual patients only as no overall benefit for macrovascular events demonstrated in trials) | Follow ADA Guidelines<br>*First line*: Metformin given overall risk/benefits among diabetic patients and per ADA guidelines<br>Other nonhypoglycemia agents and insulin as required to reach targets | ± | Same recommendations<br>More aggressive $HbA_{1c}$ goals of "as close to 6% as possible" per TASC II recommendations are not goals we advocate based on trials (see text) |
| Hypertension | *All patients*: <140/90 mm Hg<br>Minimal trial evidence to support lower targets (even with CKD or diabetes). Not recommended except in select and individual cases (see text) | *First line*: ACEI + amlodipine combination therapy recommended for most patients (see text)<br>β-Blocker not contraindicated due to PAD or IC alone if required for other reasons (eg, heart failure) | Hypertension treatment (+)<br>ACEI (possibly ++) | Same recommendations<br>Except a goal <130/80 mm Hg (goals we do not advocate based on trials) is adopted for patients with CKD or diabetes<br>Thiazide diuretics or an ACEI are first-line single agents recommended: we propose using ACEI + amlodipine |
| Hyperlipidemia | *All patients*: LDL-C <70 mg/dL; non-HDL-C <100 mg/dL<br>Meta-analyses strongly support a log-linear relation between LDL-C and cardiovascular events without a threshold at 100 mg/dL. The lowest LDL-C level safely attainable should be targeted | *First line*: Statins<br>Diet and other medications in addition to statins (or alone if statin not tolerated) as required to achieve targets<br>Add fenofibrate to a statin if triglycerides and HDL-C remain abnormal (particularly if diabetic per ACCORD trial). Consider fenofibrate alone or together with a statin to reduce amputation rates among diabetics | Cholesterol-lowering (+)<br>Statins (++) | Same recommendations<br>Except the goal is less aggressive for LDL-C <100 mg/dL; non–HDL-C <130 mg/dL for all patients<br>Lower goals (LDL-C <70 and non–HDL-C <100 mg/dL) were deemed reasonable for those with concomitant CAD. We advocate these aggressive targets for all PAD patients if possible based on trials and meta-analyses (see text) |

| | | | | |
|---|---|---|---|---|
| Antiplatelet therapy | *Consider*: aspirin treatment in PAD patients without CAD on an individual basis (see text)<br>Carefully weigh the risks (bleeding) versus benefits for each patient. No mandate to use aspirin in all PAD patients (ie, those without other indications such as CAD)<br>We recommend treatment with aspirin for all PAD patients with CAD or other indications (stroke, carotid disease) | No antiplatelet treatment required for PAD alone (consideration only)<br>*First line*: Aspirin 81 mg/d in patients with other indications (eg, CAD, stents, stroke). Higher dose not required or proven more effective<br>*Consider*: clopidogrel instead of aspirin in high-risk patients with symptomatic PAD; or if aspirin not tolerated<br>No combination antiplatelet treatments proven worthwhile with PAD unless required for other reasons (eg, coronary stent)<br>No treatment with oral anticoagulants (warfarin) recommended | ±<br>+<br>+<br>–<br>– | Aspirin for patients with carotid or coronary disease (same as our recommendations)<br>However, all symptomatic PAD patients are recommended aspirin and consideration given for those without symptoms by TASC II (which we do not advocate based on trials)<br>Clopidogrel recommended in patients with symptomatic PAD |
| Emerging risk factors | Homocysteine<br>Elevated Lp(a) >50 mg/dL<br>C-reactive protein | No treatment (ie, folic acid, B vitamins) based on negative clinical trials<br>*Consider*: Niacin treatment (see text)<br>No recommendations | –<br>± | Same recommendations<br>No recommendations given for Lp(a) treatment<br>Same recommendations |

*Abbreviations:* ACEI, angiotension-converting enzyme inhibitors; ADA, American Diabetes Association; CAD, coronary artery disease; CKD, chronic kidney disease; $HbA_{1c}$, hemoglobin $A_{1c}$; HDL-C, high-density lipoprotein cholesterol; LDL-C, low-density lipoprotein cholesterol; Lp(a), lipoprotein (a).

[a] +++, Treatment improves PAD complications/symptoms and cardiovascular events; ++, possible improvement in PAD complications and proven cardiovascular disease protection by treatment; +, no proven reduction in PAD complications/symptoms but reduces the cardiovascular events by treatment; ±, data mixed or require further studies; –, no benefit or harmful.

among patients with CKD, do not support lowering systolic BP to less than 130 mm Hg compared with standard goals for nephroprotection.[38] Therefore, even among diabetic and CKD patients, a systolic BP lower than 130 mm Hg cannot be universally recommended at this time based on clinical trial data. We therefore support a target systolic BP of lower than 140 mm Hg for all patients; and perhaps less than 135 mm Hg among diabetics given the results of the ADVANCE trial demonstrating a benefit from lowering BP down to this level.[39] Given that this issue remains controversial regarding the optimal goal BP and that there are ongoing studies investigating this issue further, a more aggressive BP target of lower than 130/80 mm Hg can be considered on an individual-level basis among patients with PAD (and has some trial evidence supporting that it can reduce strokes among diabetics as long as serious side effects are monitored closely).

Although the specific choice of antihypertensive medication depends on other underlying diseases (ie, ACEI for diabetic patients, CKD, or proteinuria), ACEIs are also considered a good choice for treatment of symptomatic or asymptomatic PAD by TASC II guidelines.[40,41] Moreover, a recent study has suggested that the ACEI ramipiril may even improve IC symptoms.[42] Thus, we believe that ACEIs are a reasonable first-choice BP-lowering agent among patients requiring only a single agent to reach BP goal. We also stress the importance from previous studies as highlighted in TASC II that β-blockers are not contraindicated exclusively due to IC symptoms or the presence of PAD. When used appropriately and if required for other indications (eg, angina), they do not significantly worsen PAD-related outcomes.

Because no study has specifically evaluated PAD-related outcomes among the hypertension trials, we believe that the optimal regimen should be selected based on its merits for reducing cardiovascular disease events when treating hypertension in patients with PAD. Recently, the ACCOMPLISH study evaluated the strategy of first-line combination therapy using amlodipine versus a thiazide diuretic added to background ACEI treatment. The composite cardiovascular outcome was reduced by in the ACEI + amlodipine group.[43] This positive outcome occurred among all patient subgroups (including diabetics and those with CKD) despite nearly identical BP levels corroborated by ambulatory monitoring. In light of these landmark findings, we believe that dual therapy with an inhibitor of the renin angiotensin system + a calcium-channel blocker should be strongly considered as first-line therapy for all PAD patients with hypertension that require 2 or more medications. However, clinical trial data demonstrate that about 75% of patients with hypertension require 2 or more agents to achieve a goal BP of less than 140/90 mm Hg.[44] Hence, this combination should be strongly considered for most patients with PAD and an elevated BP, regardless of hypertension stage (unless contraindicated or not tolerated). This combination provides the best CHD event reduction as proved by available clinical trials and a potential improvement of IC symptoms derived from the ACEI component (as described above), along with superior goal BP attainment than single-drug therapy. Additional antihypertensive agents should be added as required to achieve target BP levels.

## *Hyperlipidemia*

According to United States national guidelines from the Adult Treatment Panel of the National Cholesterol Education Program III (NCEP ATP III), patients with PAD are considered a "CHD risk equivalent." Hence, they require aggressive lipid management to optimal levels whenever possible.[12] The most recent meta-analysis[45] confirms that regardless of the initial lipid values among patients with atherosclerosis, the lower the LDL-C is treated (ie, more aggressive therapy) the lower the CHD event rate achieved even to values of less than 50 mg/dL. This situation occurs without evidence of excess noncardiovascular morbidity or mortality (eg, no excess cancer event rate). The landmark Heart Protection Study demonstrated that PAD patients with a pretreatment LDL-C at 100 mg/dL still benefited from statin treatment. Indeed, the recent meta-analysis also demonstrated that initial pretreatment LDL-C (even below 100 mg/dL) did not obviate the benefits derived from statin therapy. However, PAD outcomes were not included in these cholesterol-lowering studies. Nonetheless, given the high CHD risk of these patients, it is reasonable to support a goal target for the lowest LDL-C possible that is safe. We therefore recommend treatment with statins as first line, given their proven efficacy and in accord with the TASC II and AHA/ACC recommendation. However, we believe that treatment should be targeted to achieve an LDL-C less than 70 mg/dL (and perhaps lower if possible) in all patients with PAD (even in the absence of previous known CHD and regardless of initial LDL-C even if between 70 and 100 mg/dL). Although studies are ongoing to prove the benefit of combination lipid-lowering therapy, the overall evidence suggests that the addition of other agents (niacin, fibrates, ezetimbine, bile acid resins) should be used as needed (or instead of in the case of statin intolerance) to achieve this aggressive goal.

Ongoing trials will assess whether raising HDL-C by medications is worthwhile. However, the recently published ACCORD study demonstrated that adding fenofibrate lowered CHD events among patients with a high TG (>220 mg/dL) and a low HDL-C who were on simvastatin and who had achieved on average an LDL-C of less than 100 mg/dL.[46] Thus, this trial suggests that in PAD patients who have LDL-C treated on a statin but continue to have a mixed dyslipidemic phenotype, the addition of fenofibrate should be strongly considered. Meta-analyses of trials with fibric acid medications support this benefit among such patients as well. Finally, a prespecified analysis of the FIELD study demonstrated that fenofibrate reduced the incidence of first amputation among all patients (hazard ratio [HR] 0.64) and minor amputations among diabetics without known PAD (HR 0.53).[47] Strong consideration should be given for using a fibric acid therapy (along among statin-intolerant patients) and perhaps in addition to a statin even if LDL-C is at target, based on this trial, to reduce amputations in diabetic patients.

In the TASC II and AHA/ACC recommendations, statins are indicated in all patients with PAD to maintain an LDL-C target level of less than 100 mg/dL. However, the more aggressive target level of 70 mg/dL is recommended only for patients with lower extremity PAD at high risk of ischemic events, including those with concomitant CAD.[2] In the updated NCEP ATP III guidelines,[48] PAD patients are stratified into two categories, "high risk" or "very high risk," depending on related risk factors. For subjects with PAD, very high risk can be described as the presence of recognized PAD plus (a) multiple major risk factors (especially diabetes), (b) severe and poorly controlled risk factors (especially continued cigarette smoking), or (c) multiple risk factors of the metabolic syndrome (especially high triglycerides [$\geq$200 mg/dL] plus non–HDL-C $\geq$130 mg/dL, and low HDL-C [$\leq$40 mg/dL]). The very high-risk patients have a goal LDL-C of less than 70 mg/dL. Our recommendations differ from the TASC II, ATP III, and AHA/ACC guidelines. We believe the evidence has grown to now support achieving the lowest possible LDL-C (ie, <70 mg/dL) and non–HDL-C (ie, <100 mg/dL as a secondary target if triglycerides are >200 mg/dL) in all high-risk patients (which includes those with PAD) if possible.[45]

Recent studies have shown that statin therapy has a positive effect on femoral atherosclerosis, rates of new cases, and deterioration of intermittent claudication, as well as improvement in walking distance and pain-free walking time.[49–51] As per the Scandinavian Simvastatin Survival Study (4S), angina or previous MI patients with total cholesterol levels between 212 and 319 mg/dL had low incidence or worsening of intermittent claudication by 38% on treatment with 20 to 40 mg/d simvastatin.[52,53] Therefore, there may be an additional underrecognized benefit of statins on improving PAD symptoms and IC in addition to reducing CHD risk overall.

Finally, the evidence is continuing to grow that statins can prevent cardiovascular events among patients undergoing vascular surgeries. Randomized trials and meta-analyses support their benefit in reducing adverse postoperative CHD outcomes. Thus, statins should be considered for routine use prior to invasive vascular procedures in patients with PAD, even among those not previously (perhaps inappropriately) being treated for hyperlipidemia.[54]

## *Antiplatelet Therapy*

Official guidelines have continued to recommend antiplatelet therapy to decrease the risk of MI, stroke, or vascular death in patients with atherosclerotic lower extremity PAD.[1,17] Doses of 75 to 325 mg per day are generally recommended.[36] Clopidogrel 75 mg/d is an effective alternative therapy.[55] Compared with aspirin treatment, clopidogrel results in a relative risk reduction of 24% for major adverse cardiovascular events compared with aspirin alone in a prespecified subgroup of PAD in the CAPRIE trial.[56]

The data for antiplatelet therapy in the primary prevention of events in the asymptomatic patient population with PAD or in those with type 2 diabetes or risk factors alone (absence of PAD) is more controversial. **Table 2** summarizes the data from trials that have attempted to address this question. Key issues with several of these trials, at least type 2 diabetes and PAD trials, is their small sample size and that a lower dose of aspirin was typically used. Ongoing clinical trials, such as A Study of Cardiovascular Events in Diabetes (ASCEND), which involves 10,000 patients with diabetes, and the Aspirin and Simvastatin Combination for Cardiovascular Events Prevention Trial in Diabetes (ACCEPT-D), may have adequate statistical power to detect a significant treatment effect of aspirin beyond contemporary background therapy. From these trials, we support that there is no indication to use systemic anticoagulation therapy in patients with PAD without bypass grafts based on the WAVE trial, which also showed increased fatal bleeding in this population.

Based on these new studies, there is insufficient evidence to firmly recommend use of aspirin or clopidogrel in all patients with PAD. We believe that this should be determined by the presence

**Table 2**
**Summary of evidence for antiplatelet and antithrombotic therapy in PAD**

| Authors | Trial | Results |
|---|---|---|
| POPADAD study[104] | 1276 patients with Type II DM and asymptomatic PAD randomized to aspirin (75–100 mg) or placebo | No evidence of benefit from aspirin on cardiovascular disease events and mortality. (HR 0.98, 95% CI 0.76–1.26) |
| AAA trial. Fowkes G, et al.[105] JAMA 2010;303:841–8 | 3350 patients with asymptomatic PAD randomized to aspirin 100 mg/d or placebo | Risk of using aspirin for primary prevention outweighed any benefit among participants at high vascular risk (HR 1.03, 95% CI 0.84–1.27) |
| Ogawa H, et al.[106] JAMA 2008;300:2134–41 | 2539 Japanese patients with type II DM randomized to aspirin (80–100 mg/d) or placebo | Aspirin did not reduce the risk of cardiovascular events (HR 0.80, 95% CI 0.58–1.10, $P = .16$) or mortality (HR 0.90, 95% CI 0.57–1.14, $P = .67$) |
| Berger, et al.[107] JAMA 2009;301:1909–19 | Meta-analysis of aspirin alone or in combination with dipyridamole among 5269 patients with PAD enrolled in 18 prospective randomized studies | No benefit of aspirin on cardiovascular events (HR 0.88, 95% CI 0.76–1.04). Inadequate evidence to support aspirin prophylaxis in patients with symptomatic PAD who do not have coronary or cerebrovascular events. No benefits established for DM |
| De Berardis G, et al.[108] BMJ 2009;339:b4531 | Meta-analysis of 6 studies that included 10,117 patients with type II DM randomized to aspirin or placebo | No reduction in major cardiovascular events (RR 0.90, 95% CI 0.81–1.0); cardiovascular mortality (HR 0.94, 95% CI 0.72–1.23) |
| Anticoagulation and antiplatelet trials | | |
| Cacoub, et al.[109] Eur Heart J 2009;30(2):192–201 | Post hoc analysis of 3096 patients with symptomatic or asymptomatic PAD from CHARISMA study | Primary end point 7.6% in the clopidogrel plus aspirin versus 8.9% in the placebo plus aspirin (HR, 0.85; 95% CI, 0.66–1.08; $P = .18$). MI and hospitalization lower in the dual antiplatelet arm than aspirin alone. Rate of major bleeds no different in groups with PAD whereas minor bleeding was increased with clopidogrel |
| WAVE trial.[110] NEJM 2007; 357:217–27 | Aspirin/ticlopidine/clopidogrel versus vitamin K antagonist + antiplatelet therapy randomly assigned to 2161 patients with PAD and carotid artery disease | Combination therapy not more effective than antiplatelet therapy alone in preventing cardiovascular events. Significant increase in major bleeding with combination therapy |
| CASPAR trial. Belch JJ, et al.[111] Vasc Surg 2010;52(4):825–33, 833.e1–2 | Clopidogrel + aspirin versus aspirin + placebo randomly assigned to PAD patients who underwent recent below-knee bypass graft | Primary end point (graft occlusion, revascularization, amputation, or death) no different in groups (HR 0.98, 95% CI 0.78–1.23). Clopidogrel plus aspirin conferred benefit in patients receiving prosthetic grafts without increase in bleeding |

*Abbreviations:* CI, confidence interval; DM, diabetes mellitus; HR, hazard ratio; MI, myocardial infarction; RR, relative risk.

and absence of other indications (eg, underlying CHD or stroke) and be chosen on an individual patient basis. There is no role for combination antiplatelet therapy (eg, aspirin and clopidogrel) for PAD alone, or for oral anticoagulation. These treatments should be given only for their other accepted indications in patients with PAD.

### *Emerging Risk Factors*

Homocysteine is an independent risk factor for the development of CAD and PAD.[57–61] However, clinical trials do not show a benefit for cardiovascular disease event reduction by treatment with folic acid or B vitamins. We agree with the TASC II guidelines that do not support measuring or treatment of homocysteine.

Lipoprotein (a) (Lp(a)) is an LDL-like particle with apoprotein (a) covalently attached to apoprotein B of the LDL particle, and is an independent risk factor in the development of PAD.[62,63] AHA/ACC guidelines have established treatment for dyslipidemia to lower LDL to less than 100 mg/dL in all patients with PAD, but no guidelines currently recommend treatment of Lp(a) in PAD patients. Recently, based on meta-analyses demonstrating a continuous increase in cardiovascular disease risk related to Lp(a) elevations, the European Atherosclerosis Society recommended to treat with niacin a level greater than 50 mg/dL among high-risk and intermediate-risk patients.[64] These guidelines would apply to patients with PAD. However, no outcome study has thus far been performed to confirm the benefit of these recommendations; therefore, we suggest that this is a viable treatment option on a case-by-case basis.

C-reactive protein (CRP) is an inflammatory marker released from the liver in response to cytokines, and has been associated with an increased risk for atherosclerosis and CAD. Similarly, CRP is associated with a higher rate of PAD and independently predicts the risk for IC in PAD patients.[65,66] However, routine screening for CRP in PAD is not well established or proven to change clinical management or outcomes. All patients with PAD mandate treatment with agents that lower CRP such as aspirin and statins.[2] We do not recommend measuring CRP levels in patients with PAD or guiding treatment intensity by these values.

## TREATMENTS TO IMPROVE IC SYMPTOMS

In addition to aggressive management of CHD risk factors, patients with symptomatic PAD should undergo trials of therapeutic modalities (outlined in **Fig. 1**) to improve their IC, quality of life, and overall functional capacity. Exercise programs remain the cornerstone of treatment. Oral medications can be used concomitantly at the onset of diagnosis with exercise or, if rehabilitation fails, 3 to 6 months later. Surgical or endovascular interventions are typically reserved for the most severe cases (ie, critical limb ischemia) and for those individuals who have not responded to initial noninvasive measures.

### *Exercise Programs*

A supervised exercise program has confirmed improvement in symptoms of claudication.[67,68] This topic has recently been reviewed in detail elsewhere.[69] Meta-analyses of randomized controlled trials showed that a supervised exercise program caused an increase in maximum walking time by 6.5 minutes, and this benefit was more than that seen with angioplasty at 6 months (mean difference 3.3 minutes).[70] Even asymptomatic patients may benefit from exercise programs with improved walking distances.[71] Of interest, several studies show that dynamic upper arm exercise can provide similar improvements in leg IC symptoms.[72] Perhaps most importantly, there is also some evidence that exercise and greater physical activity during daily life may substantially improve overall survival among patients with PAD.[73]

An exercise rehabilitation program includes the use of a motorized treadmill or track to allow monitoring of a patient's symptoms of claudication. The patient follows multiple sessions, each lasting for 45 to 60 minutes. In ideal settings, each patient attends 3 sessions per week for more than 3 months under the supervision of an exercise physiologist, nurse, or physical therapist, who monitors the patient's claudication threshold and cardiovascular limitation.[74,75] Most patients show improvement in 2 months; however, these advantages of exercise dissipate once training is stopped.

An unsupervised exercise program may also be beneficial. There are limitations for supervised exercise programs, such as availability, cost, and transportation. A meta-analysis, comparing supervised and unsupervised exercise programs for a 3-month period, showed that the supervised exercise program had significantly better improvement of nearly 150 m. A few observational studies showed that patients who performed a self-directing walking exercise for more than 3 times a week had a decline in 6-minute walking distance compared with those who did the same once or twice a week.[70,76–78] We therefore recommend the use of supervised exercise programs, if possible, and prescribed unsupervised regimens for all other patients. This recommendation accords with official TASC II and AHA/ACC guidelines.

### Pharmacologic Therapy

#### Cilostazol

Cilostazol, a phosphodiesterase-3 inhibitor, is the most effective available medication to improve IC and should be first-line medical therapy for treatment of lower extremity symptoms due to PAD. Besides its vasodilator effects, its antiplatelet and antiproliferative activity may also have additional properties that may be beneficial. The most recent review supported that cilostazol is associated with a 50.7% improvement in maximal walking distance (42.1 m) versus placebo over a mean of 20.4 weeks. Although benefits are observed within 4 weeks, the therapeutic effect is stable as symptoms continued to improve with longer treatment. In addition, all subgroups of patients showed improvement. However, there is no evidence for a reduction in all-cause mortality provided by cilostazol.[79] A study comparing cilostazol with pentoxifylline showed that cilostazol alone is more effective than pentoxifylline, but less effective than exercise.[80–84]

We therefore agree with the AHA/ACC and TASC II recommendations that support the use of cilostazol, 100 mg, twice a day as the first-line treatment to improve symptoms and increase walking distance in patients with IC. In the absence of systolic dysfunction and congestive heart failure of any severity (a contraindication), a therapeutic trial of cilostazol for 3 to 6 months is indicated in all patients with lifestyle-limiting IC.

The most common and important side effects of cilostazol are headache, diarrhea, dizziness, and palpitations. Cilostazol should be taken 30 minutes before or 2 hours after a meal, as high-fat food increases its absorption. Diltiazem, omeprazole, and grapefruit juice increase the serum concentration of cilostazol if taken simultaneously.[83,84] There is also evidence that it can be taken safely with antiplatelet agents such as aspirin without excess bleeding events.

#### Second-line agents for claudication

Pentoxifylline, a methylxanthine derivative, is approved by the Food and Drug Administration (FDA) for the treatment of IC; however, it is less effective than cilostazol. The possible mechanisms of action include antiplatelet effects, the lowering of plasma fibrinogen, and improving the deformability of red blood cells and white cells.[85] The few available trials have showed approximately a 12% improvement in maximal treadmill walking distance; however, further studies have showed no improvement in maximal treadmill walking distance or functional status when assessed by questionnaires in comparison with placebo.[86] A meta-analysis showed a gross benefit of 44 m in maximal distance walked on treadmill with a 95% confidence interval of 14 to 74.[87] Other systematic studies and meta-analyses showed that pentoxifylline has little effect on walking ability.[22] We agree with the ACC/AHA guidelines that its usage can be considered as a second-line agent after cilostazol (if it fails or is not tolerated).

Naftidrofuryl is a 5-hydroxytryptamine-2 receptor antagonist that may act by improving muscle metabolism/glucose uptake, thus increasing adenosine triphosphate levels in the skeletal muscle. It may also reduce erythrocyte and platelet aggregation. Meta-analyses demonstrate improvements in walking time; therefore the TASC II document recommended the use of naftidrofuryl (600 mg/d orally) for the treatment of IC.[1,88] It is available in Europe and not in the United States.

Prostaglandins and prostacyclins have vasodilatory and antiplatelet actions. Though of potential benefit for improving walking distance as observed in meta-analyses, the intravenous formulations are not suitable for most patients.[89,90] Oral prostacyclins such as Iloprost and Beraprost have shown some improvement in walking distance[91]; however, due to indeterminate results in other studies, they are not formally recommended by the ACC/AHA for the treatment of PAD.[2]

Other agents that may have some promise for improving PAD symptoms that require more investigation and/or that are not available in the United States include verapamil, antichlamydophila treatment with antibiotics, defibrotide, the $\alpha$-blocker buflomedil, mesoglycan, intravenous glutathione, investigational phosphodiesterase inhibitors, and hemodilution therapy. Ineffective treatment options that should not be considered include testosterone, estrogen hormone replacements, chelation therapy with ethylenediamine tetraacetic acid, and vitamin E.

#### Angiogenic growth factors

Angiogenic growth factors such as vascular endothelial growth factor (VEGF), basic fibroblast growth factor (bFGF), and hypoxia-inducible factor 1 have been investigated as potential therapeutic agents for PAD. These agents have been effective in animal studies by improving collateral blood vessel formation and increasing the flow to the ischemic limb.[92,93] These growth factors showed significant improvement in walking distance in a few trials, such as bFGF in the TRAFFIC trial. However, other studies including the RAVE trial reported no benefit from intramuscular VEGF. Thus, use of these potential therapeutic modalities remains experimental at present.[94,95]

### *Complementary Therapies*

The most recent TASC II and ACC/AHA guidelines do not formally support the use of any complementary treatments for IC. However, a few treatments have been shown to provide at least some potential benefit and might be considered on a case-by-case basis. Propionyl-L-carnitine acts as a cofactor in skeletal muscle metabolism and supplementation of L-carnitine to ischemic tissues in PAD has improved maximal walking distance by 50% to 73%. PAD patients with walking capacity less than 250 m before treatment showed maximum benefit with a suggested dose of propionyl-L-carnitine 1 g twice daily.[96–98] It therefore might be considered on a case-by-case basis. L-Arginine may act as a vasodilator by releasing nitric oxide.[99] Although there was initial enthusiasm for supplementing L-arginine up to 8 g twice daily to improve pain-free and maximum walking distance,[100,101] recent studies show a lack of benefit and possible harm during longer-term treatment.[102] Thus, its usage is not recommended. Gingko Biloba is a herb that contains flavonoids and gingkolides. Gingko decreases blood viscosity and red cell aggregation, and acts as an inhibitor of platelet activating factor; it inhibits platelet aggregation, is antioxidant, inhibits vascular injury, and thereby has a protective mechanism in atherosclerosis. When given to patients with PAD in a dose of 120 to 160 mg daily for 12 to 24 weeks, patients have shown significant improvement in walking distance.[103] Gingko can be considered as a possible alternative agent for treatment of PAD, but as yet there is no single prospective trial to support this potential benefit. Therefore, as with the other complementary therapies, the AHA/ACC has not yet formally recommended its use in PAD.

Finally, when aggressive risk factor optimization, the use of cilostazol (or alternative medical agents), and lifestyle medications (exercise programs, smoking cessation) have failed to improve IC or cannot be successfully adhered to over the long term, surgical and/or endovascular revascularization should be considered. Other indications include patients with continued or progressive life-limiting IC, worsening PAD (eg, nonhealing ulcers), and the development of critical limb ischemia (rest pain). Many options are now available and should be tailored for the individual patient based on the anatomy of the PAD. This matter is discussed in more detail in other articles elsewhere in this issue.

## SUMMARY

The medical approach to IC includes reducing cardiovascular events via risk factor optimization, preventing progression of the underlying PAD (eg, limb loss), and improving symptoms through exercise regimen programs, pharmacotherapy, and surgical/endovascular interventions when required.

## REFERENCES

1. Norgren L, Hiatt WR, Dormandy JA, et al. Inter-society consensus for the management of peripheral arterial disease (TASC II). J Vasc Surg 2007; 45(Suppl S):S5–67.
2. Hirsch AT, Haskal ZJ, Hertzer NR, et al. ACC/AHA 2005 guidelines for the management of patients with peripheral arterial disease (lower extremity, renal, mesenteric, and abdominal aortic). a collaborative report from the American Association for Vascular Surgery/Society for Vascular Surgery, Society for Cardiovascular Angiography and Interventions, Society for Vascular Medicine and Biology, Society of Interventional Radiology, and the ACC/AHA Task Force on Practice Guidelines (Writing Committee to Develop Guidelines for the Management of Patients With Peripheral Arterial Disease). J Am Coll Cardiol 2006;47:e1–121.
3. Creager MA, White CJ, Hiatt WR, et al. Atherosclerotic peripheral vascular disease symposium II: executive summary. Circulation 2008;118(25): 2811–25.
4. White C. Clinical practice. Intermittent claudication. N Engl J Med 2007;356(12):1241–50.
5. McDermott MM, Mehta S, Greenland P. Exertional leg symptoms other than intermittent claudication are common in peripheral arterial disease. Arch Intern Med 1999;159:387–92.
6. McDermott MM, Greenland P, Liu K, et al. Leg symptoms in peripheral arterial disease. JAMA 2001;286(13):1599–606.
7. Dormandy JA, Rutherford RB. Management of peripheral artery disease (PAD). J Vasc Surg 2000;31(1 Pt 2):S1–296.
8. Hirsch AT, Criqui MH, Treat-Jacobson D, et al. Peripheral arterial disease detection, awareness, and treatment in primary care. JAMA 2001;286: 1317–24.
9. Criqui MH, Vargas V, Denenberg JO, et al. Ethnicity and peripheral arterial disease: the San Diego Population Study. Circulation 2005;112(17):2703–7.
10. Criqui MH, Langer RD, Fronek A, et al. Mortality over a period of 10 years in patients with peripheral arterial disease. N Engl J Med 1992;326:381–6.
11. Criqui MH. Systemic atherosclerosis risk and the mandate for intervention in atherosclerotic peripheral arterial disease. Am J Cardiol 2001;88:43J–7J.
12. Expert Panel on Detection, Evaluation, and Treatment of High Blood Cholesterol in Adults. Executive summary of the Third Report of the National

Cholesterol Education Program (NCEP) Expert panel on detection, evaluation, and treatment of high blood cholesterol in adults (Adult Treatment Panel III). JAMA 2001;285:2486–509.
13. Shamoun F, Sural N, Abela G. Peripheral artery disease: therapeutic advances. Expert Rev Cardiovasc Ther 2008;6(4):539–53.
14. Aboyans V, Lacroix P, Postil A, et al. Subclinical peripheral arterial disease and incompressible ankle arteries are both long-term prognostic factors in patients undergoing coronary artery bypass grafting. J Am Coll Cardiol 2005;46(5):815–20.
15. Criqui MH, Denenberg JO, Bird CE, et al. The correlation between symptoms and non-invasive test results in patients referred for peripheral arterial disease testing. Vasc Med 1996;1:65–71.
16. McKenna M, Wolfson S, Kuller L. The ratio of ankle and arm arterial pressure as an independent predictor of mortality. Atherosclerosis 1991;87(2–3): 119–28.
17. Olin JW, Allie DE, Belkin M, et al. ACCF/AHA/ACR/SCAI/SIR/SVM/SVN/SVS 2010 performance measures for adults with peripheral artery disease. A Report of the American College of Cardiology Foundation/American Heart Association Task Force on Performance Measures, the American College of Radiology, the Society for Cardiac Angiography and Interventions, the Society for Interventional Radiology, the Society for Vascular Medicine, the Society for Vascular Nursing, and the Society for Vascular Surgery (Writing Committee to Develop Clinical Performance Measures for Peripheral Artery Disease) Developed in Collaboration With the American Association of Cardiovascular and Pulmonary Rehabilitation; the American Diabetes Association; the Society for Atherosclerosis Imaging and Prevention; the Society for Cardiovascular Magnetic Resonance; the Society of Cardiovascular Computed Tomography; and the PAD Coalition Endorsed by the American Academy of Podiatric Practice Management. J Vasc Surg 2010;52(6):1616–52.
18. Faulkner KW, House AK, Castleden WM. The effect of cessation of smoking on the accumulative survival rates of patients with symptomatic peripheral vascular disease. Med J Aust 1983;1:217–9.
19. Jonason T, Bergstrom R. Cessation of smoking in patients with intermittent claudication: effects on the risk of peripheral vascular complications, myocardial infarction and mortality. Acta Med Scand 1987;221:253–60.
20. Quick CR, Cotton LT. The measured effect of stopping smoking on intermittent claudication. Br J Surg 1982;69(Suppl):S24–6.
21. Gardner AW. The effect of cigarette smoking on exercise capacity in patients with intermittent claudication. Vasc Med 1996;1:181–6.
22. Girolami B, Bernardi E, Prins MH, et al. Treatment of intermittent claudication with physical training, smoking cessation, pentoxifylline, or nafronyl: a meta-analysis. Arch Intern Med 1999;159(4): 337–45.
23. Frey P, Waters DD, DeMicco DA, et al. Impact of smoking on cardiovascular events in patients with coronary disease receiving contemporary medical therapy (from the Treating to New Targets [TNT] and the Incremental Decrease in End Points Through Aggressive Lipid Lowering [IDEAL] trials). Am J Cardiol 2011;107(2):145–50.
24. Hennrikus D, Joseph AM, Lando HA, et al. Effectiveness of a smoking cessation program for peripheral artery disease patients: a randomized controlled trial. J Am Coll Cardiol 2010;56(25):2105–12.
25. Jorenby DE, Leischow SJ, Nides MA, et al. A controlled trial of sustained-release bupropion, a nicotine patch, or both for smoking cessation. N Engl J Med 1999;340:685–91.
26. Tsai ST, Cho HJ, Cheng HS, et al. A randomized, placebo-controlled trial of varenicline, a selective alpha4beta2 nicotinic acetylcholine receptor partial agonist, as a new therapy for smoking cessation in Asian smokers. Clin Ther 2007;29(6):1027–39.
27. Reiber GE, Pecoraro RE, Koepsell TD. Risk factors for amputation in patients with diabetes mellitus: a case-control study. Ann Intern Med 1992;117: 97–105.
28. Gerstein HC, Riddle MC, Kendall DM, et al. Glycemia treatment strategies in the Action to Control cardiovascular risk in diabetes (ACCORD) trial. Am J Cardiol 2007;99(12A):34i–43i.
29. Effect of intensive diabetes management on macrovascular events and risk factors in the Diabetes Control and Complications Trial. Am J Cardiol 1995;75(14):894–903.
30. The effect of intensive treatment of diabetes on the development and progression of long-term complications in insulin-dependent diabetes mellitus. The Diabetes Control and Complications Trial Research Group. N Engl J Med 1993;329:977.
31. Intensive blood-glucose control with sulphonylureas or insulin compared with conventional treatment and risk of complications in patients with type 2 diabetes (UKPDS 33). UK Prospective Diabetes Study (UKPDS) Group. Lancet 1998;352:837.
32. Skyler JS, Bergenstal R, Bonow RO, et al. Intensive glycemic control and the prevention of cardiovascular events: implications of the ACCORD, ADVANCE, and VA diabetes trials: a position statement of the American Diabetes Association and a scientific statement of the American College of Cardiology Foundation and the American Heart Association. Circulation 2009;119(2):351–7.
33. Ray KK, Seshasai SR, Wijesuriya S, et al. Effect of intensive control of glucose on cardiovascular

outcomes and death in patients with diabetes mellitus: a meta-analysis of randomised controlled trials. Lancet 2009;373(9677):1765–72.
34. Nathan DM, Buse JB, Davidson MB, et al. Medical management of hyperglycemia in type 2 diabetes: a consensus algorithm for the initiation and adjustment of therapy: a consensus statement of the American Diabetes Association and the European Association for the Study of Diabetes. Diabetes Care 2009;32(1):193–203.
35. Chobanian AV, Bakris GL, Black HR, et al. Seventh report of the Joint National Committee on prevention, detection, evaluation, and treatment of high blood pressure. Hypertension 2003;42(6):1206–52.
36. ACCORD Study Group, Cushman WC, Evans GW, et al. Effects of intensive blood-pressure control in type 2 diabetes mellitus. N Engl J Med 2010; 362(17):1575–85.
37. Bloch MJ, Basile JN. Is there accord in ACCORD? Lower blood pressure targets in type 2 diabetes does not lead to fewer cardiovascular events except for reductions in stroke. J Clin Hypertens (Greenwich) 2010;12(7):472–7.
38. Appel LJ, Wright JT Jr, Greene T, et al. Intensive blood-pressure control in hypertensive chronic kidney disease. N Engl J Med 2010;363(10):918–29.
39. Patel A, ADVANCE Collaborative Group, MacMahon S, et al. Effects of a fixed combination of perindopril and indapamide on macrovascular and microvascular outcomes in patients with type 2 diabetes mellitus (the ADVANCE trial): a randomised controlled trial. Lancet 2007;370:829–40.
40. Yusuf S, Sleight P, Pogue J, et al. Effects of an angiotensin-converting-enzyme inhibitor, ramipril, on cardiovascular events in high-risk patients. The Heart Outcomes Prevention Evaluation Study Investigators. N Engl J Med 2000;342:145–53 [erratum appears in N Engl J Med 2000;342: 1376; erratum appears in N Engl J Med 2000; 342:748].
41. Gould AL, Rossouw JE, Santanello NC, et al. Cholesterol reduction yields clinical benefit: impact of statin trials. Circulation 1998;97:946–52.
42. Ahimastos AA, Lawler A, Reid CM, et al. Brief communication: ramipril markedly improves walking ability in patients with peripheral arterial disease: a randomized trial. Ann Intern Med 2006; 144(9):660–4.
43. Jamerson KA, Jamerson K, Weber MA, et al. Benazepril plus Amlodipine or Hydrochlorothiazide for hypertension in high-risk patients. N Engl J Med 2008;359:2417–28.
44. Gradman AH, Basile JN, Carter BL, et al. ASH Position Article. Combination therapy in hypertension. J Am Soc Hypertens 2010;4:42–50.
45. Cholesterol Treatment Trialists' (CTT) Collaboration, Baigent C, Blackwell L, Emberson J, et al. Efficacy and safety of more intensive lowering of LDL cholesterol: a meta-analysis of data from 170,000 participants in 26 randomised trials. Lancet 2010; 376(9753):1670–81.
46. The ACCORD Study Group. Effects of combination lipid therapy in type 2 diabetes mellitus. N Engl J Med 2010;362:1563–74.
47. Rajamani K, Colman PG, Li LP, et al. Effect of fenofibrate on amputation events in people with type 2 diabetes mellitus (FIELD study): a prespecified analysis of a randomised controlled trial. Lancet 2009;373(9677):1780–8.
48. Grundy SM, Cleeman JI, Bairey Merz CN, et al. Implications of recent clinical trials for the National Cholesterol Education Program Adult Treatment Panel III Guidelines. Circulation 2004;110:227–39.
49. Mohler ER 3rd, Hiatt WR, Creager MA. Cholesterol reduction with atorvastatin improves walking distance in patients with peripheral arterial disease. Circulation 2003;108:1481.
50. Mondillo S, Ballo P, Barbati R, et al. Effects of simvastatin on walking performance and symptoms of intermittent claudication in hypercholesterolemic patients with peripheral vascular disease. Am J Med 2003;114:359.
51. Aronow WS, Nayak D, Woodworth S, et al. Effect of simvastatin versus placebo on treadmill exercise time until the onset of intermittent claudication in older patients with peripheral arterial disease at six months and at one year after treatment. Am J Cardiol 2003;92:711.
52. de Groot E, Jukema JW, Montauban van Swijndregt AD, et al. B-mode ultrasound assessment of pravastatin treatment effect on carotid and femoral artery walls and its correlations with coronary arteriographic findings: a report of the Regression Growth Evaluation Statin Study (REGRESS). J Am Coll Cardiol 1998;31:1561.
53. Pedersen TR, Kjekshus J, Pyörälä K, et al. Effect of simvastatin on ischemic signs and symptoms in the Scandinavian simvastatin survival study (4S). Am J Cardiol 1998;81:333.
54. Winchester DE, Wen X, Xie L, et al. Evidence of pre-procedural statin therapy a meta-analysis of randomized trials. J Am Coll Cardiol 2010;56(14): 1099–109.
55. CAPRIE Steering Committee. A randomised, blinded, trial of clopidogrel versus aspirin in patients at risk of ischaemic events (CAPRIE). Lancet 1996;348:1329–39.
56. Antithrombotic Trialists', Collaboration. Collaborative meta-analysis of randomised trials of antiplatelet therapy for prevention of death, myocardial infarction, and stroke in high risk patients. BMJ 2002;324:71.
57. Hankey GJ, Eikelboom JW. Homocysteine and vascular disease. Lancet 1999;354:407–13.

58. Taylor LM Jr, DeFrang RD, Harris EJ Jr, et al. The association of elevated plasma homocyst(e)ine with progression of symptomatic peripheral arterial disease. J Vasc Surg 1991;13:128–36.
59. Welch GN, Loscalzo J. Homocysteine and atherothrombosis. N Engl J Med 1998;338(15):1042–50.
60. Graham IM, Daly LE, Refsum HM. Plasma homocysteine as a risk factor for vascular disease. The European Concerted Action Project. JAMA 1997; 277(22):1775–81.
61. Smith P, Arnesen H, Holme I. The effect of warfarin on mortality and reinfarction after myocardial infarction. N Engl J Med 1990;323(3):147–52.
62. Kroon AA, van Asten WN, Stalenhoef AF. Effect of apheresis of low-density lipoprotein on peripheral vascular disease in hypercholesterolemic patients with coronary artery disease. Ann Intern Med 1996;125:945–54.
63. Kullo IJ, Gau GT, Tajik AJ. Novel risk factors for atherosclerosis. Mayo Clin Proc 2000;75:369–80.
64. Nordestgaard BG, Chapman MJ, Ray K, et al. Lipoprotein(a) as a cardiovascular risk factor: current status. Eur Heart J 2010;31(23):2844–53.
65. Ross R. Mechanisms of disease: atherosclerosis: an inflammatory disease. N Engl J Med 1999;340: 115–26.
66. Ridker PM, Stampfer MJ, Rifai N. Novel risk factors for systemic atherosclerosis: a comparison of c-reactive protein, fibrinogen, homocysteine, lipoprotein(1), and standard cholesterol screening as predictors of peripheral arterial disease. JAMA 2001;285:2481–5.
67. Gardner AW, Skinner JS, Bryant CX, et al. Stair climbing elicits a lower cardiovascular demand than walking in claudication patients. J Cardiopulm Rehabil 1995;15:134.
68. Zwierska I, Walker RD, Choksy SA, et al. Upper vs lower-limb aerobic exercise rehabilitation in patients with symptomatic peripheral arterial disease: a randomized controlled trial. J Vasc Surg 2005; 42:1122.
69. Hamburg NM, Balady GJ. Exercise rehabilitation in peripheral artery disease: functional impact and mechanisms of benefits. Circulation 2011;123(1): 87–97.
70. Bendermacher BL, Willigendael EM, Teijink JA, et al. Supervised exercise therapy versus non-supervised exercise therapy for intermittent claudication. Cochrane Database Syst Rev 2006;2: CD005263.
71. McDermott MM, Ades P, Guralnik JM, et al. Treadmill exercise and resistance training in patients with peripheral arterial disease with and without intermittent claudication: a randomized controlled trial. JAMA 2009;301(2):165–74.
72. Treat-Jacobson D, Bronas UG, Leon AS. Efficacy of arm-ergometry versus treadmill exercise training to improve walking distance in patients with claudication. Vasc Med 2009;14(3):203–13.
73. Garg PK, Tian L, Criqui M, et al. Physical activity during daily life and mortality in patients with peripheral arterial disease. Circulation 2006;114: 242–8.
74. Stewart KJ, Hiatt WR, Regensteiner JG, et al. Exercise training for claudication. N Engl J Med 2002; 347:1941.
75. Brendle DC, Joseph LJ, Corretti MC, et al. Effects of exercise rehabilitation on endothelial reactivity in older patients with peripheral arterial disease. Am J Cardiol 2001;87:324.
76. Gustafsson T, Kraus WE. Exercise-induced angiogenesis-related growth and transcription factors in skeletal muscle, and their modification in muscle pathology. Front Biosci 2001;6:D75.
77. Hiatt WR, Regensteiner JG, Wolfel EE, et al. Effect of exercise training on skeletal muscle histology and metabolism in peripheral arterial disease. J Appl Physiol 1996;81:780.
78. Ernst EE, Matrai A. Intermittent claudication, exercise, and blood rheology. Circulation 1987;76:1110.
79. Pande RL, Hiatt WR, Zhang P, et al. A pooled analysis of the durability and predictors of treatment response of cilostazol in patients with intermittent claudication. Vasc Med 2010;15(3):181–8.
80. Dawson DL, Cutler BS, Hiatt WR, et al. A comparison of cilostazol and pentoxifylline for treating intermittent claudication. Am J Med 2000;109(7):523–30.
81. Dawson DL, Cutler BS, Meissner MH, et al. Cilostazol has beneficial effects in treatment of intermittent claudication: results from a multicenter, randomized, prospective, double-blind trial. Circulation 1998;98:678.
82. Beebe HG, Dawson DL, Cutler BS, et al. A new pharmacological treatment for intermittent claudication: results of a randomized, multicenter trial. Arch Intern Med 1999;159:2041.
83. Pratt CM. Analysis of the cilostazol safety database. Am J Cardiol 2001;87(12A):28D–33D.
84. Regensteiner JG, Ware JE Jr, McCarthy WJ, et al. Effect of cilostazol on treadmill walking, community-based walking ability, and health-related quality of life in patients with intermittent claudication due to peripheral arterial disease: meta-analysis of six randomized controlled trials. J Am Geriatr Soc 2002;50:1939.
85. Samlaska CP, Winfield EA. Pentoxifylline. J Am Acad Dermatol 1994;30(4):603–21.
86. Jaff MR. Pharmacotherapy for peripheral arterial disease: emerging therapeutic options. Angiology 2002;53(6):627–33.
87. Hood SC, Moher D, Barber GG. Management of intermittent claudication with pentoxifylline: meta-analysis of randomized controlled trials. CMAJ 1996;155(8):1053–9.

88. Spengel F, Clément D, Boccalon H, et al. Findings of the Naftidrofuryl in quality of life (NIQOL) European study program. Int Angiol 2002;21(1):20–7.
89. Belch JJ, Bell PR, Creissen D, et al. Randomized, double-blind, placebo-controlled study evaluating the efficacy and safety of AS- 013, a prostaglandin E1 prodrug, in patients with intermittent claudication. Circulation 1997;95:2298–302.
90. Diehm C, Balzer K, Bisler H, et al. Efficacy of a new prostaglandin E1 regimen in outpatients with severe intermittent claudication: results of a multicenter placebo-controlled double- blind trial. J Vasc Surg 1997;25:537–44.
91. Lievre M, Morand S, Besse B, et al. Oral Beraprost sodium, a prostaglandin I(2) analogue, for intermittent claudication: a double-blind, randomized, multicenter controlled trial. Beraprost et Claudication Intermittente (BERCI) Research Group. Circulation 2000;102:426–31.
92. Yang HT, Deschenes MR, Ogilvie RW, et al. Basic fibroblast growth factor increases collateral blood flow in rats with femoral arterial ligation. Circ Res 1996;79:62–9.
93. Takeshita S, Zheng LP, Brogi E, et al. Therapeutic angiogenesis: a single intraarterial bolus of vascular endothelial growth factor augments revascularization in a rabbit ischemic hind limb model. J Clin Invest 1994;93:662–70.
94. Rajagopalan S, Trachtenberg J, Mohler E, et al. Phase I study of direct administration of a replication deficient adenovirus vector containing the vascular endothelial growth factor cDNA (CI- 1023) to patients with claudication. Am J Cardiol 2002;90:512–6.
95. Rajagopalan S, Mohler ER 3rd, Lederman RJ, et al. Regional angiogenesis with vascular endothelial growth factor in peripheral arterial disease: a phase II randomized, double-blind, controlled study of adenoviral delivery of vascular endothelial growth factor 121 in patients with disabling intermittent claudication. Circulation 2003;108:1933–8.
96. Brevetti G, Diehm C, Lambert D. European multicenter study on propionyl-L-carnitine in intermittent claudication. J Am Coll Cardiol 1999;34:1618–24.
97. Brevetti G, Perna S, Sabba C, et al. Propionyl-L-carnitine in intermittent claudication: double-blind, placebo-controlled, dose titration, multicenter study. J Am Coll Cardiol 1995;26:1411–6.
98. Hiatt WR, Regensteiner JG, Creager MA, et al. Propionyl-L-carnitine improves exercise performance and functional status in patients with claudication. Am J Med 2001;110:616–22.
99. Cooke JP, Creager MA. Hypercholesterolemia, atherosclerosis, and the NO synthase pathway. In: Vallance PJ, Webb DJ, editors. Vascular endothelium in human physiology and pathophysiology. Amsterdam: Harwood Academic Publishers; 2000. p. 147–70.
100. Boger RH, Bode-Boger SM, Thiele W, et al. Restoring vascular nitric oxide formation by L-arginine improves the symptoms of intermittent claudication in patients with peripheral arterial occlusive disease. J Am Coll Cardiol 1998;32:1336–44.
101. Maxwell AJ, Anderson BE, Cooke JP. Nutritional therapy for peripheral arterial disease: a double-blind, placebo-controlled, randomized trial of HeartBar. Vasc Med 2000;5:11–9.
102. Wilson AM, Harada R, Nair N, et al. L-arginine supplementation in peripheral arterial disease: no benefit and possible harm. Circulation 2007; 116(2):188–95.
103. Pittler MH, Ernst E. Ginkgo biloba extract for the treatment of intermittent claudication: a meta-analysis of randomized trials. Am J Med 2000; 108:276–81.
104. Belch J, MacCuish A, Campbell I, et al. The prevention and progression of arterial disease and diabetes (POPADAD) trial: factorial randomized placebo controlled trial of aspirin and antioxidants in patients with diabetes and asymptomatic peripheral arterial disease. BMJ 2008. DOI:10.1136/bmj.a1840.
105. Fowkes FG, Price JF, Stewart MC, et al. Aspirin for prevention of cardiovascular events in a general population screened for a low ankle brachial index: a randomized controlled trial. JAMA 2010;303(9): 841–8.
106. Ogawa H, Nakayama M, Morimoto T, et al. Low-dose aspirin for primary prevention of atherosclerotic events in patients with type 2 diabetes: a randomized controlled trial. JAMA 2008; 300(18):2134–41.
107. Berger JS, Krantz MJ, Kittelson JM, et al. Aspirin for the prevention of cardiovascular events in patients with peripheral artery disease: a meta-analysis of randomized trials. JAMA 2009; 301(18):1909–19.
108. De Berardis G, Sacco M, Strippoli GF, et al. Aspirin for primary prevention of cardiovascular events in people with diabetes: meta-analysis of randomised controlled trials. BMJ 2009;339:b4531.
109. Cacoub PP, Bhatt DL, Steg PG, et al. CHARISMA Investigators. Patients with peripheral arterial disease in the CHARISMA trial. Eur Heart J 2009; 30(2):192–201.
110. Warfarin Antiplatelet Vascular Evaluation Trial investigators. Oral anticoagulant and antiplatelet therapy and peripheral arterial disease. N Engl J Med 2007;357:217–27.
111. Belch JJ, Dormandy J, Biasi GM, et al. CASPAR Writing Committee. Results of the randomized, placebo-controlled clopidogrel and acetylsalicylic acid in bypass surgery for peripheral arterial disease (CASPAR) trial. J Vasc Surg 2010;52(4): 825–33.

# Recent Advances in Percutaneous Management of Iliofemoral and Superficial Femoral Artery Disease

Sanjay Gandhi, MD, FSCAI[a], Rahul Sakhuja, MD, MPP, MSc[a], David Paul Slovut, MD, PhD[b,*]

**KEYWORDS**

- Peripheral arterial disease • Endovascular treatment
- Iliac artery • Superficial femoral artery
- Percutaneous transluminal angioplasty • Stent

Unrevascularized lower-extremity peripheral arterial disease (PAD) is the most common cause of lower-extremity amputation.[1] Over the past decade, the number of endovascular procedures has nearly quadrupled for patients with critical limb ischemia (CLI). This increase in procedural volume has fortunately coincided with a decrease in amputation rates.[2] Improvements in device technology and the skill-sets of the interventionist have facilitated the treatment of complex lesions, including long-segment chronic occlusions. The goal of this article is to describe the latest advances in endovascular therapy of aortoiliac and femoral arteries and to review the clinical outcomes and costs associated with the use of these treatments.

## ADVANCES IN ENDOVASCULAR TREATMENT FOR AORTOILIAC DISEASE

Endovascular revascularization of infrarenal aortic and iliac obstructive disease can be performed with a high rate of technical success and with lower morbidity and mortality than open bypass surgery (**Fig. 1**). Traditionally, endovascular therapy was the preferred modality for treatment of patients with Trans-Atlantic Inter-Society Consensus Document (TASC) II type A and B lesions, whereas surgical revascularization was preferred for patients with TASC type C and D lesions.[1] However, in contemporary practice, surgery is reserved for failure of endovascular approach.

### *Advances in Stent Technology for Aortoiliac Disease*

The design of both balloon-expandable and self-expanding bare metal stents has remained fairly constant over the past decade with little impact from stent architecture and composition on restenosis rate in location.[3] Bare metal stents such as the Zilver (Cook Inc, Bloomington, IN, USA) placed in the common and external iliac artery demonstrate a 2-year patency rate of 90% by duplex ultrasound.[4] Covered stents use expanded polytetrafluoroethylene (ePTFE), a synthetic material that may reduce the incidence of restenosis by acting as barrier to neointimal proliferation.[5] The iCAST stent (Atrium Medical Corp, Hudson, NH, USA),

Financial Disclosures: None of the authors has anything to disclose.
[a] Section of Vascular Medicine, Cardiology Division, Massachusetts General Hospital, 55 Fruit Street, GRB 8-852K, Boston, MA 02114, USA
[b] Division of Cardiology, Department of Cardiovascular and Thoracic Surgery, Montefiore Medical Center, Bronx, NY, USA
* Corresponding author. Montefiore Medical Center, 1825 Eastchester Road, Bronx, NY 10467.
*E-mail address:* dslovut@montefiore.org

Cardiol Clin 29 (2011) 381–394
doi:10.1016/j.ccl.2011.04.005
0733-8651/11/$ – see front matter 

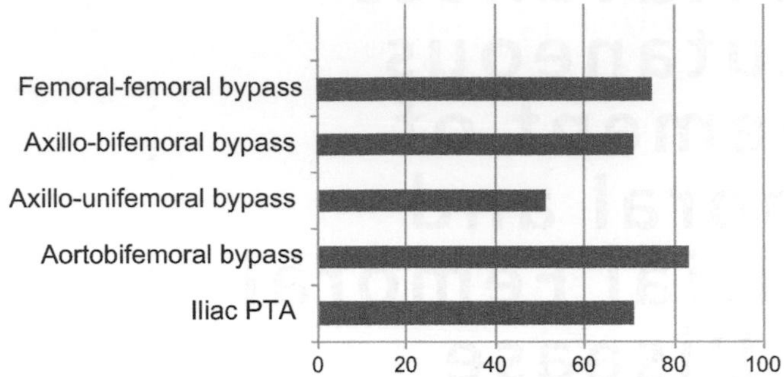


**Fig. 1.** Five-year patency (%) of aortoiliac revascularization. (*Data from* Norgren L, Hiatt WR, Dormandy JA, et al. Inter-society Consensus for the Management of Peripheral Arterial Disease (TASC II). J Vasc Surg 2007; 45(Suppl S):S5–67.)

a balloon-expandable stent made of 316 L stainless steel covered with microporous PTFE, is being evaluated in the Atrium iCAST Iliac Stent Pivotal Study (NCT00593385).

## *Advances in Treatment of Aortoiliac Occlusions*

The inability to cross an occlusion with a guidewire or to reenter the true lumen beyond the occlusion remains the most common cause for technical failure in interventions of chronic total occlusions (CTOs). A number of devices have been introduced to improve the technical success in patients with long-segment arterial occlusions in the aortoiliac and femoropopliteal segments.

### *FrontRunner device*

The FrontRunner XP CTO catheter (J & J Cordis, New Brunswick, NJ, USA) uses small, hinged jaws for controlled microdissection through a chronic occlusion. The device was evaluated prospectively in 36 patients with 44 CTOs, mainly in the iliac and femoral arteries.[6] The mean occlusion length was 9.5 plus or minus 7 cm. Angiographic success was achieved in 40 (91%) of the CTOs. Fourteen (35%) of the recanalizations required a reentry catheter to regain the true lumen. There were no complications related to the device itself. In a recent retrospective study,[7] the FrontRunner was used in CTOs located in the aortoiliac (11 arteries, 13%), infrainguinal (72 arteries, 83%), and infrapopliteal (4 arteries, 5%) arteries. The mean lesion length was 14.2 plus or minus 8 cm. The technical success rate of the procedure was 84%. The mean time required to cross the occlusive lesion was 6.7 minutes. In 53% of cases, use of the FrontRunner device alone was successful for lesion traversal and reentry, whereas the remaining 47% of cases required use of a wire or reentry device. The FrontRunner may be used as an adjunctive means of crossing a CTO when the usual guidewire techniques have failed.

### *Crosser catheter*

The Crosser device (Flowcardia Inc, Sunnyvale, CA, USA) delivers vibrational energy to mechanically recanalize the CTO. The catheter tip measures 1.6 mm and is delivered over a 0.014-in wire. In a series of 25 patients[8] with 27 CTOs, the success rate of crossing the CTO after failed conventional wiring was only 41% with one small perforation directly attributable to the use of Crosser catheter. Recent data from the PATRIOT trial suggest a higher success rate, but the results have not yet appeared in the peer-reviewed literature.

### *Reentry devices*

In treatment of CTO, a subintimal angioplasty technique is commonly used in which the guidewire is redirected from the subintimal space into the true lumen distal to the site of occlusion. Two devices are available to facilitate reentry into the true lumen.

The Outback LTD reentry catheter (J & J, Cordis New Brunswick, NJ, USA) is a single lumen 6F-compatible catheter that can be tracked over a 0.014-in guide wire. Reentry is achieved with a 21-gauge needle guided by a marker at the tip (**Fig. 2**). In iliofemoral interventions, the catheter has been successful in regaining the true lumen in 88% to 100% of cases.[6,9] The Pioneer catheter (Medtronic, Menlo Park, CA, USA) is a 6.2 F rapid exchange catheter integrated with a 20 MHz phased-array intravascular ultrasound (IVUS) transducer at the catheter tip. Under IVUS guidance, the true lumen is punctured with a 24-gauge needle that allows delivery of a second 0.014-in wire. In most cases, the average time to recanalize the occluded vessel is less than 10 minutes.[10,11] In a recent retrospective study, the true lumen could not be regained in 23 of 87 patients with CTO of iliac or femoral artery using standard catheter wire technique.[10] The Pioneer catheter (n = 20) or Outback catheter (n = 3) was used successfully to reenter the true lumen. Bleeding at the site of

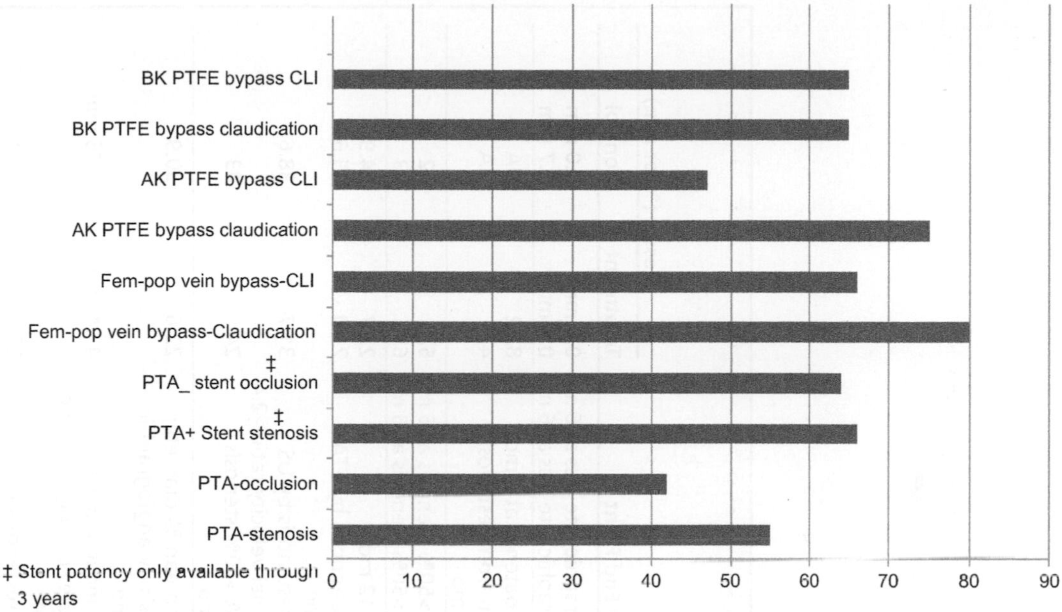


**Fig. 2.** Five-year patency (%) of femoral popliteal revascularization. (*Data from* Norgren L, Hiatt WR, Dormandy JA, et al. Inter-society Consensus for the Management of Peripheral Arterial Disease (TASC II). J Vasc Surg 2007;45(Suppl S):S5–67.)

recanalization during the procedure was seen in four patients (28%); it was controlled with placement of bare metal stent in two patients and covered stents in two patients. Compared with the Outback, the Pioneer catheter offers the advantage of IVUS to visualize the artery, but at the expense of increased catheter size and rigidity, increased cost and the need for an IVUS machine. In contrast, the Outback catheter provides ease of use but with less controlled needle deployment. Overall, both catheters demonstrate comparable success rates.

## ADVANCES IN ENDOVASCULAR TREATMENT FOR SUPERFICIAL FEMORAL ARTERY DISEASE

Although success rates for femoral-popliteal intervention have improved, the durability of both percutaneous transluminal angioplasty (PTA) and self-expanding stents remain limited (**Fig. 3**). Several new modalities are being evaluated in an effort to improve long-term patency. It is recommended that the reader keep certain caveats in mind when interpreting results of the studies described below and in **Table 1**. The first and

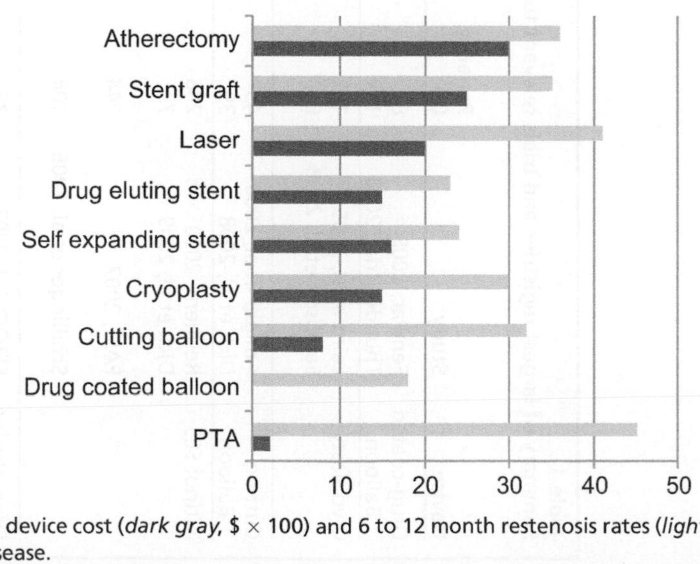


**Fig. 3.** Approximate device cost (*dark gray*, \$ × 100) and 6 to 12 month restenosis rates (*light gray*, %) for femoral arterial occlusive disease.

**Table 1**
**Summary of largest registries and trials relevant to peripheral endovascular devices**

| Device | Study | Patients (n) | Treatment/ Control | CLI (%) | Mean Lesion Length (cm) | Primary End Point | Result (% or mm) Treatment | Result (% or mm) Control |
|---|---|---|---|---|---|---|---|---|
| Drug-coated Balloon | FemPac, 2008 | 87 | 45/42 | 6 | 5.7 | Angiographic late loss at 6 mo | **0.5 mm** | **1.0 mm** |
| | Thunder trial, 2008 | 154 | 48/54 | [a] | 7.4 | Angiographic late loss at 6 mo | **0.4 mm** | **1.7 mm** |
| Cryoplasty | Laird et al, 2005 | 102 | Registry | 0 | 4.7 | Clinical patency at 9 mo | 82.2 | NA |
| | Sampson et al, 2008 | 64 | Registry | 23 | 3.9 | Freedom from restenosis at 12 mo | 47 | NA |
| Cutting Balloon | Amighi et al, 2008 | 43 | 22/21 | 19 | 2.5 | Duplex >50% stenosis at 6 mo | **62** | **32** |
| | Dick et al, 2008 | 39 | 17/22 | 20 | 8.0 | Duplex >50% stenosis at 6 mo | 65 | 73 |
| Nitinol SES | Resilient, 2010 | 206 | 134/72 | 0 | 6.7 | TLR[b] at 12 mo | **22.7** | **54.9** |
| | Dick et al, 2009 | 73 | 34/39 | 4 | 8.0 | >50% restenosis by CTA at 6 mo | **21.9** | **55.6** |
| | FAST, 2007 | 244 | 123/121 | 2.8 | 4.5 | Binary restenosis by US proximal velocity ratio≥2.4 | 31.7 | 38.6 |
| | Schillinger et al, 2006 | 104 | 51/53 | 12.5 | 13 | CTA/DSA >50% stenosis at 6 mo | **24** | **43** |
| Drug-eluting Stents | SIROCCO I, 2002 | 36 | 18/18 | [d] | 8.5 | In-stent mean % diameter stenosis by angiographic at 6 mo | 22.6 | 30.9 |
| | SIROCCO II, 2005 | 57[c] | 29/8 | [d] | 8.2 | In-stent mean luminal diameter by angiographic at 6 mo | 4.94 mm | 4.76 mm |
| | SIROCCO pooled, 2006 | 93 | 47/46 | [d] | 8.3 | Duplex restenosis rate at 24 mo | 22.9 | 21.1 |

| | | | | | | | | |
|---|---|---|---|---|---|---|---|---|
| Bioabsorbable Stent | PERSEUS trial[e] | 45 | Single arm | 0 | 4.5 | Feasibility restenosis at 6 mo | 30 | NA |
| Stent Graft | McQuade et al, 2010 (Stent vs surgery) | 86 (100 limbs) | 40/46 | 28 | 25.6 | Primary patency at 1–4 y | 72% at 1 y and 59% at 4 y | 76% at 1 y and 58% at 4 y |
| | Saxon et al, 2008 (Stent graft vs PTA) | 197 | 97/100 | 11 | 7 | Primary patency at 1 y by duplex | **65%** | **40%** |
| | Lenti et al, 2007 | 150 (166 limbs) | Registry | 44.6[f] | 10.7 | Primary patency at 12, 24, and 36 mo | 64%–12 59%–24 59%–36 | NA |
| | Kedora et al, 2007 (Stent graft vs surgery) | (100 limbs) | 40/46 | 30 | 25.6 | Primary patency at 1 y by duplex | 73.5[g] | 74.2 |
| Excimer Laser | Scheinert et al, 2001 | 318 (411 lesions) | Retrospective data | 6.8 | 19.4 | 1 y primary patency | 33.6 | NA NA |
| | CELLO registry, 2009 | 65 | Registry | 0 | 5.6 | Primary patency at 12 mo by duplex | 54 | NA |
| Atherectomy | Zeller et al, 2006 | 84 (131 lesions)[h] | Prospective study | NA | 9 | Primary patency at 1 y by duplex | 64.1 | NA |
| | Mckinsey et al, 2008 | 275 (579 lesions) | Prospective database | 63.3 | NA | Primary patency at 18 mo | 52 | NA |
| | Korabathina et al, 2010 | 98 (200 lesions) | Database | 47 | 7.2 | Procedural success 30 d MAE | 84.5 2.2 | NA |
| | Zeller et al, 2009 | 172 (210 lesions) | Registry | NA | NA | 30 d MAE 1 y restenosis by duplex | 38.2 1 | |

*Abbreviations:* AE, major adverse events; CTA, computed tomography angiogram; DSA, digital subtraction angiogram; TLE, target lesion revascularization; SES, self-expanding stent.
Statistically significant results are in bold.

[a] Mean Rutherford stage 3.3.
[b] 40.3% bailout stent counted as TLR in PTA group.
[c] Failed to recruit planned sample size of 74.
[d] Rutherford 3 + 4 = 47% in SIROCCO I and 52.6% in SIROCCO II.
[e] Unpublished data.
[f] 30% underwent surgery.
[g] 13 graft thrombosis at mean of 5 mo.
[h] 84% for de novo lesions 54% for restenosis.

foremost is to understand the patient population being studied. Patients with CLI have more advanced disease than patients with claudication. Thus, baseline anatomic characteristics such as lesion length, degree of calcification, and number of patent run-off vessels are often less favorable in CLI patients than for claudicants. It is important to recognize that most studies report high rates of procedural (ie, technical) success. In many instances, this success is achieved only after adjunctive use of balloons and stents. The Society for Vascular Surgery and the Society of Interventional Radiology have proposed reporting standards for clinical evaluation of new devices.[12] However, few clinical trials adhere to these guidelines. Most studies report technical end points such as late loss or target lesion revascularization, which are less relevant than clinical outcomes such as changes in treadmill-measured, pain-free walking distance; maximum walking distance; or quality of life. It is also useful to consider the economic impact of intervention and to determine whether the benefit of "novel" revascularization methods justifies their added cost. According to Medicare data from 1999 to 2005, the use of PTA declined from 35.1% to 30.1%, and the use of stents alone or in combination with other endovascular techniques increased from 28.2% to 39.2%.[13] The per-patient, risk-adjusted costs in the treatment quarter and four subsequent quarters was significantly higher for those requiring additional endovascular interventions ($18,591 for PTA plus stent alone vs $28,038 stent plus other endovascular interventions). **Fig. 4** highlights the usual retail cost of devices in our region in relation to outcomes observed in clinical trials.

## *Advances in Balloon Angioplasty-Based Approaches*

PTA continues to play an important role in endovascular revascularization for patients with PAD. However, the efficacy of PTA without additional adjunctive measures for maintaining long term-patency is limited, especially in patients with CLI, diffuse disease, diabetes or chronic total occlusions.[14–17] Newer angioplasty balloons have been developed with the hope of improving procedural success and long-term patency.

### *Drug-coated balloons*

Local delivery of an antiproliferative drug using a balloon catheter may lower the incidence of restenosis without the presence of stents, polymer, or prolonged exposure to the drug.[18] Paclitaxel is the most commonly used agent for drug-coated balloons (DCBs) owing to its ability to achieve

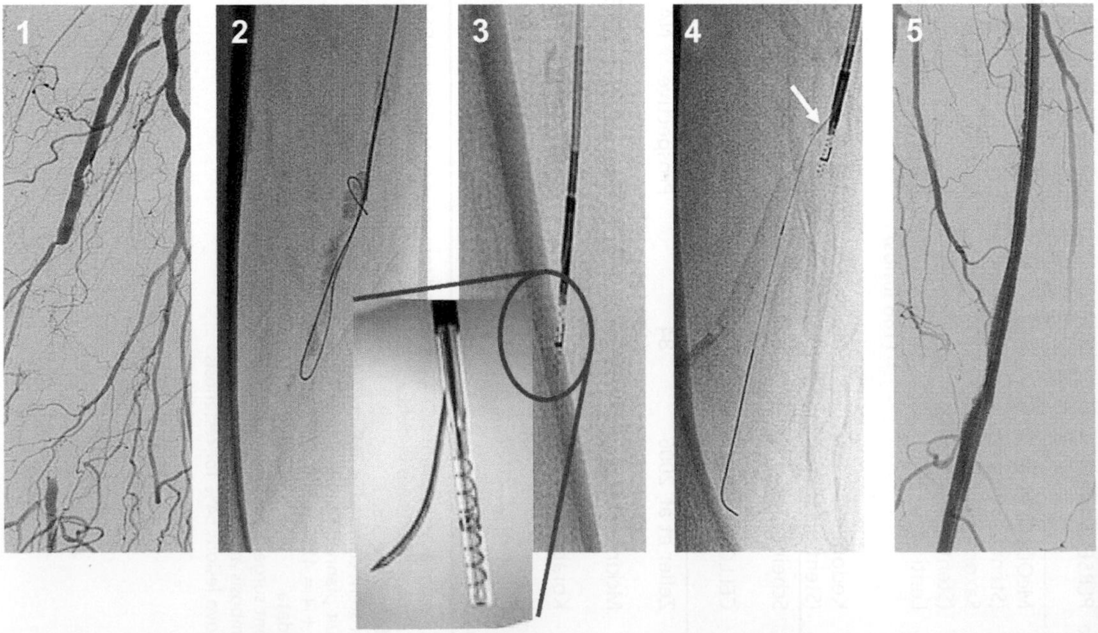


**Fig. 4.** Case demonstrating steps using the Outback reentry catheter (J&J, Cordis, New Brunswick, NJ, USA). Occluded SFA (*panel 1*). The guidewire is positioned in the subintimal space; the operator was unable to reenter the true lumen (*panel 2*). After advancing reentry device to occlusion (*panel 3*), the intima is pierced using the reentry device and the wire is navigated into the true lumen distal to the occlusion (*panel 4*) shows needle for reentry (*white arrow*). Blood flow is restored following stent implantation (*panel 5*). (*Adapted from* Rogers JH. Overview of new technologies for lower extremity revascularization. Circulation 2007;116:2083; with permission.)

high local drug concentration and diminish neointimal proliferation following brief exposure during balloon inflation.[18] DCBs have been approved for human use in Europe, but not the United States. The balloons are coated with paclitaxel 3 ug/mm$^2$ in a manner that allows rapid and almost complete release of drug after a single balloon inflation.

Two trials have examined the efficacy of paclitaxel-coated balloons. The FemPac study[19] randomized 87 patients with femoropopliteal PAD to uncoated (n = 42) versus paclitaxel-coated (n = 45) balloon catheters, while the Thunder trial[16] randomized 154 patients to percutaneous intervention with paclitaxel-coated balloons (n = 48), uncoated balloons with paclitaxel dissolved in the contrast media (n = 52), or uncoated balloons without paclitaxel (n = 54). Patients treated with the paclitaxel-coated balloon had lower late loss and angiographic restenosis at 6-month follow-up (17% vs 44% in the Thunder study; 19% vs 47% in FemPac). Addition of paclitaxel to the angiographic contrast had no significant effect. Although the results of these trials are encouraging, both studies are limited by small patient numbers, heterogeneity of patients treated, significant attrition rate in follow-up, use of surrogate end points, and short follow-up.

### *Cryoplasty*

Cryoplasty combines angioplasty with simultaneous delivery of cold thermal energy to the arterial wall (PolarCath, Boston Scientific, Natick, MA, USA). It has been proposed that cryoplasty may induce apoptosis and decrease elastic recoil following angioplasty, thereby leading to less vessel dissection and need for adjunctive stenting.[20] There are no randomized control trials comparing cryoplasty with balloon angioplasty alone. In a prospective registry of 102 patients with SFA and popliteal stenosis of less than 10 cm, the technical success rate was 85% after cryoplasty.[21] Significant dissection occurred in 6.9% patients, with bail-out stents used in 8.8% of patients. Primary patency as determined by duplex ultrasound was 70.1% at 9 months. These results compare favorably with patency rates of 40% to 59% at 1 year with conventional balloon angioplasty of the SFA. However, in a single center experience reported by Samson and colleagues,[22] the freedom from restenosis following cryoplasty was only 47% and 32% at 12 and 24 months, respectively. The cryoballoon added $1700 to the cost of the procedure without yielding any advantage over conventional balloon angioplasty. In particular, calcified lesions did extremely poorly with cryoplasty. In summary, although the principle of cryoplasty is appealing, there is insufficient data to support its routine use or justify the additional cost over conventional balloon angioplasty.

### *Cutting balloons*

The use of Peripheral Cutting balloon (Boston Scientific, Natick, MA, USA), which uses balloon-mounted microsurgical blades, has been explored in resistant stenosis associated with hemodialysis access and vascular graft intragraft or anastomotic stenosis.[23] Two small, randomized trials showed no advantage of cutting balloon angioplasty (CBA) over conventional PTA in patients with infrainguinal disease.[24,25] In a single center series of 135 limbs (claudication 19, CLI 116) with 203 infrainguinal lesions treated with CBA, primary patency rates at 12 and 24 months were 64.4% and 51.9%, respectively, with limb salvage rates of 84.2% and 76.9%.[26] Based on current data, CBA offers no advantage over PTA in the intermediate term in native vessel disease or in-stent restenosis.

The Angiosculpt balloon (Angioscore, Inc, Fremont, CA, USA), which uses spiral nitinol elements mounted on a semicompliant balloon, is more flexible than the cutting balloon and may be delivered more easily to the target lesion. There is limited short-term single center data for use of the Angiosculpt in treatment of infrapopliteal disease in CLI patients, and no data for use in the SFA.[27,28] The device was recently subject to a Class I US Food and Drug Administration recall because of retained device fragments or significant arterial injury.

## *Advances in Stent Technology*

Stent deployment solves the acute problems of elastic recoil, residual stenosis, and flow-limiting dissections after PTA. However, despite leading to higher procedural success rates, routine stenting of the SFA has not been consistently shown to reduce the rate of restenosis or target vessel revascularization.[29] This has led to interest in developing newer stent technology.

### *Nitinol self-expanding stents*

The 1-year patency of nitinol stents ranges from 63% to 87% (see **Table 1**). In a randomized trial of 104 patients[30] with severe claudication or chronic limb ischemia and SFA stenosis, primary stenting led to a lower rate of restenosis by angiography at 6 months (24% vs 43%, *P* = .05) and by duplex at 12 months (37% vs 63%, *P* = .01) than PTA. Patients in the stent group were able to walk farther on a treadmill than were those in the angioplasty group at 6 months (average distance, 363 m vs 270 m; *P* = .04) and 12 months (average distance, 387 m vs 267 m; *P* = .04).

A multicenter retrospective study of 511 patients (639 limbs) showed that the primary patency of nitinol stents in the femoropopliteal segment was 79.8%, 66.7%, and 63.1% at 1, 3, and 5 years, respectively.[31]

Owing to complex mechanical forces from leg movement, stents in the SFA are subject to fracture, delayed malapposition, and poor endothelialization resulting in stent thrombosis.[32] Stent fractures have been graded in severity from type I with single fracture to type V with spiral fracture of the stent struts.[33] Increased stent length and multiple stents increase the risk of fracture.[34] In study by Scheinert and colleagues,[35] stent fracture was seen in 24.5% of 93 patients treated with nitinol stents at 10.7 months follow-up. Fracture occurred in 13.2% of patients with stent length less than 8 cm and in 52% of patients with stent length greater than 16 cm. Stent fractures increase the risk for restenosis by 1.5 times[31] and reduce primary patency at 1 (68% vs 83%) and 2 years (65% vs 75%).[34] More resilient and flexible nitinol stents are being developed to decrease the chance of strut fracture. The Lifestent (Edwards Life sciences, Irvine, CA, USA) has a helical design that allows for high radial strength and bending or twisting without kinking. In the RESILIENT study,[15] 206 patients with SFA and proximal popliteal artery stenosis were randomized to PTA (n = 72) or nitinol self-expanding stent (n = 134). Procedural success, defined as less than 30% residual stenosis (95.8% vs 83.9%) and duplex-derived primary patency at 12 months was significantly higher in the stent group compared with PTA through 12 months (81.3% vs 36.7%); fractures were observed in only 3.1% of stents. Another stent, Supera (IDEV Technologies, Inc, Webster, TX, USA), is a nitinol stent with 6 pairs of super-elastic nitinol wires interwoven in a helical pattern with closed cell geometry. This design is postulated to provide superior radial strength while preserving longitudinal flexibility. The stent is being evaluated in clinical trials in the iliac artery compared with historical controls (I-WIN trial NCT00613418) and in femoral arteries compared with PTA (SUPERB trial NCT00933270).

### *Drug-eluting stents*

The success of drug-eluting stents (DES) in the coronary arteries has not been replicated in the infrainguinal vessels. The Sirolimus Coated Cordis Self-expandable Stent (SIROCCO) I and II trials[36,37] compared the use of DES to the Cordis SMART nitinol bare metal stent in total of 93 patients with SFA stenosis or occlusion. In a pooled analysis of both studies,[38] angiographic stenosis at 6 months (0% vs 10.8%, p = not significant [NS]) and duplex ultrasound in-stent restenosis at 24 months (22.9% vs 21.1%, p = NS) were low and similar between groups. For both type of stents, improvement in ankle-brachial index and relief from claudication symptoms were maintained at 24 months. The stent fracture rate by radiography at 18 months was 36% in the sirolimus stent versus 20% in the bare metal stent group ($P$ = .245). Two other drug-eluting stents are under investigation for SFA disease: the Zilver PTX paclitaxel-eluting stent (Cook Medical, Bloomington, IN, USA; Zilver PTX registry NCT 01,094,678) and Dynalink E everolimus-eluting stents (Abbot Vascular, Abbot Park, IL, USA; STRIDES registry NCT 00,475,566). Results from these registries have not yet been published in peer-reviewed manuscripts. From the data available so far, drug-eluting stents do not provide a significant advantage over bare metal stents.

### *Bioabsorbable stents*

In addition to risk for strut fracture and restenosis, the presence of permanent metallic stents may complicate future surgical revascularization. Bioabsorbable polymer stents have the potential advantage of providing short-term vessel scaffolding combined with drug or gene delivery capability, without the long-term drawbacks of permanent stent placement. The ideal bioabsorbable stent would be deployed reliably, invoke minimal degree of inflammation, and degrade into nontoxic byproducts.[39]

Available bioabsorbable stents are either polymer-based (eg, Igaki-Tamai poly-L-lactic acid [PLLA] stent [Igaki Medical Planning Company, Kyoto, Japan]) or corrodible metal-based (eg, Biotronik, Biotronik Inc, Lake Oswego, OR, USA). In the PERSEUS trial, the Igaki-Tamai stent was deployed in 45 patients with Rutherford class 2 to 3 and de novo SFA lesions up to 6 to 7 cm.[40] The primary technical success was 100%. The angiographic restenosis rate at 6 months, defined as greater than 50% stenosis, was 30% with a 91% primary-assisted patency rate at 9 months.

The bioabsorbable magnesium alloy stent by Biotronik AG was compared with PTA in 117 patients with CLI and infrapopliteal disease in the AMS Insight study.[41] The primary end point of absence of major amputation or death at 30 days was similar in both groups (5.3% in PTA alone vs 5.0% in PTA plus AMS). However 6-month angiographic patency rate of lesions treated with AMS was only 31.8% versus 58% for those treated with PTA alone ($P$ = .013). There are no data for patients with SFA disease.

Polymeric biodegradable stents in their current iteration have several limitations including low radial strength resulting in early recoil, thick stent struts with larger crossing profile, radiolucency, local inflammatory response, and slow bioabsorption rate. Further research is required before biodegradable stents can substitute for conventional stents. By controlling the ideal absorption time and rate, they may be useful for other applications such as angiogenesis and gene transfer.

### *Nitinol stent grafts and covered stents*

Although vein bypass is still considered the "gold standard" in surgical treatment of severe atherosclerotic disease, ePTFE surgical graft is commonly used for bypass from femoral to above-knee in patients with limited autogenous conduit.[42] Fabric-covered stent grafts were designed with the idea of replicating the excellent success achieved with synthetic bypass grafts.

The Viabahn Endoprosthesis (WL Gore & Associates, Inc, Flagstaff, CA, USA) is a self-expanding helical nitinol stent mounted to the outside surface of a tube of ePTFE that is approved for treatment of SFA lesions in 4.8 to 7.5 mm diameter vessels. In a premarket approval trial,[43] 197 patients were randomized to PTA (n = 100) or stent graft (n = 97) placement. Patients with de novo or restenotic SFA stenosis or occlusion up to 13 cm in length who had claudication or chronic critical limb ischemia were included in the study. The technical success rate was 95% in the stent-graft group versus 66% for PTA-only group. There was no difference in the treatment arms in early or late adverse events. Hematoma and pain were observed more frequently in the stent graft group. At 12-month follow-up, primary patency by duplex ultrasound was 65% for the stent-graft group versus 40% for the PTA patients ($P$ = .0003). Of note, owing to the inability to record exact PTA site, the study modified the primary end point to define total SFA patency by ultrasound (absent flow or >2 times peak systolic velocity) rather than lesion patency. This change in definition may explain the lower patency rates observed in this study compared with the studies below.

Stent grafts have been compared with surgical bypass from femoral to above-knee in 100 patients in a randomized prospective study.[44] At 12 months, primary patency (74.2% vs 73.5%) and secondary patency (83.7% vs 83.9%) were similar in both groups. In another randomized trial, McQuade and colleagues[45] evaluated ePTFE-nitinol self-expanding stent versus open surgical prosthetic bypass in 86 patients (100 limbs) with mean lesion length of 25.6 cm. The investigators found that the primary and secondary patency rates were similar to bypass surgery at up to 4 years. These studies included active surveillance of the stent grafts similar to that of surgical bypass with duplex ultrasound.

The aSpire stent (Vascular Architects Inc, San Jose, CA, USA) is made of nitinol shaped in a double spiral and fully encapsulated with a thin layer of ePTFE. In a prospective, multicenter registry[46] of patients with Rutherford stage 3 to 6, who had SFA or above-knee popliteal stenosis or occlusion greater than 3 cm and vessel diameter 5 to 10 mm, technical and clinical success was obtained in 97.6% of procedures. Procedure-related complications occurred in 22 out of 166 procedures including 6 cases of embolization, 2 hemorrhages, 1 vessel rupture, 6 vessel dissections and 7 cases of intraoperative thrombosis. Primary patency rates at 12, 24, and 36 months were 64%, 59%, and 59%, respectively.

Stent grafts may cover the collateral vessels and cannot be deployed across vessel bifurcations. There is also a concern for stent thrombosis. In one study, abrupt stent thrombosis occurred in 6 out of 57 (10%) patients within 30 days of the procedure.[47] Stent graft thrombosis leads to acute limb ischemia, a vascular emergency that may require mechanical or pharmacologic lysis or in some instances, surgical bypass. Although the latest generation of Viabahn stent grafts is coated with heparin, it remains unclear whether the heparin bonding will lead to a decrease in abrupt graft closure. Available data suggest no advantage of covered stent grafts compared with bare metal stents. The value of a surveillance program to monitor for impending stent-graft failure has not been adequately studied.

## *Advances in Plaque Removal or Debulking*

### *Excimer laser*

Excimer laser causes plaque and thrombus excision by photochemical and photomechanical interaction with the tissue. Use of intravascular saline has reduced the incidence of thermal injury reported in earlier series. Scheinert and colleagues[48] analyzed results of 318 patients (411 SFA occlusions with average length of 19.4 cm) using excimer laser-assisted recanalization. Although there was high initial success rate of 90.5%, the primary and secondary patency rates were dismal at 33% and 75.9% at 1 year. Similar disappointing results were noted in the PELA randomized trial of PTA versus laser, with ultrasound-defined primary patency of 48% for laser versus 58% for the PTA arm at 1 year.[49] The newer version of laser catheter, TURBO-Booster (Spectranetics Corporation, Colorado Springs, CO, USA) allows the laser to directionally ablate to obtain a larger lumen. In the CELLO study,[50] a prospective registry of 65 patients, patency rates (percent diameter stenosis <50%) were 59% and 54% at 6 and 12 months, respectively. Target lesion revascularization was required in 23.1% of CELLO participants within the 1-year follow-up period. Due to these disappointing results, the excimer laser has a limited role in clinical practice.

### *Excisional and rotational atherectomy*

Atherectomy devices debulk and remove atherosclerotic plaque without subjecting the arterial wall to stretch injury observed following PTA. The introduction of SilverHawk atherectomy catheter (FoxHollow Technologies, Redwood City, CA, USA) in 2003 led to renewed interest in this technique. There are no randomized clinical trials of SilverHawk Atherectomy versus balloon angioplasty alone or stenting. In a single center series[51] of 131 limbs in 84 patients with Rutherford 2 to 5 ischemia, technical success rate (defined as <30% stenosis) was 76% with atherectomy alone and increased to 100% after use of adjunctive therapy. Adjunctive balloon angioplasty was used in 59% and stents were placed in 6% of patients. The primary patency rate at 18 months by duplex was 73% for de novo stenosis, 42% for native vessel restenosis, and 49% for in-stent restenosis. Several studies have shown high incidence of distal embolization with the SilverHawk device.[52–54] For example, in the PROTECT registry,[54] clinically significant macro debris (≥2 mm in diameter) was found in 27.6% of the PTA or stent patients and 90.9% of the atherectomy patients.

The Diamondback Orbital Atherectomy System (Cardiovascular Systems, St Paul, MN, USA) features an abrasive crown that when rotated at high speed, moves eccentrically in the vessel to create a lumen that is larger than the diameter of the crown. The device generates particles with mean size of 1.9 um, which is smaller than the size of red blood cells. In a single-center study[55] of 98 patients with Rutherford 2 to 6 ischemia treated with this device, the procedural success was 86.3% for SFA, 64.7% for popliteal, and 92.5% for tibial lesions. There were 39 angiographic complications including 31 (15.5%) dissections; 54% of the dissections required stent placement. Laboratory evidence of hemolysis was noted in 46 (33.8%) cases. Adjunctive stents were used in 24.8% of patients and PTA in 34% of patients. Three subjects (2.2%) developed acute pancreatitis that resolved within 24 hours. No cases of acute renal failure requiring dialysis were observed. Long-term clinical outcomes with this device use are not available.

The Pathway System (Pathway Medical Technologies, Redmond, WA, USA) employs a fluted, differentially cutting catheter tip that remains at a defined nominal diameter (2.1 mm) when spinning clockwise but expands to a defined maximum diameter (3.0 mm) when rotating counterclockwise (**Fig. 5**). The excised material is aspirated via ports in the fluted tip into the catheter lumen and transported to a collection bag located on the device console. In a study of 172 patients with 210 lesions in patients with Rutherford class 2 to 5 ischemia,[56] device success was 99% (208 of 210 lesions). One percent of patients experienced a major adverse event at day 30. Clinically driven target lesion revascularization rates at 6 and 12 months were 15% (25:172) and 26% (42:162), respectively. The 1-year restenosis rate was 38.2% based on duplex imaging.

Distal embolization during atherectomy is an important consideration in patients with single-vessel run-off, who may suffer limb-threatening ischemia if run-off is compromised. A prospective study identified evidence of distal embolization in 22% (8 of 36) of patients who underwent atherectomy with the Pathway or Diamondback device.[57] However, embolization was easily reversible and had no effect on limb salvage and patency rates at follow up. Given risk for distal embolization, use of distal protection devices should be strongly considered during atherectomy. Long-term outcomes following atherectomy need further scrutiny in randomized studies.

## MANAGEMENT OF COMMON FEMORAL ARTERY DISEASE

Obstructive disease of the common femoral artery (CFA) occurs frequently in association with disease in the other vascular territories. Surgical endarterectomy with or without patch angioplasty remains the standard treatment. This approach has high technical success rate but postoperative morbidity is observed in about 15% of patients. In a series of 58 patients who underwent CFA endarterectomy, there was no mortality. There were nine complications including three (5%) major complications requiring reintervention (early failure secondary to untreated inflow lesion, hematoma, and wound infection).[58] The average hospital stay was 3.2 days postprocedure.

Percutaneous management of obstructive CFA disease may lower the morbidity associated with surgery, shorten hospital stay, and allow for a quicker recovery to functional status. However, "bail-out" stent placement in this location is considered problematic due to bifurcation disease, risk of stent fracture, and potential compromise of

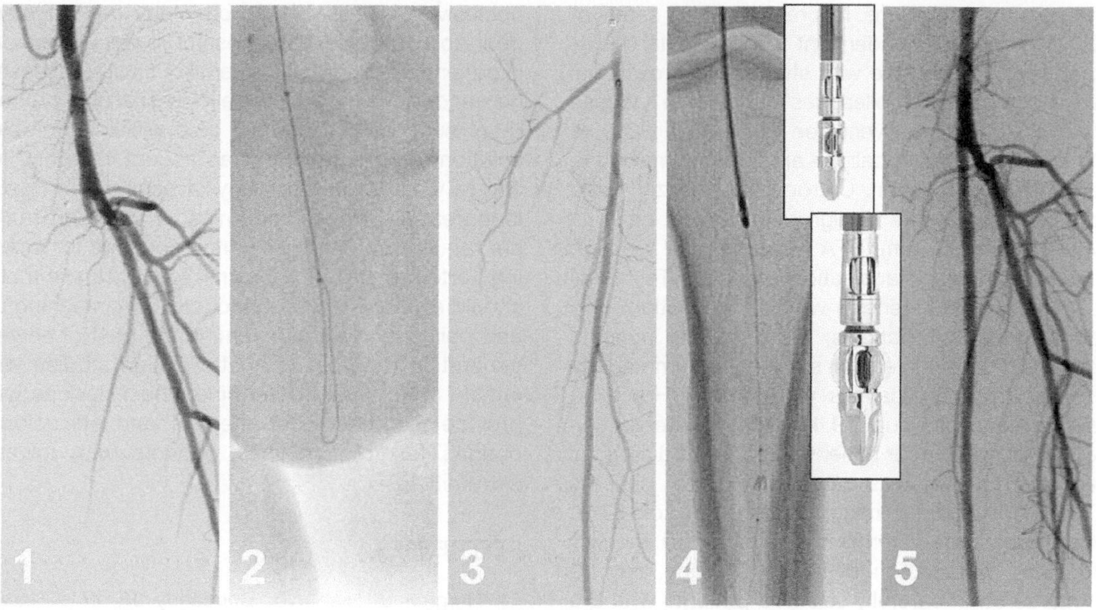


**Fig. 5.** Occluded proximal SFA in a patient with critical limb ischemia (*panel 1*) traversed with GlidewireTM and support catheter (*panel 2*) and confirmed to be intraluminal (*panel 3*). The wire was exchanged for a 0.014-in wire. With distal embolic protection in place, the Pathway JetStream device was used to facilitate recanalization of long occlusion (*panel 4*) with excellent result after further balloon angioplasty and stenting (*panel 5*). Insets: Pathway JetStream device "blades down" ~2.1 mm channel (*upper*) and "blades up" enlarged ~3.0 mm channel (*lower*). (*Courtesy of* Pathway Medical Inc, Redmond, WA, USA; with permission.)

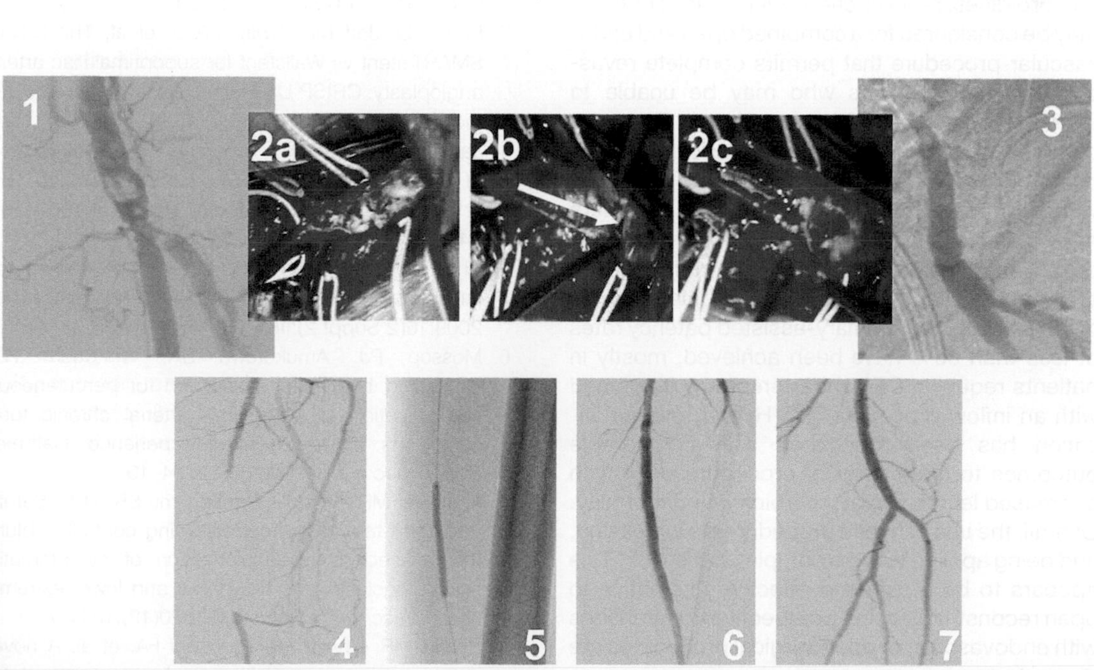


**Fig. 6.** Hybrid approach to CFA and SFA disease. The severe CFA disease (*panel 1*) was treated by an open surgical endarterectomy, with longitudinal incision revealing diffuse atheromatous disease in the CFA (*white arrow*, panel 2b), which was removed (*panel 2b*) with little residual plaque (*panel 2c*) and patched with good result (*panel 3*). The residual focal SFA lesion (*panel 4*) was treated by an endovascular approach with an antegrade puncture, balloon angioplasty (*panel 5*), and self-expanding stent, with an excellent result (*panel 6*) and preserved run-off (*panel 7*). (*Courtesy of* Dr Christopher Kwolek.)

future surgical options. In a retrospective series of 20 patients who underwent endovascular treatment of CFA disease with strategy of provisional stenting, Silva and colleagues[59] showed a success rate of 95% and event-free survival of 90% at 11 months. Cutting balloon angioplasty may have a role in this location. Cotroneo and Iezzi[60] used cutting balloons in 18 high-risk surgical patients with focal (<3 cm) CFA disease and severe, lifestyle-limiting claudication or CLI. Technical success (<30% stenosis with no dissection) was achieved in all patients; none of the patients required bailout stent or surgery. No immediate in-hospital complications were noted. However, over a mean follow up of 9.4 months, reintervention was required in four patients (25.9%) and surgical endarterectomy was needed in two patients (11%) for a total reintervention rate of 37%. Although surgery remains the standard therapy for CFA disease, endovascular therapy may be considered in carefully selected patients who are high surgical risk.

## BRIDGING THE GAP: ROLE OF HYBRID PROCEDURES

Treatment of multilevel peripheral arterial occlusive disease, particularly in older patients with several comorbidities, remains challenging. These patients may be considered for a combined open and endovascular procedure that permits complete revascularization in patients who may be unable to tolerate an extensive open procedure.[61] The most common examples of hybrid procedures include common femoral artery endarterectomy combined with angioplasty of the iliac or SFA (**Fig. 6**). There have been many reports of hybrid procedures, though they are all small single-arm retrospective analyses. At 2 and 3 years, primary patency rates of 70% to 80% and primary-assisted patency rates of less than 85% have been achieved, mostly in patients requiring CFA endarterectomy combined with an inflow procedure.[62,63] Hybrid revascularization has been associated with comparable outcomes to open surgical procedures, but with decreased length of stay, morbidity, and mortality. Overall, the use of hybrid procedures is increasing, and being applied to more complex patients.[64] This appears to be a safe and effective alternative to open reconstruction, but prospective comparisons with endovascular or open surgical procedures are warranted.

## SUMMARY

Significant advances have been made in the endovascular treatment of lower extremity arterial occlusive disease. New technology has enabled operators to achieve successful revascularization in patients with complex arterial occlusive disease. Newer devices must provide more than just procedural success. They must also provide durable solutions to the patient at an acceptable cost. In an era where pubic scrutiny of health care costs is increasing, more randomized, controlled trials are required to compare various options for treating aortoiliac and SFA lesions. Ideally, these trials should evaluate well-defined, clinically meaningful end points, as well as examine the cost of newer generation devices. Ultimately, such studies will enable clinicians to determine which devices will provide the most cost-effective and efficacious options for treating their patients with lower-extremity PAD.

## REFERENCES


1. Norgren L, Hiatt WR, Dormandy JA, et al. Inter-Society Consensus for the Management of Peripheral Arterial Disease (TASC II). J Vasc Surg 2007; 45(Suppl S):S5–67.
2. Egorova NN, Guillerme S, Gelijns A, et al. An analysis of the outcomes of a decade of experience with lower extremity revascularization including limb salvage, lengths of stay, and safety. J Vasc Surg 2010;51(4):878–85, 885.e1.
3. Ponec D, Jaff MR, Swischuk J, et al. The Nitinol SMART stent vs Wallstent for suboptimal iliac artery angioplasty: CRISP-US trial results. J Vasc Interv Radiol 2004;15(9):911–8.
4. Jaff MR, Katzen BT. Two-year clinical evaluation of the Zilver vascular stent for symptomatic iliac artery disease. J Vasc Interv Radiol 2010;21(10): 1489–94.
5. Ansel GM, Lumsden AB. Evolving modalities for femoropopliteal interventions. J Endovasc Ther 2009;16(2 Suppl 2):II82–97.
6. Mossop PJ, Amukotuwa SA, Whitbourn RJ. Controlled blunt microdissection for percutaneous recanalization of lower limb arterial chronic total occlusions: a single center experience. Catheter Cardiovasc Interv 2006;68(2):304–10.
7. Thatipelli MR, Misra S, Sanikommu SR, et al. Safety and short-term outcomes following controlled blunt microdissection revascularization of symptomatic arterial occlusions of the pelvis and lower extremities. J Vasc Interv Radiol 2009;20(12):1541–7.
8. Khalid MR, Khalid FR, Farooqui FA, et al. A novel catheter in patients with peripheral chronic total occlusions: a single center experience. Catheter Cardiovasc Interv 2010;76(5):735–9.
9. Beschorner U, Sixt S, Schwarzwalder U, et al. Recanalization of chronic occlusions of the superficial femoral artery using the outback re-entry

catheter: a single centre experience. Catheter Cardiovasc Interv 2009;74(6):934–8.
10. Jacobs DL, Motaganahalli RL, Cox DE, et al. True lumen re-entry devices facilitate subintimal angioplasty and stenting of total chronic occlusions: initial report. J Vasc Surg 2006;43(6):1291–6.
11. Scheinert D, Braunlich S, Scheinert S, et al. Initial clinical experience with an IVUS-guided transmembrane puncture device to facilitate recanalization of total femoral artery occlusions. EuroIntervention 2005;1(1):115–9.
12. Sacks D, Marinelli DL, Martin LG, et al. Reporting standards for clinical evaluation of new peripheral arterial revascularization devices. J Vasc Interv Radiol 2003;14(9 Pt 2):S395–404.
13. Jaff MR, Cahill KE, Yu AP, et al. Clinical outcomes and medical care costs among Medicare beneficiaries receiving therapy for peripheral arterial disease. Ann Vasc Surg 2010;24(5):577–87.
14. Bosch JL, Hunink MG. Meta-analysis of the results of percutaneous transluminal angioplasty and stent placement for aortoiliac occlusive disease. Radiology 1997;204(1):87–96.
15. Laird JR, Katzen BT, Scheinert D, et al. Nitinol stent implantation versus balloon angioplasty for lesions in the superficial femoral artery and proximal popliteal artery: twelve-month results from the RESILIENT randomized trial. Circ Cardiovasc Interv 2010;3(3):267–76.
16. Tepe G, Zeller T, Albrecht T, et al. Local delivery of paclitaxel to inhibit restenosis during angioplasty of the leg. N Engl J Med 2008;358(7):689–99.
17. Adam DJ, Beard JD, Cleveland T, et al. Bypass versus angioplasty in severe ischaemia of the leg (BASIL): multicentre, randomised controlled trial. Lancet 2005;366(9501):1925–34.
18. Gray WA, Granada JF. Drug-coated balloons for the prevention of vascular restenosis. Circulation 2010;121(24):2672–80.
19. Werk M, Langner S, Reinkensmeier B, et al. Inhibition of restenosis in femoropopliteal arteries: paclitaxel-coated versus uncoated balloon: femoral paclitaxel randomized pilot trial. Circulation 2008;118(13):1358–65.
20. Yiu WK, Cheng SW, Sumpio BE. Vascular smooth muscle cell apoptosis induced by "supercooling" and rewarming. J Vasc Interv Radiol 2006;17(12):1971–7.
21. Laird J, Jaff MR, Biamino G, et al. Cryoplasty for the treatment of femoropopliteal arterial disease: results of a prospective, multicenter registry. J Vasc Interv Radiol 2005;16(8):1067–73.
22. Samson RH, Showalter DP, Lepore M Jr, et al. CryoPlasty therapy of the superficial femoral and popliteal arteries: a reappraisal after 44 months' experience. J Vasc Surg 2008;48(3):634–7.
23. Vikram R, Ross RA, Bhat R, et al. Cutting balloon angioplasty versus standard balloon angioplasty for failing infra-inguinal vein grafts: comparative study of short- and mid-term primary patency rates. Cardiovasc Intervent Radiol 2007;30(4):607–10.
24. Amighi J, Schillinger M, Dick P, et al. De novo superficial femoropopliteal artery lesions: peripheral cutting balloon angioplasty and restenosis rates–randomized controlled trial. Radiology 2008;247(1):267–72.
25. Dick P, Sabeti S, Mlekusch W, et al. Conventional balloon angioplasty versus peripheral cutting balloon angioplasty for treatment of femoropopliteal artery in-stent restenosis: initial experience. Radiology 2008;248(1):297–302.
26. Canaud L, Alric P, Berthet JP, et al. Infrainguinal cutting balloon angioplasty in de novo arterial lesions. J Vasc Surg 2008;48(5):1182–8.
27. Scheinert D, Peeters P, Bosiers M, et al. Results of the multicenter first-in-man study of a novel scoring balloon catheter for the treatment of infra-popliteal peripheral arterial disease. Catheter Cardiovasc Interv 2007;70(7):1034–9.
28. Bosiers M, Deloose K, Cagiannos C, et al. Use of the AngioSculpt scoring balloon for infrapopliteal lesions in patients with critical limb ischemia: 1-year outcome. Vascular 2009;17(1):29–35.
29. Kasapis C, Henke PK, Chetcuti SJ, et al. Routine stent implantation vs. percutaneous transluminal angioplasty in femoropopliteal artery disease: a meta-analysis of randomized controlled trials. Eur Heart J 2009;30(1):44–55.
30. Schillinger M, Sabeti S, Loewe C, et al. Balloon angioplasty versus implantation of nitinol stents in the superficial femoral artery. N Engl J Med 2006;354(18):1879–88.
31. Soga Y, Iida O, Hirano K, et al. Mid-term clinical outcome and predictors of vessel patency after femoropopliteal stenting with self-expandable nitinol stent. J Vasc Surg 2010;52(3):608–15.
32. Bates MC, Campbell JR, Campbell JE. Late complication of stent fragmentation related to the "lever-arm effect". J Endovasc Ther 2008;15(2):224–30.
33. Jaff M, Dake M, Pompa J, et al. Standardized evaluation and reporting of stent fractures in clinical trials of noncoronary devices. Catheter Cardiovasc Interv 2007;70(3):460–2.
34. Iida O, Nanto S, Uematsu M, et al. Influence of stent fracture on the long-term patency in the femoropopliteal artery: experience of 4 years. JACC Cardiovasc Interv 2009;2(7):665–71.
35. Scheinert D, Scheinert S, Sax J, et al. Prevalence and clinical impact of stent fractures after femoropopliteal stenting. J Am Coll Cardiol 2005;45(2):312–5.
36. Duda SH, Pusich B, Richter G, et al. Sirolimus-eluting stents for the treatment of obstructive superficial femoral artery disease: six-month results. Circulation 2002;106(12):1505–9.
37. Duda SH, Bosiers M, Lammer J, et al. Sirolimus-eluting versus bare nitinol stent for obstructive

superficial femoral artery disease: the SIROCCO II trial. J Vasc Interv Radiol 2005;16(3):331–8.
38. Duda SH, Bosiers M, Lammer J, et al. Drug-eluting and bare nitinol stents for the treatment of atherosclerotic lesions in the superficial femoral artery: long-term results from the SIROCCO trial. J Endovasc Ther 2006;13(6):701–10.
39. Brown DA, Lee EW, Loh CT, et al. A new wave in treatment of vascular occlusive disease: biodegradable stents—clinical experience and scientific principles. J Vasc Interv Radiol 2009;20(3):315–24 [quiz: 325].
40. Biamino G, Schmidt A, Scheinert D. Treatment of SFA lesions with PLLA biodegradable stents: results of PERSEUS study. J Endovas Ther 2005;12(Suppl I):5.
41. Bosiers M, Peeters P, D'Archambeau O, et al. AMS INSIGHT—absorbable metal stent implantation for treatment of below-the-knee critical limb ischemia: 6-month analysis. Cardiovasc Intervent Radiol 2009;32(3):424–35.
42. Daenens K, Schepers S, Fourneau I, et al. Heparin-bonded ePTFE grafts compared with vein grafts in femoropopliteal and femorocrural bypasses: 1- and 2-year results. J Vasc Surg 2009;49(5):1210–6.
43. Saxon RR, Dake MD, Volgelzang RL, et al. Randomized, multicenter study comparing expanded polytetrafluoroethylene-covered endoprosthesis placement with percutaneous transluminal angioplasty in the treatment of superficial femoral artery occlusive disease. J Vasc Interv Radiol 2008;19(6):823–32.
44. Kedora J, Hohmann S, Garrett W, et al. Randomized comparison of percutaneous Viabahn stent grafts vs prosthetic femoral-popliteal bypass in the treatment of superficial femoral arterial occlusive disease. J Vasc Surg 2007;45(1):10–6 [discussion: 16].
45. McQuade K, Gable D, Pearl G, et al. Four-year randomized prospective comparison of percutaneous ePTFE/nitinol self-expanding stent graft versus prosthetic femoral-popliteal bypass in the treatment of superficial femoral artery occlusive disease. J Vasc Surg 2010;52(3):584–90 [discussion: 590–1, 591.e1–e7].
46. Lenti M, Cieri E, De Rango P, et al. Endovascular treatment of long lesions of the superficial femoral artery: results from a multicenter registry of a spiral, covered polytetrafluoroethylene stent. J Vasc Surg 2007;45(1):32–9.
47. Fischer M, Schwabe C, Schulte KL. Value of the hemobahn/viabahn endoprosthesis in the treatment of long chronic lesions of the superficial femoral artery: 6 years of experience. J Endovasc Ther 2006;13(3): 281–90.
48. Scheinert D, Laird JR Jr, Schroder M, et al. Excimer laser-assisted recanalization of long, chronic superficial femoral artery occlusions. J Endovasc Ther 2001;8(2):156–66.
49. Laird JR. Peripheral excimer laser angioplasty (PELA) trial. Washington, DC: TCT; 2002.
50. Dave RM, Patlola R, Kollmeyer K, et al. Excimer laser recanalization of femoropopliteal lesions and 1-year patency: results of the CELLO registry. J Endovasc Ther 2009;16(6):665–75.
51. Zeller T, Rastan A, Sixt S, et al. Long-term results after directional atherectomy of femoro-popliteal lesions. J Am Coll Cardiol 2006;48(8):1573–8.
52. Suri R, Wholey MH, Postoak D, et al. Distal embolic protection during femoropopliteal atherectomy. Catheter Cardiovasc Interv 2006;67(3):417–22.
53. Lam RC, Shah S, Faries PL, et al. Incidence and clinical significance of distal embolization during percutaneous interventions involving the superficial femoral artery. J Vasc Surg 2007;46(6):1155–9.
54. Shammas NW, Dippel EJ, Coiner D, et al. Preventing lower extremity distal embolization using embolic filter protection: results of the PROTECT registry. J Endovasc Ther 2008;15(3):270–6.
55. Korabathina R, Mody KP, Yu J, et al. Orbital atherectomy for symptomatic lower extremity disease. Catheter Cardiovasc Interv 2010;76(3):326–32.
56. Zeller T, Krankenberg H, Steinkamp H, et al. One-year outcome of percutaneous rotational atherectomy with aspiration in infrainguinal peripheral arterial occlusive disease: the multicenter pathway PVD trial. J Endovasc Ther 2009;16(6):653–62.
57. Shrikhande GV, Khan SZ, Hussain HG, et al. Lesion types and device characteristics that predict distal embolization during percutaneous lower extremity interventions. J Vasc Surg 2011;53(2):347–52.
58. Kang JL, Patel VI, Conrad MF, et al. Common femoral artery occlusive disease: contemporary results following surgical endarterectomy. J Vasc Surg 2008;48(4):872–7.
59. Silva JA, White CJ, Quintana H, et al. Percutaneous revascularization of the common femoral artery for limb ischemia. Catheter Cardiovasc Interv 2004; 62(2):230–3.
60. Cotroneo AR, Iezzi R. The role of "cutting" balloon angioplasty for the treatment of short femoral bifurcation steno-obstructive disease. Cardiovasc Intervent Radiol 2010;33(5):921–8.
61. Slovut DP, Sullivan TM. Combined open and endovascular revascularization. Ann Vasc Surg 2009; 23(3):414–24.
62. Antoniou GA, Sfyroeras GS, Karathanos C, et al. Hybrid endovascular and open treatment of severe multilevel lower extremity arterial disease. Eur J Vasc Endovasc Surg 2009;38(5):616–22.
63. Nishibe T, Kondo Y, Dardik A, et al. Hybrid surgical and endovascular therapy in multifocal peripheral TASC D lesions: up to three-year follow-up. J Cardiovasc Surg (Torino) 2009;50(4):493–9.
64. Ebaugh JL, Gagnon D, Owens CD, et al. Comparison of costs of staged versus simultaneous lower extremity arterial hybrid procedures. Am J Surg 2008;196(5):634–40.

# Percutaneous Management of Chronic Critical Limb Ischemia

Aravinda Nanjundappa, MD, FSCAI, RVT[a,*], Akhilesh Jain, MD[b], Kevin Cohoon, MD, RPVI[c], Robert S. Dieter, MD, RVT[d]

**KEYWORDS**

• Critical limb ischemia • Stent • Occlusion • Angioplasty

Critical limb ischemia (CLI) is primarily a disease of advanced atherosclerosis but may occur in the setting of other causes. CLI is defined by the TransAtlantic Inter-Society Consensus (TASC) as persistent recurring ischemic rest pain requiring opiate analgesics for at least 14 days, ulceration or gangrene of the foot or toes, ankle-brachial index (ABI) less than 0.4, toe pressure less than 30 mm Hg, systolic ankle pressure less than 50 mm Hg, flat pulse volume waveform, and absent pedal pulses.[1,2] There are 2 widely used methods for classifying the symptoms of peripheral arterial disease (PAD), the Rutherford-Becker and the Fontaine systems.[3] Both of these classifications categorize the spectrum of PAD from asymptomatic to advanced tissue loss (**Tables 1** and **2**).

CLI develops when the blood flow does not meet the metabolic demands of the tissue at rest. It has been estimated that 150,000 patients require lower-limb amputation for CLI in the United States annually.[4] The prognosis after amputation is even worse. In some series, the perioperative mortality is 5% to 10% for below-the-knee amputation and 15% to 20% for above-the-knee amputation.[5] When these patients survive, nearly 40% die within 2 years of their first major amputation. A second amputation is required in 30% of cases, and full mobility is achieved in only 50% of patients who have below-the-knee amputation and 25% of those who have above-the-knee amputation.[5] It is essential for the treating physician to understand the complexity of patients with CLI and the appropriate and emerging treatment approaches in this patient population. The authors provide a comprehensive review of the percutaneous endovascular management of CLI in this article.

## GOALS OF MANAGEMENT

The primary goals of treatment of CLI are to relieve ischemic pain, heal ischemic ulcers, improve patient function and quality of life, and prolong survival. A multidisciplinary effort among cardiology, vascular medicine physicians, podiatry, wound care experts, plastic surgery, and endovascular interventionalists/vascular surgeons may be often required for optimal outcomes. Basics

Dr Nanjundappa would like to dedicate this section to late Ms M. Lakshmidevamma, beloved mother, who was the inspiration and motivation to his life.

[a] Division of Vascular Surgery, West Virginia University, 3100 McCorkle Avenue SE, Charleston, WV 25304, USA
[b] Vascular and Endovascular Surgery, Section of Vascular Surgery, Yale University School of Medicine, 333 Cedar Street - FMB 137, New Haven, CT 06510, USA
[c] Division of Cardiology, Loyola University, 260 South Summit Avenue, Oakbrook Terrace, IL 60181, USA
[d] Vascular & Endovascular Medicine, Interventional Cardiology, Loyola University Medical Center, VA Hospital, 5000 South 5th Avenue, Hines, IL 60141, USA
* Corresponding author.
*E-mail address:* dappamd@yahoo.com

Cardiol Clin 29 (2011) 395–410
doi:10.1016/j.ccl.2011.04.008
0733-8651/11/$ – see front matter 

**Table 1**
**Classification of PAD: Fontaine's stages**

| Stage | Clinical Description |
|---|---|
| I | Asymptomatic |
| IIa | Mild claudication |
| IIb | Moderate-to-severe claudication |
| III | Rest pain |
| IV | Ulceration or gangrene |

of wound care, such as twice-a-day saline dressing, leg elevation to prevent dependent blood transfusion in severe anemia, and cessation of smoking and nutritional status evaluation, should be implemented after initial assessment. The patient, family members, and caregivers should be educated on wound care, the natural history of CLI, risk of amputation, death, myocardial infarction, or stroke. Assessment of general nutritional status should be performed with assessment of serum albumin level, hemoglobin level, and platelet counts. Adequate protein and oxygenated blood assist in wound healing. Adjuvant antibiotics and wound debridement or cleaning is pivotal to prevent secondary infections and bacteremia. Deep infections, such as osteomyelitis, should be assessed using radiography, magnetic resonance imaging, or bone scan. Adequate hydration for renal prophylaxis is imperative in patients with elevated serum creatinine levels. Baseline images of the wound or ulcer aid in follow-up and prognosis before and after revascularization.

## MEDICAL MANAGEMENT OF RISK FACTORS

The risk factors associated with CLI include age older than 65 years, diabetes mellitus, cigarette smoking, and hyperlipidemia. Smoking is the most important risk factor and is correlated more closely with developing PAD than any other risk factor.[6] Cessation of cigarette smoking reduces the progression of disease, as shown by lower rates of amputation and lower incidences of rest ischemia in patients who quit, and the risks of myocardial infarction and death from other vascular causes.[7] Cessation of smoking is the single most important preventable risk factor, and it is vital for health care providers to educate patients on the importance of cessation. Of those patients who are 60 years and older with hypertension, 25% have been found to have an ABI less than 0.9. Systolic blood pressure is strongly correlated with PAD and reflects arterial stiffness and increased pulse pressures.[8] Diabetes mellitus is strongly associated with outcomes and CLI. Patients with PAD with diabetes are approximately 10 times more likely to require amputation than those without diabetes. Also, patients with PAD with diabetes mellitus typically require amputations at younger ages than those without diabetes. The Edinburgh Artery Study shows that patients with diabetes and glucose intolerance have a higher risk for PAD.[9]

Several large clinical trials have demonstrated the benefits of lipid-lowering therapy in patients with PAD who have coexisting coronary and cerebral arterial diseases.[10–13] Simvastatin has been shown to drastically reduce the rates of cardiovascular ischemic events in a large PAD subgroup, despite initial low-density lipoprotein (LDL) levels. Lipid normalization has been shown to reduce disease progression and the severity of claudication. LDL cholesterol directly correlates with the risk of PAD, and the smaller the total LDL particles, the higher the risk of PAD. C-reactive protein, lipoprotein(a), and homocysteine concentrations have all been associated with atherosclerotic vascular disease. High-density lipoprotein cholesterol seems to be inversely related to the development of PAD. Antiplatelet therapy with aspirin has been shown to substantially decrease the risk of myocardial infarction, stroke, and death in patients with peripheral vascular disease and also reduces the rate of arterial reocclusion after angioplasty or bypass grafting.[14] Antiplatelet drugs have been shown to reduce the risk of systemic vascular events in all patients with PAD.

**Table 2**
**Classification of PAD: Rutherford classification**

| Grade | Category | Clinical Description |
|---|---|---|
| 0 | 0 | Asymptomatic |
| I | 1 | Mild claudication |
| I | 2 | Moderate claudication I |
| I | 3 | Severe claudication |
| II | 4 | Rest pain |
| III | 5 | Minor tissue loss ulceration or gangrene |
| IV | 6 | Major tissue loss |

## DIAGNOSTIC APPROACH

Conventional angiography is still preferred by many peripheral interventionalists, particularly at the time of intervention. Approaches such as magnetic resonance angiography and computed tomographic angiography are used increasingly frequently to diagnose CLI and to plan revascularization strategies.

During x-ray contrast angiography, both the inflow and outflow territories need to be evaluated, and all inflow lesions should be defined in orthogonal views. Use of full-strength contrast material is preferable to optimize images. In patients with reduced glomerular filtration rate, diluted contrast can be used. Femoral angiography of the contralateral limb is the most common modality for obtaining an angiogram in 90% of CLI cases. Patients with difficult anatomy, such as a narrow bifurcation of the aortoiliac artery, benefit from antegrade femoral artery puncture. Segmental angiograms of the iliac arteries, femoropopliteal arteries, and tibioperoneal vessels assist in optimum visualization of the lower extremities. Patients with tissue loss have significant leg pain, and movement during image acquisition can impair the image quality. Hence, the role of adequate sedation in these patients cannot be overemphasized. Angiography further enables appropriate planning for percutaneous revascularization such as antegrade access or popliteal access and pedal arterial access. Contrast injections should be administered with a power injector with at least 600 to 900 psi for adequate visualization. However, before power injection, the catheter position at the center of the arterial lumen must be confirmed by both fluoroscopy and hemodynamic arterial pressure waveform evaluation.

## PRINCIPLES OF ANGIOPLASTY/STENTING

Patients with CLI need a straight-line flow to 1 or 2 tibioperoneal arteries to provide rapid wound healing. Inflow lesions should always be treated first, and a good outflow distal to the site of revascularization is vital to maintain durability of intervention. Because of the multisegment nature of their disease, patients with CLI may need more than 1 procedure to achieve straight in-line flow.

## ANGIOPLASTY AND STENTING IN CLI

Balloon angioplasty of an arterial atherosclerotic lesion results in irreversible stretching of the arterial wall and intentional dissection and/or fracture of the intima.[15] This process results in compression of the plaque and further intimal-medial dehiscence and stretching of the tunica adventitia. Postangioplasty vascular inflammation results in initiation of intimal hyperplasia, which eventually leads to restenosis. The level of inflammation after balloon angioplasty is higher than after stenting, which may be the reason for less restenosis with the latter.[16]

Vascular access is the key to successful revascularization in patients with CLI. Vascular access of the common femoral artery (CFA) under fluoroscopy is quintessential to prevent high or low sticks resulting in retroperitoneal bleed or pseudoaneurysm/atrioventricular fistula formation. Alternative options of antegrade puncture may need ultrasound guidance to ensure proper entry of the percutaneous needle into the CFA. The atypical access sites for the management of CLI include the popliteal artery under fluoroscopy, pedal access by direct puncture or a cut down, and radial or brachial access for iliac occlusions rarely. Careful vascular access and vascular closure reduce most vascular access complications.

A 5F pigtail catheter is typically placed in the distal aorta, and the aortoiliac arteries are imaged. This angiogram in the anteroposterior (AP) view shows common, internal, and external iliac arteries. If the external iliac arteries are not well visualized in the AP view, then contralateral views should be used. For example, left external iliac artery is best imaged in the right anterior oblique 30°. The CFA is imaged by placing a 5F multipurpose catheter in the contralateral side after crossing the contralateral CFA with an angled glide wire. The ostium of the superficial femoral artery (SFA) and the profunda femoris artery are best imaged in the ipsilateral 30° angulation. The mid-distal SFA and the popliteal are best visualized in the AP view. The tibioperoneal vessels are seen well in an ipsilateral 10° angulation, whereas the pedal arch vessels are imaged in the contralateral 10° angulations.

## AORTOILIAC INTERVENTION IN CLI

As discussed earlier, patients with CLI frequently have multilevel involvement. Aortoiliac disease in such a population tends to be diffuse (TASC C or D) with the involvement of CFAs in association with infrainguinal disease. In the absence of significant CFA occlusive disease, aortoiliac disease can typically be treated with percutaneous approaches to improve perfusion to the lower extremities sufficiently to resolve the rest pain or heal ischemic ulceration. Patients with significant CFA disease burden, however, need either open surgery or a combination of femoral artery endarterectomy and patch angioplasty with simultaneous aortoiliac stenting. Endovascular therapy is the recommended first-line therapy for TASC A and B lesions and also select TASC C lesions in hands of experienced operators. High-risk patients with TASC C and D disease and CLI having multiple advanced comorbidities leading to an unacceptable surgical risk may be offered endovascular therapy as a palliative therapy. Ipsilateral retrograde access via the CFA is the standard approach for nonocclusive common iliac lesions. For the external iliac lesions, a contralateral crossover technique allows better purchase and also an ability to extend the therapy to proximal CFA distally, if needed. Patients with chronic total occlusions (CTOs) are preferentially approached by a contralateral crossover technique to avoid dissections involving distal aorta. (See section on "Chronic Total Occlusions" later.) Lesions at the aortic bifurcation are generally treated by bilateral kissing balloons or kissing stents to protect the contralateral vessel from subsequent stenosis.

The CRISP-US (Cordis Randomized Iliac Stent Project—United States) is a multicenter randomized clinical iliac stent trial sponsored by Cordis performed in the United States. In this study, 203 patients were treated with shape memory alloy recoverable technology (SMART; Cordis, Johnson & Johnson, Bridgewater, NJ, USA) nitinol stents and stainless steel Wallstents (Boston Scientific, Minneapolis, MN, USA) after a suboptimal angioplasty of the iliac artery obstructive disease. The procedural success rates were higher with SMART stents than with Wallstents, 94.7% and 91%, respectively. The primary patency at 1 year was 94.7% and 91.1% for the SMART stents and Wallstents, respectively. The primary end point of target vessel revascularization and restenosis at 9 months and death at 30 days for SMART stents and Wallstents were 6.9% versus 5.9%. Functional and hemodynamic improvements were similar between the 2 stents.[17]

## FEMOROPOPLITEAL INTERVENTION IN CLI

SFA CTO can be crossed via true lumen crossing using a 5F multipurpose catheter and a combination of straight stiff wire and angled glide wires of 0.035-in caliber. All total occlusion crossing should be confirmed by pressure tracing and contrast injection via the crossing catheter. After successful crossing, balloon inflation of SFA is usually performed with a 4- or 5-mm balloon. Prolonged balloon inflations usually provide an acceptable balloon angioplasty result (100% to <50%). If there is a flow-limiting dissection or a residual lesion of more than 50%, the SFA may need stenting with self-expanding stents. An alternative method to cross the SFA CTO is to use the subintimal technique. Here an angled glide wire with a small leading edge loop is used to create a deliberate subintimal loop. A firm catheter to support the short loop can cross most SFA CTOs. At the site of reconstitution of the occluded artery, a straight still wire or an angled stiff wire maybe used. Plain balloon angioplasty may suffice in some cases, but most need stenting to ensure patency.

Mewissen[18] published the results of use of SMART nitinol stents in SFA in patients with CLI. A total of 137 patients with CLI in 122 limbs were treated with SFA stents. The procedural successes were 98%, and the mean follow-up period was 302 days. The primary stent patency rate was 92%, 76%, 66%, and 60% at 6, 12, 18, and 24 months, respectively. The role of drug-eluting stents in SFA was addressed by Duda and colleagues.[19] The SMART nitinol stents coated with a polymer impregnated with sirolimus versus uncoated SMART stents were tested. This study included 36 patients with CLI with SFA occlusions. The mean in-stent lumen diameter was better and larger with sirolimus-impregnated SMART stent than with uncoated SMART stents (4.95 vs 4.31 mm, $P = .047$). The study further demonstrated the safety of sirolimus-coated stents with no major adverse events.

## INFRAGENICULATE INTERVENTION IN CLI

Below-knee interventions can be performed with a retrograde or an antegrade technique. If the SFA is disease free, then longer-length guides are usually used, and the catheter tip is kept close to the distal popliteal artery. Adequate anticoagulation with heparin is a must to prevent thrombosis of the tibioperoneal vessels. A smaller caliber guide is placed in a telescoping manner to provide added support before crossing the occluded tibioperoneal vessels. The use of road map technology assists in visualizing the occluded arteries. Intra-arterial nitroglycerin prevents spasm, and the use of 0.018-in wire is beneficial to prevent spasm. After successful crossing via true lumen or in a subintimal manner with reentry, balloon angioplasty with long 2- to 3-mm balloons is generally adequate. The role of short-segment self-expanding stents in the proximal segment has been replaced largely by short balloon-expandable coronary bare-metal stents. Drug-eluting coronary stents (DES) in the proximal tibioperoneal trunk may have increased patency. For current data on infrapopliteal angioplasty and/or stents, see **Tables 3** and **4**.

## ATHERECTOMY IN CLI

Lasers as a mode of atherectomy were evaluated and abandoned for peripheral arterial use in the late 1980s secondary to the high complications caused by thermal damage. The last few years

**Table 3**
**Results of angioplasty in infrapopliteal territory in patients with CLI**

| Primary Treatment | Investigators | N | CLI (%) | Procedural Success (%) | Follow-Up (mo) | Limb Salvage (%) | Survival (%) |
|---|---|---|---|---|---|---|---|
| Percutaneous Transluminal Angioplasty | Romiti et al[32] | 2557 | 94.7 | 89 | 36 | 82.4 | 68.4 |
| Cryoplasty | Das et al[33] | 108 | 100 | 97.3 | 6 | 93.4 | 95.4 |
| Cutting Balloon | Ansel et al[34] | 73 | 71 | 100 | 12 | 89.5 | 84 |
| Drug-Eluting Balloon | Schmidt[35] | 107 | N/R | N/R | 3 | Results pending | 93 |

*Abbreviation:* N/R, not reported.

have, however, seen a resurgence of interest in a variety of laser-based and mechanical atherectomy devices, such as SilverHawk (FoxHollow Technologies, Redwood City, CA, USA), and excimer laser atherectomy catheters (CliRpath; Spectranetics Corp, Colorado Springs, CO, USA). These devices have been promoted as a minimally invasive alternative to a major surgical bypass and can be used as an isolated technique or as a facilitator of adjunctive procedures such as angioplasty and stents. Results, thus far, have demonstrated their ability to treat a variety of different lesions, including severe long-segment stenoses and occlusions, with variable success.[20,21] The following sections review each of the devices used in CLI with the caveat that although each of these adjunctive therapies add substantially to the cost of intervention, none seem superior to percutaneous transluminal angioplasty (PTA) and/or stenting alone.

## *Laser Atherectomy in CLI*

The 308-nm excimer laser uses flexible fiber optic catheters to deliver intense bursts of ultraviolet energy in short pulse durations. This type of laser has a short penetration depth of 50 μm and breaks molecular bonds directly by a photochemical rather than a thermal process. Potential advantages of laser atherectomy include the ability to treat long occlusions and complex disease effectively, thereby providing a better angiographic result with a lesser risk of distal embolization and decreased need for adjuvant stenting. The excimer laser has also been used to facilitate crossing of CTOs using the step-by-step technique in which the guidewire is advanced just proximal to the lesion and the excimer laser catheter is brought into contact with the occlusion.

The use of excimer laser in patients with CLI was studied in the LACI (Laser Angioplasty for Critical Limb Ischemia) trial.[22] This trial was a prospective registry of 15 sites in the United States and Germany, which enrolled 145 patients (155 critically ischemic limbs) with CLI who were poor candidates for bypass surgery. The reasons for ruling out surgical options in this cohort included diffuse distal disease, poor targets for bypass, the absence of venous conduit, or significant medical or cardiac comorbidities placing the

**Table 4**
**Stents in infrapopliteal disease**

| Primary Treatment | Investigators | N | CLI (%) | Procedural Success (%) | Follow-Up (mo) | Limb Salvage (%) | Survival (%) |
|---|---|---|---|---|---|---|---|
| Balloon-Expandable | | | | | | | |
| BMS | Feiring[36] | 82 | 68 | 94 | 12 | 87 | 100 |
| DES | | | | | | | |
| Paclitaxel | Siablis[37] | 29 | 100 | 96.6 | 6 | 100 | 96.6 |
| Sirolimus | Scheinert[38] | 30 | 65 | N/A | 9 | 100 | 100 |
| Self-Expanding | Kickuth[39] | 35 | 46 | 100 | 6 | 100 | 89 |
| Bioabsorbable | Bosiers[40] | 20 | 100 | 100 | 24 | 94.7 | 95 |
| Meta-Analysis | Biondi-Zoccai[41] | 640 | N/A | N/A | 12 | 96.4 | N/A |

*Abbreviations:* BMA, bare-metal stent; N/A, not applicable.

patient at high risk for complications from surgery. A total of 423 lesions were treated in the SFA (41%), popliteal (15%), and infrapopliteal (41%) arteries. Occlusions were present in 92% of limbs. Mean treatment length was about 16 cm. At a 6-month follow-up, limb salvage was achieved in 110 (92%) of 119 surviving patients or 118 (93%) of 127 limbs. Adjunctive stents were implanted in 45% of limbs.

### *Mechanical Atherectomy in CLI*

The SilverHawk device is a forward-cutting excisional atherectomy device, which uses a high-speed rotating blade to shave off the obstructing plaque while a nose cone at the tip of catheter collects the debris. Absence of barotrauma to the arterial wall, potentially complete removal of the plaque, and ability to handle below-knee lesions are the proposed advantages of this system. The SilverHawk system, however, has limited effectiveness against heavily calcified lesions, which reduces its usefulness in patients with CLI. Various complications of excisional atherectomy include distal embolization, thrombosis, and vessel wall perforation. There are, however, no randomized controlled trials comparing the efficacy of this atherectomy device. Much of the evidence comes from retrospective reviews/registries involving a small number of patients. Kandzari and colleagues[23] compared the results of SilverHawk-based excisional atherectomy with surgery or angioplasty with stent placement in 69 patients (76 limbs with 160 lesions) with CLI. Adjunctive PTA or stents were used in 17% of patients undergoing atherectomy. The procedure was considered a technical success in 99% of patients. At a 6-month follow-up of the cohort, clinical improvement in 66% of patients, with 13% undergoing major amputation, and a mortality rate of 14% were reported. However, the lack of objective criteria to define the patients' need for amputation, clinical improvement, and candidacy for endovascular revascularization by other means limited the usefulness of the study. Zeller and colleagues[24] reviewed their experience with femoropopliteal excisional atherectomy. The investigators treated 131 lesions in 100 limbs in 84 patients presenting with Rutherford category 2 to 5 ischemia. Forty-five lesions were de novo (group 1, 34%), 43 were native vessel restenoses (group 2, 33%), and 43 were in-stent restenoses (group 3, 33%). The technical success rates were 86% for atherectomy alone and 100% after adjunctive therapies. The only independent predictor of restenosis was treatment of restenotic lesions. A prospective randomized clinical trial comparing SilverHawk atherectomy with the gold standard of surgical bypass (PROOF trial [Plaque Removal vs Open Bypass Surgery for Critical Limb Ischemia]), sponsored by FoxHollow Technologies, was initiated in 2007. This trial was, however, terminated by the company in 2008 for unknown reasons. Other atherectomy systems currently in use include the Pathway PV system (Pathway Medical Technologies, Redmond, WA, USA), which has expandable rotating scraping blades (flutes) with ports between the flutes that allow flushing and aspiration of plaque material or thrombus, and the Orbital Atherectomy System (Cardiovascular Systems, St Paul, MN, USA), which incorporates an eccentric diamond-coated abrasive crown rotating at high speeds.

In an effort to determine the efficacy of atherectomy for limb salvage compared with open bypass in CLI, Loor and colleagues[25] reviewed 99 patients with TASC C and D lesions who were treated with surgical bypass (n = 59) and atherectomy using the SilverHawk device (n = 33). Even though bypass and atherectomy achieved similar 1-year primary patency (64% vs 63%; $P = .2$), patients in whom bypass was performed had greater 1-year limb salvage rates than those in whom atherectomy was performed (87% vs 69%; $P = .004$). The investigators concluded that patients with CLI do better with open bypass than with atherectomy as first-line therapy for limb salvage.

## CTO

CLI and claudication typically arise in the presence of CTOs. The ability to successfully traverse and recanalize these CTOs is therefore imperative in CLI. Attempts at recanalization of these often heavily calcified lesions fail in about 20% of cases using traditional guidewire and balloon technology. The management of CTO in CLI is dealt under 3 headings, namely, technique, crossing devices, and lumen reentry devices.

### *Technique of Crossing CTOs*

Chronic occlusive lesions of the iliac territory differ somewhat from those in the SFA. Occlusions of SFA are typically very long and generally begin in the proximal third of the artery, whereas occlusions of iliac arteries may consist of a short or a long segment. The access to the SFA is typically via a retrograde puncture of the CFA, although contralateral crossover technique can be used as well. In difficult cases, use of an antegrade puncture may provide better catheter support and increase the chances of wire crossing because the distal plaque is typically less calcified. If the occluded SFA reconstitutes in its distal segment, as is commonly

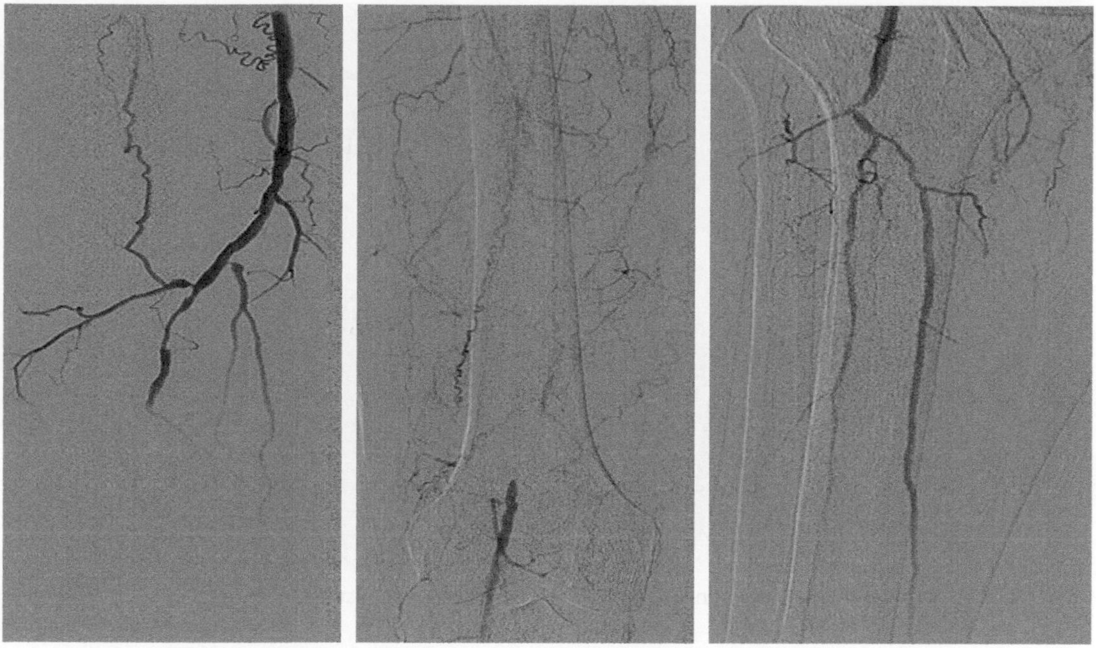

Fig. 1. Baseline angiogram of a 55-year-old man with nonhealing right great toe ulcer showing CTO of the right distal SFA. Note the reconstituted popliteal artery with a distal runoff. Repeated attempts to cross the SFA in a retrograde manner had failed.

seen, and an intact popliteal artery is noted, then the popliteal arterial puncture is preferred. Popliteal artery access requires the patient to be placed on the belly, and the access is performed using ultrasound guidance (**Figs. 1–3**). Rarely, access of pedal arteries, such as dorsal pedis and posterior tibial artery, can be attempted (**Figs. 4** and **5**). Such atypical access routes are reserved for difficult cases of CTOs.

The recommended approach to CTO of iliac arteries is the crossover approach to minimize the risk of extensive dissection involving the distal

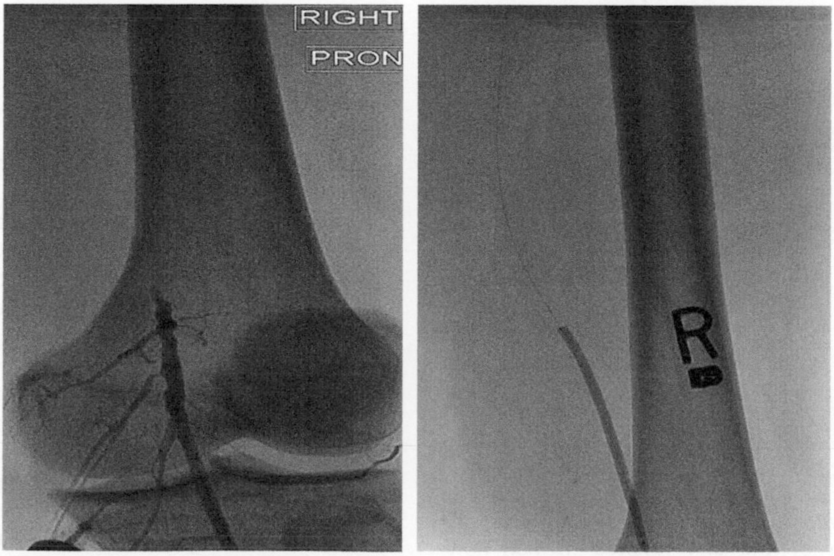


Fig. 2. Antegrade puncture of the patent popliteal artery and successful crossing of the native SFA and balloon angioplasty in the patient shown in **Fig. 1**.

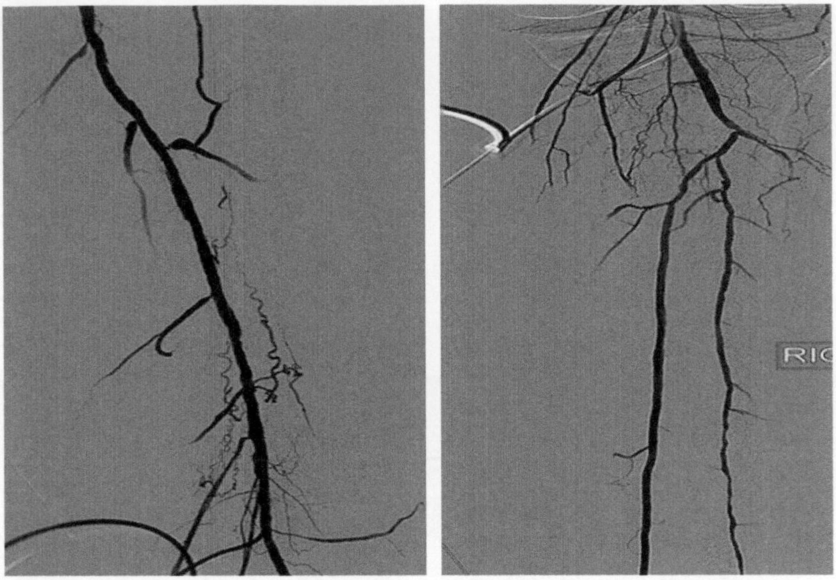

Fig. 3. Final angiogram of the patient in **Fig. 1** showing patent SFA and distal runoff.

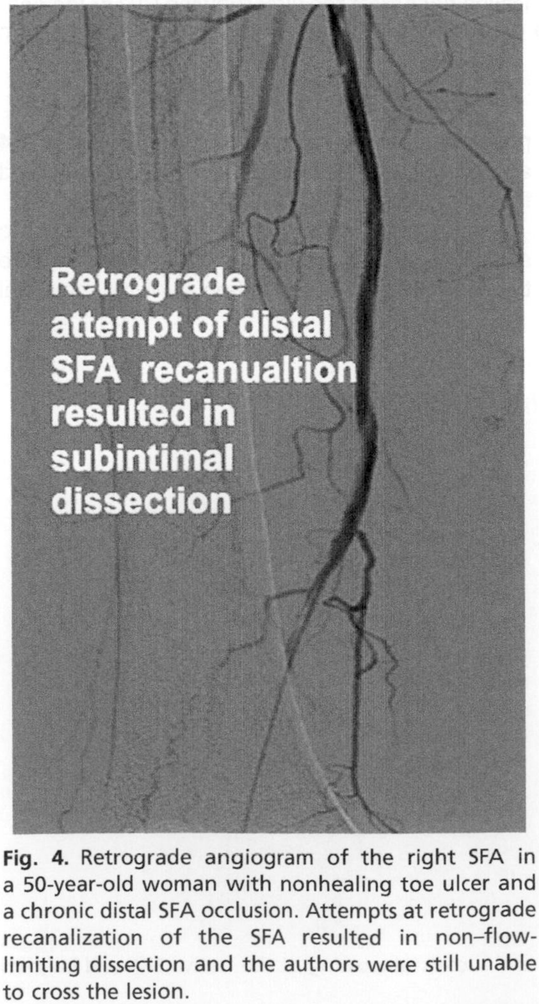

Retrograde
attempt of distal
SFA recanualtion
resulted in
subintimal
dissection


Fig. 4. Retrograde angiogram of the right SFA in a 50-year-old woman with nonhealing toe ulcer and a chronic distal SFA occlusion. Attempts at retrograde recanalization of the SFA resulted in non–flow-limiting dissection and the authors were still unable to cross the lesion.

aorta. This approach, however, is not suitable for ostial iliac occlusions secondary to poor purchase in this location.

Acute or chronic occlusion of prosthetic femoropopliteal prosthetic grafts is a common cause of recurrent acute limb ischemia after a surgical bypass. A retrograde or an antegrade technique can be used to access and cross the occluded bypass graft. Because of significant thrombus burden in such cases, thrombolysis is usually recommended. Postthrombolysis angiography is performed to identify and treat the precipitating lesion, which usually is located in the inflow or outflow native vessels (**Figs. 6–8**).

The most common method for crossing occlusions of the native vessels uses hydrophilic wires and catheters, often, if not always, in the subintimal plane for a portion of the occlusion. A successful crossing of any CTO should always be confirmed by using pressure tracing and contrast injection through the crossing catheter. Although recanalization through a CTO is often challenging, the primary limitation to successful treatment of CTOs stems from the inability to cross a lesion or the inability to reenter the distal true lumen from a subintimal location.[26,27] An additional limitation in some cases is that the true lumen reentry is not achieved until subintimal passage to a site significantly remote from the level of vessel lumen patency, causing subintimal angioplasty, stenting, or both to extend beyond the occluded segment. This extension places additional segments of the vessel at the risk of complications of angioplasty (**Figs. 9–13**).

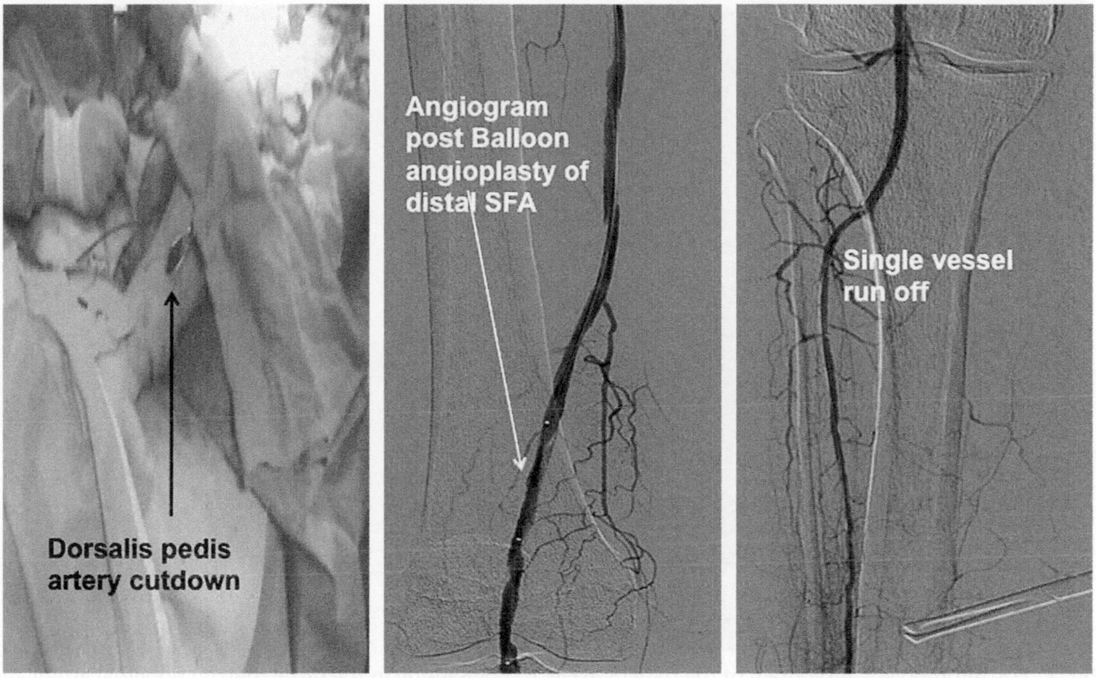


**Fig. 5.** Cutdown and access of the anterior tibial artery with successful recanalization and balloon angioplasty of the occluded SFA in the patient shown in **Fig. 4**.

## *Crossing Devices*

### *CROSSER catheter*

The CROSSER CTO recanalization system (FlowCardia Inc, Sunnyvale, CA, USA) uses high-frequency mechanical vibrations (20,000 cycles per second to a depth of 20 μm) propagated through a nitinol core wire to a stainless steel tip. The vibrational mechanical impact and cavitation

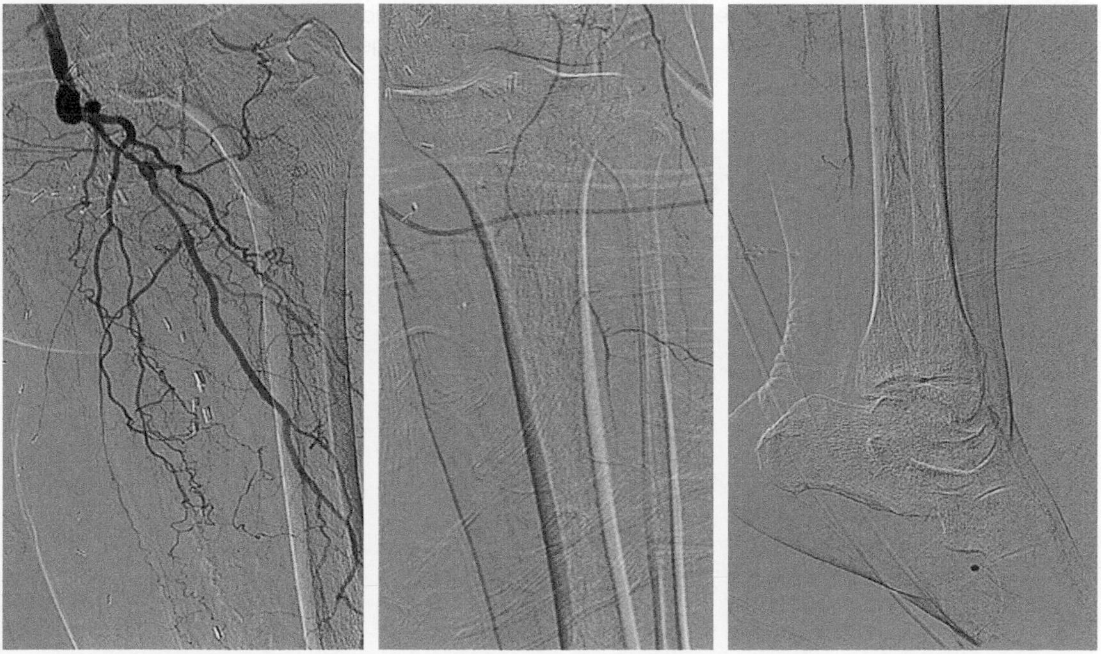

**Fig. 6.** Angiogram of a 59-year-old woman presenting with new-onset resting pain in her left leg. The patient had undergone a revision of her left leg prosthetic femoropopliteal bypass about 10 years earlier for Rutherford Stage 5 limb ischemia. Baseline ABI is 0.10.

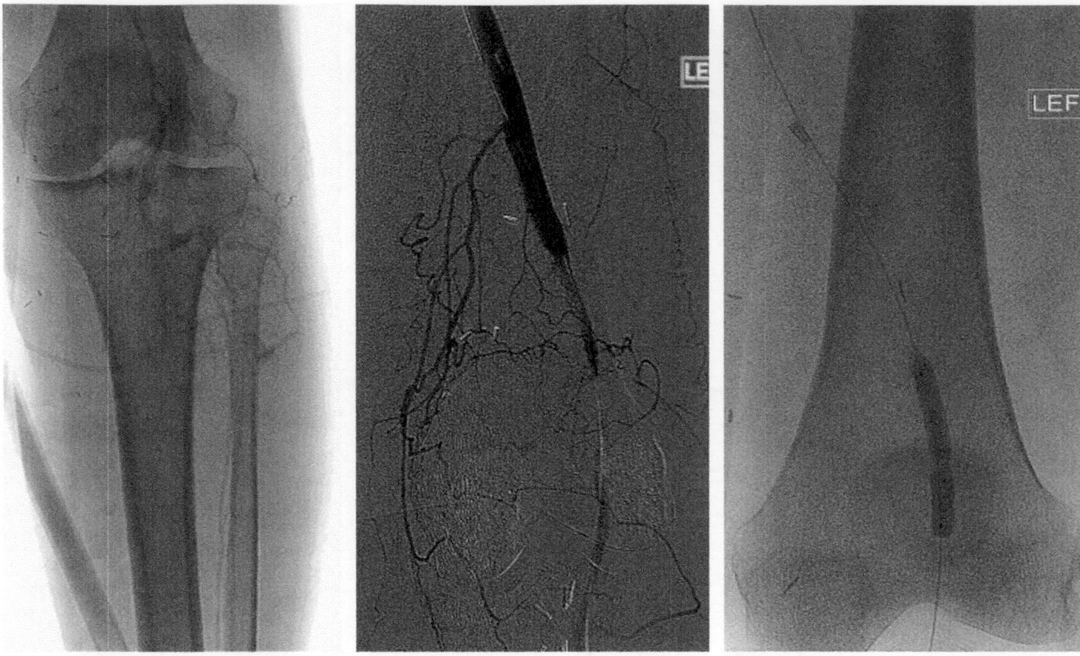

Fig. 7. Postthrombolysis angiogram of the patient in Fig. 6 shows lesion in the distal (native) popliteal artery and angioplasty.

effects result in the penetration of the occluded artery. Although there are no maximum recommendations for vessel size, a minimum diameter of 2.5 mm is recommended. Although the infusion lumen of the CROSSER is too small to aspirate blood, it is possible to inject diluted contrast to confirm true-lumen position.

### *FRONTRUNNER XP CTO catheter*

The FRONTRUNNER XP CTO catheter (Cordis, Johnson & Johnson, Bridgewater, NJ, USA) works on the principle of controlled blunt microdissection, which refers to the ability to perform catheter-based microdissection using a pair of miniature hinged jaws that can be actuated from

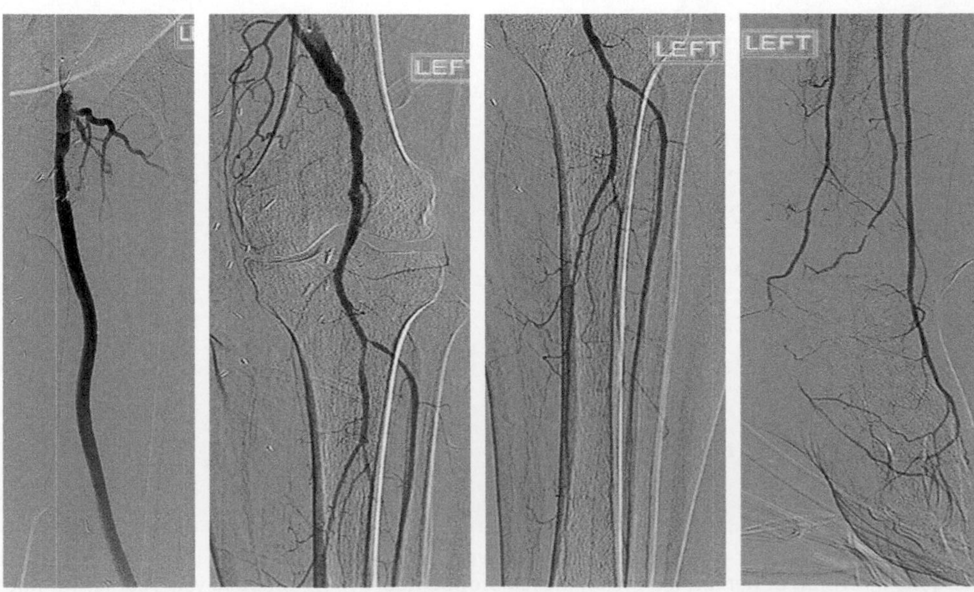


Fig. 8. Successful revascularization of the bypass and the distal runoff in the patient shown in Fig. 6.

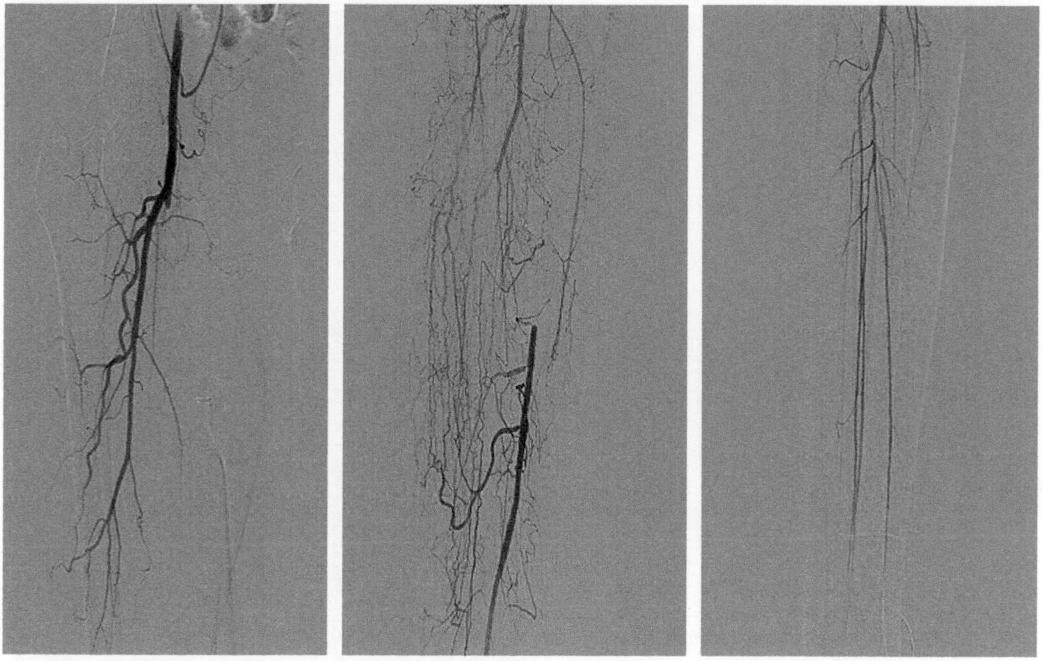

**Fig. 9.** A 54-year-old woman with a nonhealing ulcer on her right foot and ABI of 0.62. The patient's baseline angiogram demonstrated a TASC D lesion of the right SFA. The same patient is shown in **Figs. 10–13**.

the catheter handle. The technique has been reported to be safe and feasible, with a success rate of 91% in treating pelvic and lower limb CTOs in 1 series of 36 patients with 44 symptomatic CTOs that had failed conventional percutaneous revascularization.[28] The device does not have a guidewire lumen, and once a lesion is crossed, a dedicated Micro Guide catheter (Cordis, Johnson & Johnson, Bridgewater, NJ, USA) is advanced over the FRONTRUNNER catheter to its tip, and the catheter is then withdrawn. A guidewire can then be placed through the Micro

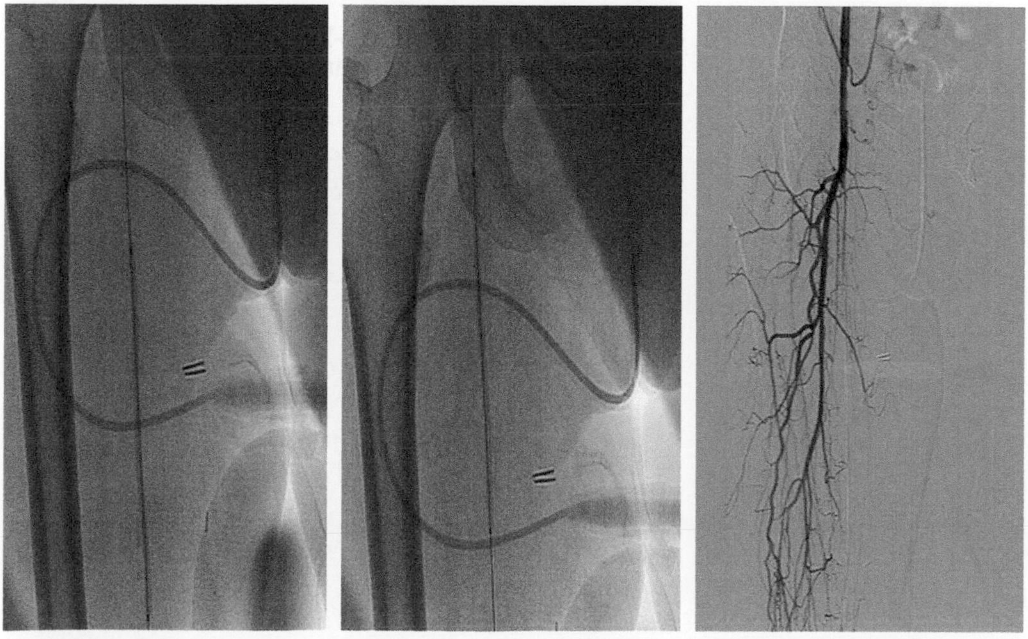

**Fig. 10.** Crossing of the native SFA within the lumen followed by balloon angioplasty. Postangioplasty angiogram shows persistent thrombus.

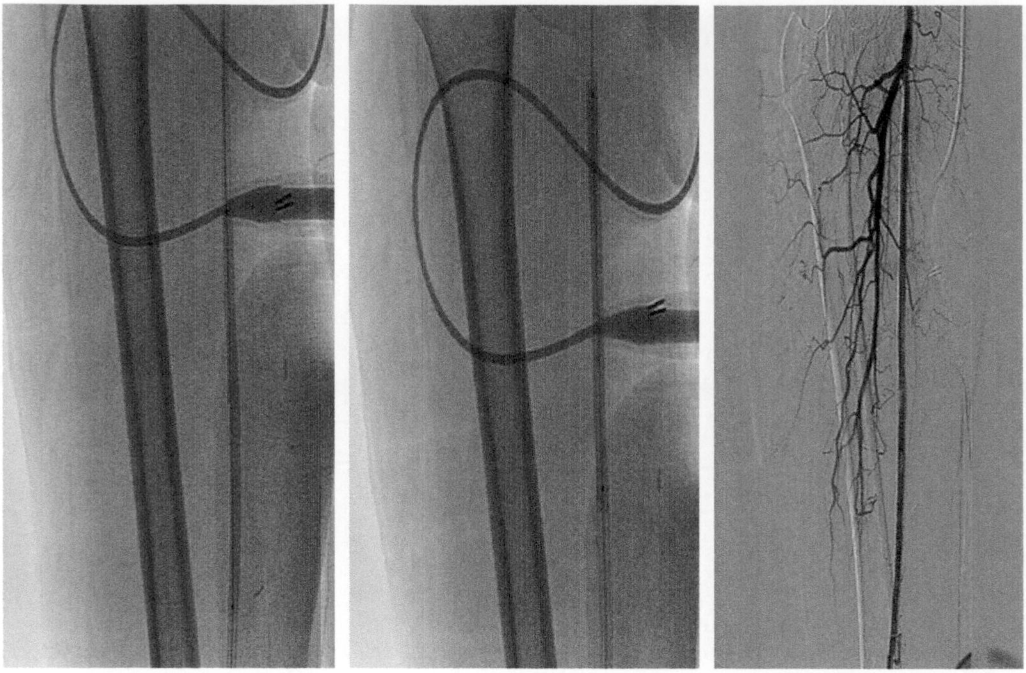

Fig. 11. Self-expanding stents placed in the native SFA. Poststent angiogram shows persistent in-stent thrombus.

Guide catheter over which further therapies, such as balloons and stents, may be delivered.

***Wildcat catheter***

Originally manufactured as a support catheter in a 0.035-in caliber system, the Wildcat catheter (AVINGER, Redwood City, CA, USA), in addition, has a rotatable tip that is manually activated by turning the device handle to which it is connected. The tip has both passive and active configurations, determined by whether the wedges at the tip of the catheter are exposed or not. The tip can be rotated

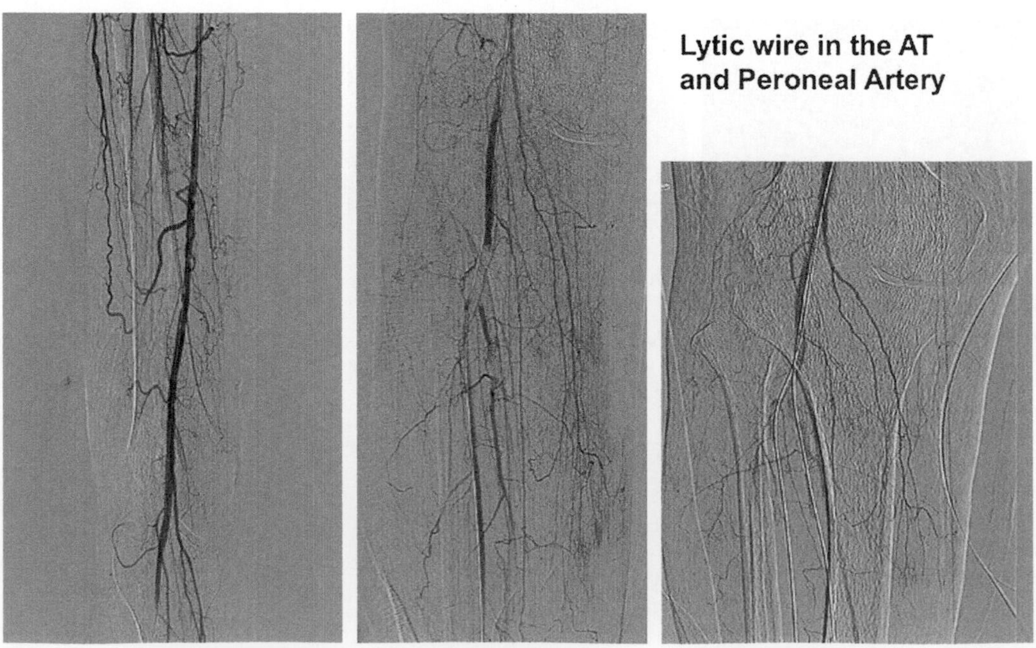


Fig. 12. Thrombotic occlusion of the popliteal artery and placement of thrombolytic wire across the thrombus. AT, anterior tibial artery.

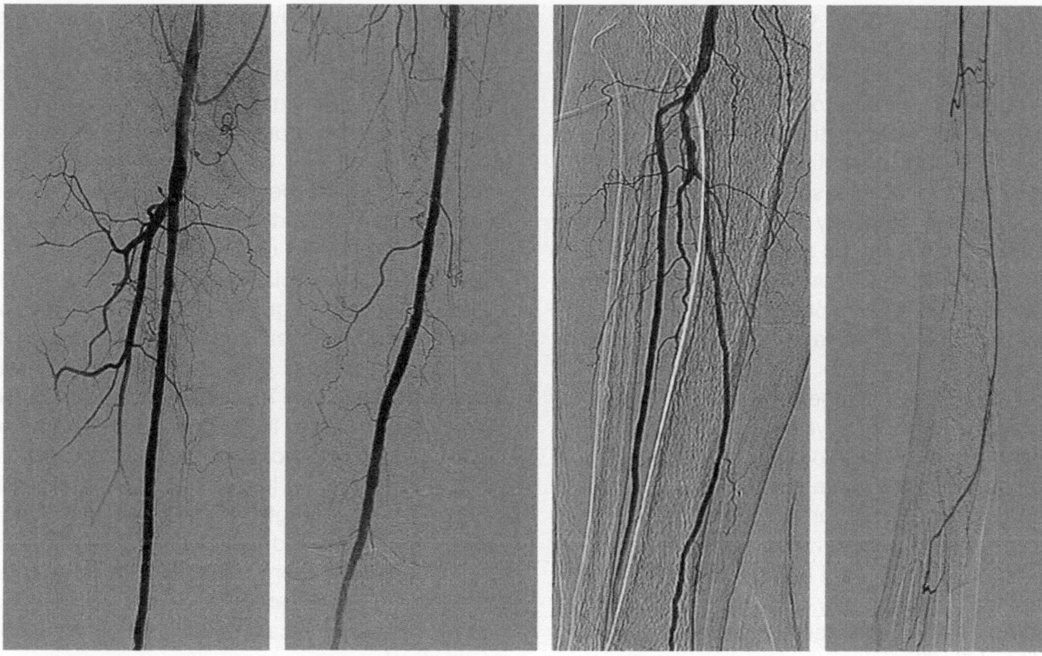

**Fig. 13.** Completion angiogram after 24 hours of thrombolysis shows patent SFA, popliteal arteries with 3 vessel runoff at the level of the ankle.

clockwise, counterclockwise, or by a combination of the 2 until the proximal cap is traversed and channeling is initiated. There is a provision for tip deflection to allow for directing of the catheter away from large collaterals just proximal to or at the CTO and back toward the occluded true lumen. The CONNECT (Chronic Total Occlusion Crossing With the Wildcat Catheter) trial is a prospective, multicenter, nonrandomized study initiated to evaluate the ability of this catheter to cross the CTOs of femoropopliteal segments. The study has recently completed its enrollment.

### *True Lumen Reentry Devices*

These devices typically cross the occlusive lesion in the subintimal plane and then aid in reentering the true lumen of the vessel immediately beyond the occlusion. The site of reentry usually needs a stent deployment to ensure adequate blood flow.

### *OUTBACK LTD Re-Entry Catheter*

The OUTBACK LTD Re-Entry Catheter (Cordis, Johnson & Johnson, Bridgewater, NJ, USA) is 120 cm in length, with a single 0.014-in wire lumen and a 5.9F profile (6F sheath compatible). The device is passed over a 0.014-in wire into the subintimal space adjacent to the desired reentry location. Orienting the catheter under fluoroscopy by means of distal L and T markers at the end of the catheter shaft aligns the cannula with the true lumen. The wire is then partially withdrawn, and the cannula is advanced into the true lumen by moving the deployment slide forward. The wire can then be advanced into the true lumen, and conventional therapies can be delivered.

#### *Pioneer catheter*

The Pioneer catheter (Medtronic, Minneapolis, MN, USA) incorporates a distal 25-gauge nitinol reentry needle with an integrated 64-element phased-array intravascular ultrasound transducer to allow directed ultrasound-guided reentry into the true lumen. This catheter is 120 cm long, accommodates two 0.014-in guidewires (1 to track the device and 1 for the reentry needle), and is compatible with a 7F sheath. The device is brought into the subintimal tract over a wire, and under intravascular ultrasound imaging, color flow is identified in the true lumen. The catheter is rotated to position the true lumen at the 12-o'clock position, after which the needle is advanced and the true lumen is wired. The Pioneer catheter can then be removed, and the intervention may proceed.

## SUBINTIMAL ANGIOPLASTY IN INFRAINGUINAL DISEASE

Subintimal angioplasty was first described in 1987 as a method of performing an endovascular arterial bypass. The subintimal space at the start of the occlusion is entered with a catheter, and a wire loop is used to cross the occlusion and reenter the vessel lumen distally. Reentry devices such as the OUTBACK LTD Re-Entry Catheter may be required in up to 15% of cases to regain the true lumen. In patients with CLI, there is evidence from prospective nonrandomized trials suggesting that the limb salvage rate for subintimal infrapopliteal angioplasty (SIA) performed primarily for SFA disease may be superior to PTA alone. In a meta-analysis of all trials with SIA performed till 2008 (37 studies, prospective and retrospective in 2810 limbs), the primary patency at 12 months was 56%, with a limb salvage rate of 89%.[29] More recent trials suggest that these rates may be even higher. A 5-year observational study comparing SIA with bypass in patients with CLI with infrainguinal disease suggested nearly comparable 5-year amputation-free survival. Compared with patients who underwent bypass, patients who underwent SIA had a shorter hospitalization, substantially lower cost, greater freedom from major adverse events, and improved quality of life.[30]

## DRUG-ELUTING STENTS IN INFRAINGUINAL DISEASE

The PARADISE (Preventing Amputations Using Drug-Eluting Stents) trial was a nonrandomized trial of 106 patients with CLI who underwent placement of DES in the infrageniculate vessels conducted in patients presenting with CLI.[31] The trial enrolled 106 patients who received balloon-expandable DES (83% received CYPHER [Cordis, Johnson & Johnson, Bridgewater, NJ], whereas 17% received TAXUS [Boston Scientific, Minneapolis, MN, USA]). The average number of stents per limb was 1.9, and 35% of limbs received overlapping DES (length of 60 mm). There were no procedural deaths, and 96% of patients were discharged within 24 hours. The 3-year cumulative incidence of amputation was 6%, survival was 71%, and amputation-free survival was 68%. Target limb revascularization occurred in 15% of patients, and repeat angiography in 35% of patients revealed a binary restenosis rate of 12%. This early study is promising but must be tested in a randomized controlled trial.

## HYBRID REVASCULARIZATION

An increasing number of patients with CLI undergo a combination of endovascular and open surgery to achieve complete revascularization. Hybrid therapy represents an attractive revascularization option in patients who are older, are frail, or have limited autologous conduit for bypass. In a hybrid procedure, the endovascular portion may consist of restoring inflow, restoring outflow, restoring both inflow and outflow, or revising a bypass graft. Endovascular repair may be performed percutaneously using the crossover technique from the contralateral CFA or via cutdown over the ipsilateral CFA, which permits reconstruction using femoral artery endarterectomy and patch angioplasty or placement of an interposition graft. The use of an endovascular inflow procedure, whether of the aortoiliac segment or the SFA, does not seem to compromise long-term patency of the downstream bypass graft. A recent series examined outcomes in 171 patients who underwent combined common femoral endarterectomy and either iliac stenting or iliac stent grafting for rest pain (32%), tissue loss (22%), or claudication (46%). Median length of hospital stay was 2 days. The 30-day mortality was 2.3%, with perioperative complications seen in 22%. The 5-year primary, primary-assisted, and secondary patencies are typically 60%, 97%, and 98%, respectively.

## THE PERSPECTIVE

Percutaneous treatment of CLI over the last few decades has seen a series of wires, catheters, balloons, stents, atherectomy devices, and crossing equipments. The key to a successful outcome for endovascular intervention for patients with CLI is at least 1 vessel runoff. More than 1 vessel runoff may provide improved wound healing and improved patency. Use of plain old balloon angioplasty with prolonged inflations seems to be the easiest, time-proven, and cheapest methodology to treat CLI. In patients with flow-limiting dissections, a self-expanding stent improves patency and wound healing.

Specialized balloons such as cutting balloon and cryoballoon (Boston Scientific corporate, Natick, MA, USA), AngioSculpt balloon (AngioScore Inc, Fremont, CA, USA), and VascuTrack (BARD Peripheral Vascular, Inc, Tempe, AZ, USA) have been used in patients with CLI. These specialized balloons have the advantages of controlled dissection and reduced chance of flow-limiting dissection and minimal plaque shift at vessel bifurcation. However, in terms of patency or improved wound healing, there are no studies demonstrating an added advantage of these specialized balloons compared with plain old balloon angioplasty.

Various atherectomy devices are used for CLI to debulk the plaque burden and modify the lesion morphology. Laser atherectomy (Spectranetics Corporation, Colorado Springs, CO, USA) has shown good data on limb salvage. Lesions that are crossed with a wire but cannot be crossed with a catheter or balloon can use atherectomy devices such as Diamondback 360 (Cardiovascular Systems Inc, St Paul, MN, USA). Significant plaque burden can be reduced using Silver hawk catheters (EV 3, Plymouth, MN, USA). However, although these devices may claim improved lumen diameter after intervention, there are limited data that this indeed improves patency or the limb salvage rates.

Difficult CTO cases in patients with CLI can be crossed using a wire and catheter support in most cases. However, complications of the device, cost, and learning curve for beginners usually make the use of accessory devices prohibitory.

## SUMMARY

CLI carries a high morbidity and mortality rate in patients who are left untreated. A multidisciplinary approach with aggressive risk factor reduction should be initiated early in the course along with referral to a vascular specialist. The last decade has seen an unprecedented rate of new device development for the treatment of peripheral arterial occlusive disease, lending us the ability to successfully treat a vast array of lesion subsets. These technologies have been associated with high acute procedure success rates; however, long-term target vessel patency after mechanical therapies remains suboptimal and unknown in many cases. The outcome criteria used in most of these studies are physician oriented and fail to reflect the actual benefit to the patient in terms of symptom relief, ambulation, and quality of life. The development of such instruments of outcome is still in infancy and needs high-quality research to better understand the cost-effectiveness and true efficacy of such interventions.

## REFERENCES

1. Norgren L, Hiatt WR, Dormandy JA, et al. Inter-Society Consensus for the Management of Peripheral Arterial Disease (TASC II). J Vasc Surg 2007; 45(Suppl S):S5.
2. TASC. Management of peripheral arterial disease (PAD). Trans-Atlantic Inter-Society Consensus (TASC). J Vasc Surg 2000;31(Suppl 1):S1–287.
3. Fontaine R, Kim M, Kieny R. Die chirurgische behandlung der peripheren durchblutungsstörungen. Helv Chir Acta 1954;5/6:199–533 [in German].
4. Dormandy JA, Thomas PR. What is the natural history of a critically ischemic patient with and without his leg? In: Greenhalgh RM, Jamieson C, Nicolaides AN, editors. Limb salvage and amputation for vascular disease. 11th edition. Philadelphia: WB Saunders; 1988. p. 11–26.
5. Second European Consensus Document on chronic critical leg ischemia. Circulation 1991;84:IV1–26.
6. Regensteiner JG, Hiatt WR. Current medical therapies for patients with peripheral arterial disease: a critical review. Am J Med 2002;112:49–57.
7. Girolami B, Bernardi E, Prins MH, et al. Treatment of intermittent claudication with physical training, smoking cessation, pentoxifylline, or nafronyl: a meta-analysis. Arch Intern Med 1999;159:337–45.
8. Krzesinski JM. Management of high blood pressure in peripheral arterial disease. Acta Chir Belg 2005; 105(6):560–6.
9. Fowkes FG, Housley E, Cawood EH, et al. Edinburgh Artery Study: prevalence of asymptomatic and symptomatic peripheral arterial disease in the general population. Int J Epidemiol 1991;20:384–92.
10. LaRosa JC, He J, Vupputuri S. Effect of statins on risk of coronary disease: a meta-analysis of randomized controlled trials. JAMA 1999;282:2340–6.
11. Ansell BJ, Watson KE, Fogelman AM. An evidence-based assessment of NCEP Adult Treatment Panel II guidelines. JAMA 1999;282:2051–7.
12. Elam MB, Hunninghake DB, Davis KB, et al. Effect of niacin on lipid and lipo-protein levels and glycemic control in patients with diabetes and peripheral arterial disease: the ADMIT study: a randomized trial. JAMA 2000;284:1263–70.
13. Heart Protection Study Collaborative Group. MRC/BHF Heart Protection Study of cholesterol lowering with simvastatin in 20,536 high-risk individuals: a randomised placebo-controlled trial. Lancet 2002; 360:7–22.
14. Golledge J. Lower-limb arterial disease. Lancet 1997;350:1459–65.
15. Castaneda-Zuniga WR, Formanek A, Tadavarthy M, et al. The mechanism of balloon angioplasty. Radiology 1980;135(3):565–71.
16. Schillinger M, Exner M, Mlekusch W, et al. Balloon angioplasty and stent implantation induce a vascular inflammatory reaction. J Endovasc Ther 2002;9(1):59–66.
17. Ponec D, Jaff MR, Swischuk J, et al, CRISP Study Investigators. The nitinol SMART stent vs Wallstent for suboptimal iliac artery angioplasty: CRISP-US trial results. J Vasc Interv Radiol 2004;15(9):911–8.
18. Mewissen MW. Self-expanding nitinol stents in the femoropopliteal segment: technique and mid-term results. Tech Vasc Interv Radiol 2004;7:2–5.
19. Duda SH, Pusich B, Richter G, et al. Sirolimus-eluting stents for the treatment of obstructive superficial femoral artery disease: six-month results. Circulation 2002;106(12):1505–9.
20. Keeling WB, Shames ML, Stone PA, et al. Plaque excision with the Silverhawk catheter: early results in patients with claudication or critical limb ischemia. J Vasc Surg 2007;45(1):25–31.
21. Yancey AE, Minion DJ, Rodriguez C, et al. Peripheral atherectomy in TransAtlantic InterSociety Consensus

type C femoropopliteal lesions for limb salvage. J Vasc Surg 2006;44(3):503–9.
22. Laird JR, Zeller T, Gray BH, et al. Limb salvage following laser-assisted angioplasty for critical limb ischemia: results of the LACI multicenter trial. J Endovasc Ther 2006;13:1–11.
23. Kandzari DE, Kiesz RS, Allie D, et al. Procedural and clinical outcomes with catheter-based plaque excision in critical limb ischemia. J Endovasc Ther 2006;13:12–22.
24. Zeller T, Rastan A, Sixt S, et al. Long-term results after directional atherectomy of femoro-popliteal lesions. J Am Coll Cardiol 2006;48:1573–8.
25. Loor G, Skelly CL, Wahlgren CM, et al. Is atherectomy the best first-line therapy for limb salvage in patients with critical limb ischemia? Vasc Endovascular Surg 2009;43:542–50.
26. Lipsitz EC, Ohki T, Veith FJ, et al. Does subintimal angioplasty have a role in the treatment of severe lower extremity ischemia? J Vasc Surg 2003;37:386–91.
27. Saket RR, Razavi MK, Padidar A, et al. Novel intravascular ultrasound-guided method to create transintimal arterial communications: initial experience in peripheral occlusive disease and aortic dissection. J Endovasc Ther 2004;11:274–80.
28. Mossop PJ, Amukotuwa SA, Whitbourn RJ. Controlled blunt microdissection for percutaneous recanalization of lower limb arterial chronic total occlusions: a single center experience. Catheter Cardiovasc Interv 2006;68:304–10.
29. Bown MJ, Bolia A, Sutton AJ. Subintimal angioplasty: meta-analytical evidence of clinical utility. Eur J Vasc Endovasc Surg 2009;38:323–37.
30. Markose G, Miller F, Bolia A. Subintimal angioplasty for femoro-popliteal occlusive disease. J Vasc Surg 2010;52:1410–6.
31. Feiring AJ, Krahn M, Wesolowski A, et al. Preventing leg amputations in critical limb ischemia with below-the-knee stents (PARADISE trial). J Am Coll Cardiol 2010;55:1580–9.
32. Romiti M, Albers M, Brochado-Neto FC, et al. Meta-analysis of infrapopliteal angioplasty for chronic critical limb ischemia. J Vasc Surg 2008;47(5):975–81.
33. Das T, McNamara T, Gray B, et al. Cryoplasty therapy for limb salvage in patients with critical limb ischemia. J Endovasc Ther 2007;14:753–6.
34. Ansel GM, Sample NS, Botti III CF Jr, et al. Cutting balloon angioplasty of the popliteal and infrapopliteal vessels for symptomatic limb ischemia. Catheter Cardiovasc Interv 2004;61:1–4.
35. Scheller B. Opportunities and limitations of drug-coated balloons in interventional therapies. Herz 2011;36(3):232–9.
36. Feiring AJ, Wesolowski AA, Lade S. Primary stent-supported angioplasty for treatment of below-knee critical limb ischemia and severe claudication: early and one-year outcomes. J Am Coll Cardiol 2004; 44(12):2307–14.
37. Siablis D, Kraniotis P, Karnabatidis D, et al. Sirolimus-eluting versus bare stents for bailout after suboptimal infrapopliteal angioplasty for critical limb ischemia: 6-month angiographic results from a nonrandomized prospective single-center study. J Endovasc Ther 2005;12(6):685–95.
38. Scheinert D, Ulrich M, Scheinert S, et al. Comparison of sirolimus-eluting vs bare-metal stents for the treatment of infrapopliteal obstructions. EuroIntervention 2006;2(2):169–74.
39. Kickuth R, Keo HH, Triller J, et al. Initial clinical experience with the 4-F self-expanding XPERT stent system for infrapopliteal treatment of patients with severe claudication and critical limb ischemia. J Vasc Interv Radiol 2007;18(6):703–8.
40. Bosiers M, Deloose K, Verbist J, et al. First clinical application of absorbable metal stents in the treatment of critical limb ischemia: 12-month results. Vasc Dis Manag 2005;2:86–91.
41. Biondi-Zoccai GG, Sangiorgi G. Commentary: Below-the-knee/ankle revascularization: tools of the trade. J Endovasc Ther 2009;16(5):613–6.

# Update on Biological Therapies for Critical Limb Ischemia

Richard J. Powell, MD

**KEYWORDS**

• Biological therapy • Critical limb ischemia • Gene
• Stem cell

Approximately 8 million Americans suffer from peripheral artery disease (PAD), which is associated with a 5-year cardiovascular death risk of 20% to 30%.[1] In its most severe form, PAD manifests as critical limb ischemia (CLI), which is defined by severely impaired hemodynamics and chronic ischemic rest pain, ulcers/tissue loss, or gangrene.[2–4] Mortality and morbidity caused by CLI is high. Up to 20% of patients with CLI die within the first 12 months after diagnosis. The 5-year mortality for CLI is in excess of 70%. As many as 40% to 50% of patients undergo major limb amputation within 12 months of diagnosis.[3] The ability of this elderly patient population with many associated comorbidities to successfully rehabilitate and maintain an independent living status following major limb amputation is poor.

The medical treatment of patients with CLI includes pharmacologic treatment of atherosclerosis with lipid-reducing agents such as statins as well as antiplatelet and antihypertensive therapies. Wound care and surgical debridement is also integral to patient care. This care frequently involves a multidisciplinary team approach. Revascularization continues to be the mainstay of therapy, and this includes either open surgical procedures or percutaneous endovascular approaches.

Up to 50% of patients with CLI are not candidates for open revascularization because of unsuitable anatomy or conduit, or associated comorbidities such as coronary disease, pulmonary disease, and renal failure.[1] Unsuitable anatomy can also preclude effective endovascular therapy for CLI. Patients with CLI who are unable to undergo successful revascularization currently have no effective treatment options. There are currently no therapies approved by the US Food and Drug Administration (FDA) for CLI. Therapy for this no-option CLI patient population is limited to management of the associated comorbidities with intensive wound care, pain control, and eventual amputation of the limb. Thus, patients with no-option CLI represent a population with a serious and life-threatening disease with unmet medical needs. Given the limitations of current therapies and high rate of mortality, CLI quality of life in this patient population has been likened to terminal cancer. The incidence of CLI is expected to increase in the next 10 to 15 years.

Pharmacologic and biological therapies have been evaluated for efficacy in the treatment of CLI. Pharmacologic therapies have largely focused on agents that result in vasodilatation, such as the prostaglandins. Recent pivotal clinical trials have failed to show significant improvement in outcome in patients treated with intravenous milepost either as a stand-alone therapy or as an adjuvant therapy combined with lower extremity bypass.[5,6] This therapy has been approved for the treatment of CLI in countries outside the United States.

Biological therapy uses various angiogenic growth factors or autologous stem cells in an attempt to improve perfusion in areas of ischemia through the development of new blood vessels from preexisting blood vessels. This process has been termed therapeutic angiogenesis and involves capillaries in the size range of 100 to 300 μm. Because of the short half-life of recombinant

Disclosures: Richard J Powell is a consultant for AnGes and Aastrom.
Section of Vascular Surgery, Dartmouth Hitchcock Medical Center, Lebanon, NH 03756, USA
*E-mail address:* richard.powell@hitchcock.org

Cardiol Clin 29 (2011) 411–417
doi:10.1016/j.ccl.2011.05.001

proteins, current clinical trials have usually approached the delivery of angiogenic factors through either a stem cell or gene therapy approach.

Recent phase II trials have shown promise both for gene therapy and stem cell therapy in the treatment of CLI. This article describes current clinical CLI trial design and methodology, reviews current trial outcomes, and identifies potential areas for improvement in future trial design.

## CLI CLINICAL TRIAL DESIGN

Because of trial design issues, there are many obstacles to the completion of CLI clinical trials.[7] The CLI patient population is widely disparate in the extent of disease, which can range from rest pain to extensive tissue loss. Patients with CLI can also present with a spectrum of wounds that vary from rapidly progressive extensive gangrene or deeply penetrating heel wounds to mild superficial skin erosions. Because of the heterogeneity of this patient population, outcomes are more variable and larger numbers of patients may be needed to obtain proof of efficacy. In addition, despite encouraging early trial results, it remains unlikely that attempts at limb revascularization using biological or pharmacologic approaches will result in the same level of improved limb perfusion as a successful lower extremity bypass or endovascular procedure.

## PATIENT POPULATION

CLI is defined as inadequate perfusion to maintain limb viability and can manifest as either ischemic rest pain (Rutherford category 4) or ischemic tissue loss (Rutherford 5). To confirm the diagnosis of CLI, patients should have supporting hemodynamic criteria. These criteria usually include an ankle pressure of less than 50 mm Hg or toe pressure of less than 30 mm Hg in patients with rest pain, and an ankle pressure less than 70 mm Hg or toe pressure less than 40 mm Hg in patients with tissue loss.[8] Patients with such severe tissue loss that it is unlikely that the limb can be salvaged (Rutherford 6) should not be included in these trials. It is reasonable to use total ulcer size to assist in preventing patients with nonsalvageable tissue loss from entering the trial.

At present, all CLI studies have enrolled no-option subjects with ischemic ulcers or rest pain; patients in whom all endovascular or open surgical options have been exhausted or are too medically high risk to undergo revascularization procedures. Biological and pharmacologic therapy within this population could potentially bias outcomes toward failure, because these patients may be biologically less likely to respond to angiogenic gene therapy compared with the general population of patients with CLI. **Box 1** shows the generally accepted inclusion and exclusion criteria for CLI trials.

## EFFICACY END POINTS

At present, time of amputation-free survival (AFS) remains the gold standard end point for a CLI pivotal trial (eg, TASC II).[9] This end point has several potential shortcomings that include the lack of any measurable effect on quality of life as well as the inclusion of death, which is a non–limb-specific end point. The event rate for AFS in the CLI population at 1 year is approximately 30% to 40%, with death occurring in 10% to 15% of subjects and major amputation in 20% to 30%.[5,7,10,11] However, this can be highly variable depending on the selection criteria used in each study. In several CLI trials, the 1-year rate of AFS in the placebo-treated patients was only 20%.[5,7,11] This rate highlights the need for blinded placebo-controlled trials in this area.

Because therapeutic angiogenesis revascularization strategies would be expected to have a modest impact on mortality in CLI, it is anticipated that the main driver of the AFS end point would be amputation.[8] As such, CLI trial design needs to be powered primarily on the anticipated rate of amputation and, as a result, needs to be large. An example of this is the Therapeutic Angiogenesis for the Management of Arteriosclerosis in a Randomized International Study (TAMARIS) trial that involved more than 500 patients and evaluated the effect of fibroblastic growth factor (FGF) plasmid on AFS in CLI.[8]

The development of end points that would be more limb specific, such as the recently reported end point suggested by the Society for Vascular Surgery major adverse limb event (MALE) that could be used in all CLI trials, would help to better define the role of future therapies for CLI.[8]

The appropriate time point for efficacy analysis remains controversial. By analyzing the outcomes of placebo control in previous CLI trials, it has been shown that patient selection can have a major impact on the time to occurrence of AFS. As such, the earliest time point that should be considered for efficacy in a pivotal CLI trial is 12 months.[8]

Additional efficacy end points could also include wound healing as measured by change in size of ulcer. Complete wound healing requires complete epithelialization of the wound for at least 2 weeks. Improved pain at rest, as measured by the visual analog score, changes in hemodynamic measurements as measured by ankle brachial index (ABI)/toe brachial index (TBI) or transcutaneous pressure of oxygen ($TcP_{O_2}$), and quality-of-life measures.

**Box 1**
**Common major inclusion and exclusion criteria used in biological therapy evaluation for CLI trials**

*Major Inclusion Criteria:*

1. Subjects need to have appropriately sized and ischemic peripheral ulcer(s) or tissue loss. Subjects need to have 1 or both of the following hemodynamic indicators of severe peripheral arterial occlusive disease:
   a. Ankle systolic pressure (in either the dorsalis pedis or posterior tibial arteries) of $\leq$70 mm Hg
   b. Toe systolic pressure $\leq$50 mm Hg
2. The subject is a poor candidate for standard revascularization treatment options for peripheral arterial disease, based on inadequate bypass conduit, unfavorable anatomy, or poor operative risk.

*Major Exclusion Criteria:*

1. Subjects who, in the opinion of the investigator, have a vascular disease prognosis that indicated they may require a major amputation (at or above the ankle) within 4 weeks of the start of treatment.
2. Subjects with a diagnosis of Buerger disease (thromboangiitis obliterans).
3. Subjects with hemodynamically significant aortoiliac occlusive disease.
4. Subjects who have had a revascularization procedure within 12 weeks before treatment initiation that remained patent. Revascularization procedures that were shown to have failed (completely occluded) for >2 weeks before treatment initiation were acceptable.
5. Subjects with history of deep ulcerations with bone or tendon exposure, or clinical evidence of invasive infection (eg, cellulitis, osteomyelitis) uncontrollable by antibiotic therapy.
6. Evidence or history of malignant neoplasm (clinical, laboratory, or imaging), except for fully resolved basal cell carcinoma of the skin. Patients who underwent successful tumor resection or radiochemotherapy for breast cancer more than 10 years before inclusion in the study, and with no recurrence, could be enrolled in the study. Patients who had successful tumor resection or radiochemotherapy for all other tumor types more than 5 years before inclusion in the study, and with no recurrence, could be enrolled in the study.
7. Subjects who have proliferative diabetic retinopathy, severe nonproliferative retinopathy, recent (within 6 months) retinal vein occlusion, macular degeneration with choroidal neovascularization, macular edema on fundus evaluation by an ophthalmologist, or intraocular surgery within 3 months.
8. Subjects with history of end-stage renal disease, defined as significant renal dysfunction shown by a creatinine of $\geq$2.5 mg/dL, or receiving chronic hemodialysis therapy.

## CURRENT CLINICAL TRIAL RESULTS

There is currently no FDA-approved medical therapy for CLI. Therapies currently used to treat CLI include endovascular therapy, open surgical revascularization, and primary amputation. Both open surgery and endovascular therapy are effective revascularization strategies.[1,8,12,13] As shown in the Bypass versus Angioplasty in Severe Ischaemia of the Leg (BASIL) Trial, open surgical options are not available in up to 50% of patients with CLI because of associated medical comorbidities, lack of suitable autogenous conduit, or distal target vessel.[1] In the absence of acceptable endovascular or surgical therapy, patients eventually require major amputation to control pain or infection.

### *Gene Therapy*

Prior studies that have attempted to use angiogenic gene therapy to treat claudication have met with disappointing results. Numerous randomized, placebo-controlled claudication trials using various vascular endothelial growth factor (VEGF) isoforms, FGF, and hypoxia-inducible factor 1$\alpha$ have failed to show a clinically meaningful improvement in peak walking time compared with placebo-treated subjects.[14,15]

However, unlike claudication, clinical trials using angiogenic gene therapy to treat CLI have had more promising results. The angiogenic gene therapy field was pioneered by Dr Jeffery Isner, whose early work using various VEGF isoforms suggested improved wound healing in patients treated with intramuscular injection of VEGF.[16,17] These early trials were open label and did not have a placebo-treated arm. This work did spark an interest in the field and laid the groundwork for future studies.

Rajagopalan and colleagues[18] published promising phase I data using adenovirus-mediated delivery of the gene for hypoxia-inducible factor 1$\alpha$ in patients with CLI. However, a subsequent pivotal trial in the claudication population failed to show any difference in peak walking time compared with placebo-treated patients.[15]

In clinical gene therapy for CLI, intramuscular injection of FGF plasmid has been the most extensively studied. The initial phase II, randomized, placebo-controlled clinical trial using plasmid-delivered FGF-1, the Talisman 201 Trial, showed a dramatic improvement in major amputation–free survival in FGF-1–treated subjects compared with placebo.[19–21] In this trial, 12-month AFS was 73% in the FGF-treated subjects compared with 48% in the subjects receiving placebo. There were no safety concerns with the FGF plasmid therapy. In a subsequent study, these investigators studied tissues from patients treated with FGF plasmid before lower extremity amputation and were able to show proof of plasmid uptake and protein expression by skeletal muscle cells in the region of FGF plasmid injection. This work showed gene therapy proof of concept in human patients suffering with CLI.[19] Recently, the results of the phase III pivotal TAMARIS FGF plasmid trial were reported (**Table 1**). Contrary to the early phase II trial, FGF gene therapy was shown to have no effect on AFS or any secondary end point compared with placebo-treated patients.[10] Potential explanations for the apparent discrepancy between the outcomes of the trials is unclear, but is likely related to a type II error, which is an important example of the importance of having an adequate number of subjects enrolled in the phase II trial.

We have recently reported the outcomes of 2 phase II trials examining the safety and efficacy of intramuscular injection of hepatocyte growth factor (HGF) in patients with CLI. The HGF-STAT trial was the initial phase I/II dose-finding trial comparing placebo with log difference in dose of intramuscular injection of HGF plasmid.[11] This trial showed that HGF gene therapy was not associated with an increase in adverse events, development of malignancy, or progression of retinopathy. In addition, the trial showed an increase in $TcPo_2$ from baseline in patients treated with high-dose HGF gene therapy compared with placebo. In a subsequent phase II trial (the HGF-0205 trial), high-dose HGF gene therapy was delivered by duplex-guided intramuscular injection.[7] This technique ensured that the plasmid was delivered into the deep intramuscular region of the lower extremity in the region of the popliteal-tibial occlusive disease. The results of this study showed improvement at 6 months in both TBI and pain as measured by visual analog score from baseline in the patients treated with HGF plasmid compared with placebo. In these 2 studies, there was no difference in major amputation between subjects treated with HGF gene therapy or placebo. This finding was not surprising for several reasons. First, given that the goal of these studies was to show safety and efficacy of the HGF plasmid therapy, the study was not powered to identify differences in an infrequent end-stage outcome measure such as major amputation. Second, the extent of tissue necrosis present in the CLI patient population was highly variable because many patients had extensive tissue loss. Because of the variation in tissue loss at presentation, there was no difference in major amputation between the groups.

A third trial using HGF gene therapy has been completed in Japan using HGF gene therapy to treat patients with small ischemic ulcers.[22] This trial was stopped early by the Data Safety Monitoring Board because of improved outcome in the patients treated with HGF plasmid. In this blinded, randomized, placebo-controlled trial, patients treated with HGF gene therapy had a 70% improvement in ulcer healing or rest pain, compared with 30% in subjects treated with placebo (**Table 2**).[8]

In summary, these 3 HGF trials have together shown an increase in limb perfusion as measured by $TcPo_2$ and TBI, as well as improvements in wound healing compared with placebo. Furthermore, there have been no safety concerns. These studies have not shown an improvement in the more clinically meaningful outcome of AFS; however, the studies were small and not powered to show such a difference.

## *Stem Cell Therapy*

Stem cell therapy using either autologous or allogenic placental stem cells is a newly developing therapy for the treatment of CLI. Since the initial isolation of endothelial progenitor cells (EPCs) from human peripheral blood by Asahara and colleagues,[23] multiple investigators have shown that EC progenitor cells can differentiate into mature

**Table 1**
**Results of the TAMARIS trial. NV1FGF plasmid versus placebo in CLI pivotal trial (n = 525)**

| 12-mo End Point | AFS | Amputation | Death |
|---|---|---|---|
| NV1FGF (%) | 63 | 26 | 18 |
| Placebo (%) | 67 | 21 | 15 |
| *P* | .48 | .31 | .53 |

**Table 2**
**Summary of Japanese phase III HGF CLI trial**

| Dose Group | Subjects Improved | Subjects Unimproved | Improvement Rate (%) |
|---|---|---|---|
| HGF | 19 | 8 | 70.37 |
| Placebo | 4 | 9 | 30.77 |
| | | | *P* = .0140 |

ECs and contribute to arteriogenesis and angiogenesis in acute hind limb ischemia animal models. In humans, it is likely that EPCs are involved in reendothelialization following arterial injury. It has been shown that circulating EC progenitors decrease in both numbers and function with aging and diabetes.

Stem cell therapy is performed through intra-arterial or intramuscular injection of stem cells into the ischemic limb.[24,25] Potential mechanisms of efficacy of stem cell therapy in humans remain unclear. It is also unclear which components of the bone marrow mononuclear cell fraction are involved in the putative beneficial effects of stem cell therapy. Many investigators currently believe that all of the progenitor cell lines together may have a synergistic role in maximizing benefits. Whether this process includes differentiation of the stem cells into mature components of the vascular wall with a direct effect on angiogenesis, which seems unlikely, or whether they serve as cytokine factories that have a paracrine effect promoting arteriogenesis, angiogenesis, and wound healing is unclear.[26]

Potential techniques to acquire autologous stem cells in sufficient numbers include direct bone marrow harvest and complex Ficoll cell separation techniques using a hematology service or, more recently, the development of rapid cell separation techniques that can be used at the point of care.[24,27] Adequate numbers of bone marrow–derived stem cells can also be generated through harvest of autologous bone marrow–derived stem cells that are then expanded within a bioreactor before intramuscular injection in to the ischemic limb.[28] Studies are also underway examining the use of bone marrow mobilization using granulocyte-macrophage colony-stimulating factor followed by plasmapheresis placental allogenic stem cells, and the use of fat-derived epidermal stem cells.[26]

Tateishi-Yayama and colleagues[29] performed the first randomized trial of bone marrow mononuclear cells (BM-MNC); the Therapeutic Angiogenesis by Cell Transplantation (TACT) study. This trial compared intramuscular injection of BM-MNC versus peripheral blood mononuclear cells in patients with CLI. AT 26 weeks, these investigators showed a significant increase in ABI and $TcPo_2$ in the patients treated with BM-MNC compared with patients treated with peripheral blood mononuclear cells. The trial was underpowered to detect differences in clinically relevant end points such as AFS or MALE.

A recent report by Iafrati and colleagues[27] has shown improvement in a composite end point in patients with CLI receiving bone marrow mononuclear therapy compared with placebo. This technique involves the harvest of 450 to 500 mL of bone that is then concentrated at the time of harvest using a proprietary centrifuge, following which the bone marrow mononuclear cells are injected into the affected extremity. This stem cell therapy technique is now undergoing pivotal trials.

We recently reported the results of a prospective, randomized, double-blinded, placebo-controlled, multicenter study (RESTORE-CLI) that was conducted at 20 centers in the United States in patients with CLI and no option for revascularization.[28] In this trial, patients underwent aspiration of 50 mL of bone marrow under local anesthesia. The aspirate was processed in a closed, automated cell manufacturing system for approximately 12 days to generate the tissue-repair cell (TRC) population of stem and progenitor cells. An average of $(136 \pm 41) \times 10^6$ total viable cells or electrolyte (control) solution were injected into 20 sites in the ischemic lower extremity. Clinical efficacy end points included major amputation–free survival and time to first occurrence of treatment failure (defined as any of the following: major amputation, death, de novo gangrene, or doubling of wound size), as well as major amputation rate.

In this trial, there was significant increase in time to treatment failure (log-rank test, $P = .0053$) and AFS in patients receiving TRC treatment, (log-rank test, $P = .038$). Major amputation occurred in 19% of TRC-treated patients compared with 43% of controls ($P = .14$, Fisher exact test).

In this trial, intramuscular injection of autologous bone marrow–derived TRCs was safe and decreased the occurrence of clinical events associated with disease progression compared with placebo in patients with lower extremity CLI and no revascularization options.

In summary, these 2 recently completed stem cell trials, although using differing harvest techniques, are promising and show beneficial effects of stem cell therapy on the clinically relevant end points of wound healing and amputation prevention. Multiple additional stem cell therapies are undergoing phase 1 trials.[26]

The potential risks and benefits of stem cell or gene therapy differ. Overall, there are fewer concerns with cell therapy regarding the risk of off-target angiogenesis compared with gene therapy. Advantages of the bone marrow harvest and preparation techniques are appealing because of the ability to provide therapy at the point of care. Disadvantages include the need to harvest a large amount of bone marrow (450–500 mL) under general anesthesia. Potential advantages of the cell expansion technique using a bioreactor include the need to collect a small amount of bone marrow under local anesthesia. Other potential advantages include that the expansion process may enrich the cell lineages that may be important for angiogenesis and neovascularization.[9]

Potential advantages of gene therapy in CLI include an off-the-shelf therapy that can be delivered at the point of contact without the need for additional procedures such as bone marrow harvest. Potential disadvantages include concern about off-target angiogenesis with resultant progression of proliferative retinopathy and occult tumor growth. However, there have been no safety concerns regarding potential tumor growth or progression of proliferative retinopathy in the previous placebo-controlled gene therapy trials conducted to date.

## FUTURE TRIAL DESIGN CONSIDERATIONS

Because of the previously mentioned trial design issues, performing CLI clinical trials using gene or stem cell therapy remains difficult; it is complicated by slow recruitment, high incidence of adverse events, and end points that do not necessarily reflect the goals of treatment. Patients with CLI represent a widely disparate population. Because of this heterogeneous patient population, outcomes are more variable and, as a result, larger numbers of patients are needed to discover proof of efficacy. Largely because of the extensive exclusion criteria, trial enrollment is difficult and large trials may take many years to enroll adequate numbers of patients. In the future, CLI trials should standardize acceptable initial wound size and wound care treatments to ensure that study populations are homogenous and comparable.

The CLI patient population is associated with a high prevalence of severe comorbidities and limited life expectancy. In the previous studies, greater than 90% of patients suffered at least 1 adverse event during the course of the study, further underscoring the extensive nature of vascular disease present in the CLI cohort.[7,11,28] At present, all CLI studies have enrolled no-option subjects with ischemic ulcers or rest pain. For these patients, all endovascular or open surgical options have been exhausted, or they are too medically high risk to undergo revascularization procedures. Gene or stem cell therapy within this population may be biased toward failure, because these patients may be biologically less likely to respond to angiogenic therapy compared with the general CLI patient population. In future CLI trials, consideration should be given to the enrollment of poor-option patients with CLI who have a higher risk for revascularization with expected decreased bypass success, such as a synthetic tibial bypass or spliced arm vein graft.[12,30]

At the present time, AFS remains the gold standard end point for a CLI trial (eg, TASC II).[9] This end point has several shortcomings that include the lack of any measurable effect on quality of life as well as the inclusion of death, which is a non–limb-specific end point. The development of end points that would be more limb specific and could be used in all CLI trials, such as the recently reported MALE end point, would help to better define the role of future therapies for CLI.[8]

## SUMMARY

Gene and stem cell therapies have been shown to be safe and well tolerated. Early trial results using these therapies have had promising results on important clinical end points such as wound healing, ischemic pain, and major amputation. Despite this, there have been no pivotal trials to date that have proved the benefit of biological therapy, although there are numerous pivotal trials in progress or about to initiate enrollment. Persistent obstacles exist with current study designs that complicate the ability to successfully perform clinical CLI trials.

## REFERENCES


1. Adam DJ, Beard JD, Cleveland T, et al. BASIL trial participants. Bypass versus angioplasty in severe ischaemia of the leg (BASIL): multicentre, randomised controlled trial. Lancet 2005;366:1925–34.
2. Criqui MH, Langer RD, Fronek A, et al. Mortality over a period of 10 years in subjects with peripheral arterial disease. N Engl J Med 1992;326:381–6.
3. Dormandy JA, Heeck L, Vig S. The fate of subjects with critical leg ischemia. Semin Vasc Surg 1999; 12:142–7.
4. Marston WA, Davies SW, Armstrong B, et al. Natural history of limbs with arterial insufficiency and chronic ulceration treated without revascularization. J Vasc Surg 2006;44:108–14.
5. Brass EP, Anthony R, Dormandy J, et al. Intensive parenteral therapy with lipo-ecraprost, a lipid-based formulation of a prostaglandin E1 analog does not alter six-month outcomes in patients with critical leg ischemia who are not candidates for revascularization. J Vasc Surg 2006;43:752–9.
6. Nehler MR, Brass EP, Anthony R, et al, Circulase investigators. Adjunctive parenteral therapy with lipo-ecraprost, a prostaglandin E1 analog, in patients with critical limb ischemia undergoing distal revascularization does not improve 6-month outcomes. J Vasc Surg 2007;45:953–61.
7. Powell RJ, Goodney P, Mendelsohn FO, et al. Safety and efficacy of patient specific intramuscular injection of HGF plasmid gene therapy on limb perfusion and wound healing in patients with ischemic lower

extremity ulceration: results of the HGF-0205 trial. J Vasc Surg 2010;52:1525–30.
8. Conte MS, Geraghty PJ, Bradbury AW, et al. Suggested objective performance goals and clinical trial design for evaluating catheter-based treatment of critical limb ischemia. J Vasc Surg 2009;50(6):1462–73.
9. Norgren L, Hiatt WR, Dormandy J, et al. Trans-Atlantic inter-society consensus for the management of peripheral arterial disease (TASC II). Eur J Vasc Endovasc Surg 2007;33(Suppl 1):s1–75.
10. Hiatt W. Results of NV1FGF gene therapy on amputation-free survival in critical limb ischemia - phase 3 randomized double-blind placebo-controlled trial. Paper presented at: 2010 American Heart Association Scientific Sessions. Chicago (IL), 2010.
11. Powell RJ, Simons M, Mendelsohn FO, et al. Results of a double-blind, placebo-controlled study to assess the safety of intramuscular injection of hepatocyte growth factor plasmid to improve limb perfusion in patients with critical limb ischemia. Circulation 2008; 118:58–65.
12. Conte M, Bandyk D, Clowes A, et al. Risk factors, medical therapies and peri-operative events in limb salvage surgery: observations from the PREVENT III multicenter trial. J Vasc Surg 2005;42:456–65.
13. Giles KA, Pomposelli FB, Hamdan AD, et al. Infrapopliteal angioplasty for critical limb ischemia: relation of transAtlantic InterSociety Consensus class to outcome in 176 limbs. J Vasc Surg 2008;48:128–36.
14. Lederman RJ, Mendelsohn FO, Anderson RD, et al, TRAFFIC Investigators. Therapeutic angiogenesis with recombinant fibroblast growth factor-2 for intermittent claudication: the TRAFFIC study. Lancet 2002;359:2053–8.
15. Mohler ER, Rajagopalan S, Olin JW, et al. Adenoviral-mediated gene transfer of vascular endothelial growth factor in critical limb ischemia: safety results from a phase I trial. Vasc Med 2003;8(1):9–13.
16. Baumgartner I, Pieczek A, Manor O, et al. Constitutive expression of phVEGF165 after intramuscular gene transfer promotes collateral vessel development in patients with critical limb ischemia. Circulation 1998;97:1114–23.
17. Isner JM, Pieczek A, Schainfeld R, et al. Clinical evidence of angiogenesis after arterial gene transfer of phVEGF165 in patient with ischaemic limb. Lancet 1996;348:370–4.
18. Rajagopalan S, Olin J, Deitcher S, et al. Use of a constitutively active hypoxia-inducible factor-1a transgene as a therapeutic strategy in no-option critical limb ischemia patients. Circulation 2007;115:1234–43.
19. Baumgartner I, Chronos N, Camerota A, et al. Local gene transfer and expression following intramuscular administration of FGF-1 plasmid DNA in patients with critical limb ischemia. Mol Ther 2009;17:914–21.
20. Comerota AJ, Throm RC, Miller KA, et al. Naked plasmid DNA encoding fibroblast growth factor type 1 for the treatment of end-stage unreconstructible lower extremity ischemia: preliminary results of a phase I trial. J Vasc Surg 2002;35:930–6.
21. Nikol S, Baumgartner I, Van Belle E, et al. Therapeutic angiogenesis with intramuscular NV1FGF improved amputation-free survival in patients with critical limb ischemia. Mol Ther 2008;16:972–8.
22. Shigematsu H, Yasuda K, Iwai T, et al. Randomized, double-blind, placebo-controlled clinical trial of hepatocyte growth factor plasmid for critical limb ischemia. Gene Ther 2010;17(9):1152–61.
23. Asahara T, Masuda H, Takahashi T, et al. Bone marrow origin of endothelial progenitor cells responsible for postnatal vasculogenesis in physiological and pathological neovascularization. Circ Res 1999;85:221–8.
24. Amann B, Luedemann C, Ratei R, et al. Autologous bone marrow cell transplantation increases leg perfusion and reduces amputations in patients with advanced critical limb ischemia due to peripheral artery disease. Cell Transplant 2009;18:371–80.
25. Sprengers RW, Moll FL, Teraa M, et al. Rationale and design of the JUVENTAS trial for repeated intra-arterial infusion of autologous bone marrow-derived mononuclear cells in patients with critical limb ischemia. J Vasc Surg 2010;51:1564–8.
26. Lawall H, Bramlage P, Aman B. Treatment of peripheral arterial disease using stem and progenitor cell therapy. J Vasc Surg 2011;53:445–53.
27. Lafrati M, Bandyk D, Benoit E, et al. Bone marrow aspirate concentrate in critical limb ischemia: results of a multicenter randomized double blind trial. J Vasc Surg 2010;52:11.
28. Powell R. Interim analysis results from the RESTORE-CLI, a randomized, double-blind multi-center phase II trial comparing expanded autologous bone marrow-derived tissue repair cells and placebo in patients with critical limb ischemia. Presented at Society for Vascular Surgery Annual Meeting. June, 2010.
29. Tateishi-Yuyama E, Matsubara H, Murohara T, et al. Therapeutic angiogenesis for patients with limb ischemia by autologous transplantation of bone-marrow cells: a pilot study and a randomized controlled trial. Lancet 2002;360:427–35.
30. Conte M, Bandyk D, Clowes A, et al. Results of PREVENT III: a multicenter, randomized trial of edifoligide for the prevention of vein graft failure in lower extremity bypass surgery. J Vasc Surg 2006;43:742–51.

# Perspectives on Optimizing Trial Design and Endpoints in Peripheral Arterial Disease: A Case for Imaging-Based Surrogates as Endpoints of Functional Efficacy

Sanjay Rajagopalan, MD*, Georgeta Mihai, PhD

**KEYWORDS**

- Surrogate • Atherosclerosis • Magnetic resonance imaging
- Peripheral arterial disease

Claudication trials over the past 3 decades have used changes in exercise performance as objective evidence of improvement. These trials have led to the successful approval of 2 drugs (pentoxifylline in the 1980s and cilostazol in the 1990s). A total of 8 randomized trials (6 positive and 2 negative) involving 2000 patients led to the submission of a new-drug application for cilostazol in 1998. Based on the collective evidence from these trials, cilostazol was approved as drug for the treatment of claudication in peripheral arterial disease (PAD). The maximum number of randomized patients in any of these individual trials in both placebo and drug groups did not exceed 500 patients. The mean difference in maximal walking distance (referred to as peak walking time [PWT]) was 65 meters, although inclusion of a ninth negative trial to the 8 submitted trials decreased the mean difference to 42 meters between placebo and treatment groups. In the cilostazol experience, the 3 trials that did not demonstrate significant differences in the primary endpoint of peak walking distance showed robust effects in the placebo groups, which were greater than those observed in the remaining 6 trials.[1] Since this initial success, there have been more than a dozen studies involving oral pharmaceuticals and injectable drugs (almost exclusively proangiogenic therapies) that have demonstrated no differences between placebo and drug.[2–14] Although the lack of treatment effect could relate simply to the fact that the vast majority of therapies tested had no merit as an efficacious treatment strategy, at least in a few examples, the drugs may have failed owing to the endpoint used, namely exercise performance.[11] The lack of a single successful therapeutic for more than a decade in the area of PAD has caused many pharmaceutical companies to abandon interest in this area with few drugs currently tested. This article considers some of

The authors have nothing to disclose.
Division of Cardiovascular Medicine, Department of Internal Medicine, The Ohio State University, 473 West 12 Avenue, Suite 200 DHLRI, Columbus, OH 43210, USA
* Corresponding author.
*E-mail address:* Sanjay.rajagopalan@osumc.edu

Cardiol Clin 29 (2011) 419–431
doi:10.1016/j.ccl.2011.04.002
0733-8651/11/$ – see front matter 

the factors that may have contributed to negative trials and provides an analysis of whether new endpoints may be required to reinvigorate interest in new therapeutic approaches. In one sense, this problem of drugs failing in trials designed to fulfill their intent is pervasive to the cardiovascular field, not just PAD, with recent examples of billion dollar losses in clinical trials involving thousands of patients over many years.[15] Although many reasons have been hypothesized for failure of drugs in PAD, it may be worthwhile to review the PAD experience and highlight aspects that may be relevant to this field.

## EXERCISE TREADMILL-BASED ENDPOINTS

As an endpoint of therapeutic effectiveness, which directly corresponds with functional limitations in walking, changes in claudication distance have been widely regarded as a highly relevant and appropriate surrogate marker of efficacy.[16] They are, therefore, considered a valid endpoint by the Food and Drug Administration (FDA) in trials evaluating therapeutic efficacy of drugs in PAD patients experiencing symptoms of claudication. The measurement of exercise performance using treadmill-based measurements has been more challenging than anticipated. Despite the enthusiasm for exercise performance endpoints in clinical trials of claudication, they have demonstrated substantial variability, even when used in the recommended context with highly standardized operating procedures and measurements. Moreover, in patients with PAD, classic claudication as a symptom is seen only in a minority of patients, leading to high screening failures.[17] Furthermore, variability in exercise performance has been an additional issue of considerable concern.[18]

Exercise performance is commonly measured using 2 metrics of performance: claudication onset time/initial claudication distance and PWT/absolute claudication distance. Both parameters are clinically relevant and can be determined using a constant treadmill protocol at 1.0 mph (3.2 km/h) at a constant 12.5% grade incline or a variable protocol wherein the patient walks initially at 2 mph at 0% grade with a subsequent 3.5% grade incline increase every 3 minutes. For constant grade treadmill protocols, time can be converted to distance, whereas the conversion from time to distance when using variable grade protocols may have to take into account changes in workload. It has been previously suggested that the reproducibility of PWT may be better when using variable grade treadmill protocols, especially with severe claudication.[16,19] Parenthetically, 6 of the cilostazol trials submitted to FDA used a constant grade protocol and only 3 used a variable grade protocol. Another issue with treadmill-based measures is the time-dependent improvement noted in the placebo limb seen for several months after randomization in clinical trials of claudication (**Tables 1** and **2**). This improvement is somewhat at odds with the observation that PAD patients with claudication generally manifest stable symptoms. This has led to the notion that perhaps factors intrinsic to exercise assessment on the treadmill may contribute to this large change in walking metrics. It has further been postulated that these factors being identified and mitigated may improve the ability to discriminate therapeutic response to a drug.[18] What are these factors and what is the evidence that these play any role in the placebo response?

### *Mechanisms of Improvement in the Placebo Arm in Treadmill Trials in PAD*

1. Entrainment with treadmill testing: The entrainment effect is seen commonly with treadmill protocols and describes an improvement in performance over time in the placebo arm of trials. Several reasons have been hypothesized as operative in this phenomenon, including familiarity with the treadmill protocol, adjustment of gait to a more favorable position, and poorly described motivational factors that may all function collectively. The aspects related to familiarity and position are expected to influence measures quickly with a plateau effect once these factors are eliminated. The fact that these measures continue to improve over several months raises the possibility of factors other than entrainment. Generally, in most claudication trials, patients are randomized after explicit instructions on walking on the treadmill and familiarity with the equipment. There is usually oversight on various aspects of conduct of the treadmill protocol to ensure that the variability in administration across patients is kept to a minimum. Thus, the first treadmill test for these patients is often not their first encounter with the machine. In a systematic study that evaluated the variance between 3 consecutive measurements in baseline treadmill, there was little evidence to suggest a bias.[18] It was far more likely for a patient to have a substantially better first treadmill than a second or third treadmill. The intrasubject coefficient of variation (CV) was 15% in this study.[18]
2. Placebo response: The effect of the placebo has been an important factor in the interpretation of claudication trials (see **Tables 1** and **2**). Historically, a figure of 35% was attributed to the

**Table 1**
**Magnitude of placebo response in intermittent claudication trials (maximum walking distance)**

| Trial | Drug/Dose | Placebo Response (Meters) | | Drug Response (Meters) | | Change Placebo (%) |
|---|---|---|---|---|---|---|
| | | Baseline | End | Baseline | End | |
| Dawson et al,[59] 1998 (N = 77) | Cilostazol/100 mg bid 12 Weeks | 169 ± 33 | 152 ± 54 | 142 ± 21 | 232 ± 37 | −9.7 |
| Beebe et al,[60] 1999 (N = 516) | Cilostazol/100 mg bid 24 Weeks | 148 | 175 | 130 | 259 | 18.2 |
| Strandness et al,[61] 2002 (N = 249) | Cilostazol/100 mg bid 24 Weeks | 120 | 141 | 119 | 196 | 17.5 |
| Money et al,[62] 1998 (N = 239) | Cilostazol/100 mg bid 16 Weeks | 219 | 268 | 211 | 307 | 22.3 |
| Dawson et al,[63] 2000 (N = 539) | Cilostazol/100 mg bid 24 Weeks | 234 ± 119 | 300 ± 180 | 241 ± 123 | 350 ± 209 | 28.2 |
| Thompson et al,[1] 2002 | Cliostazol/100 mg bid Varied weeks | — | — | — | — | 21.4[a] |
| Dawson et al,[63] 2000 (N = 539) | Pentoxifylline/400 mg tid 24 Weeks | 234 ± 119 | 300 ± 180 | 238 ± 119 | 308 ± 183 | 28.2 |
| Lindgarde et al,[64] 1989 (N = 150) | Pentoxifylline/400 mg tid 24 Weeks | 155 ± 95 | 200 ± 107 | 132 ± 78 | 198 ± 105 | 29.0 |
| Ernst et al,[65] 1992 (N = 40) | Pentoxifylline/600 mg bid 12 Weeks | 151 ± 58 | 420 ± 229 | 166 ± 58 | 504 ± 257 | 178 |
| Brevetti et al,[2] 1999 (N = 114) | Propionyl levocarnitine/2000 mg daily 52 Weeks | 176 ± 7 | 263 ± 21 | 159 ± 7 | 300 ± 33 | 46 |

Data are absolute change by least squares mean (SD).
*Abbreviation:* ΔPWT, change in PWT.
[a] Data is least-squares mean percent change.

**Table 2**
**Trials in angiogenesis involving patients with claudication and exercise endpoints**

| | Drug | Placebo Response (ΔPWT) (Minutes) | Drug Response (ΔPWT) (Minutes) | *P* Value |
|---|---|---|---|---|
| Lederman et al,[11] 2002 (N = 190) | bFGF protein (intra-arterial) | 0.60 | 1.66[a] | .08 |
| Rajagopalan et al,[12] 2003 (N = 105) | Adenovirus VEGF-121 (AdVEGF121) | 1.80 | 1.55[b] | NS |
| Grossman et al,[13] 2007 (N = 105) | Poloxamer-mediated Del-1 (VLTS-589) | 1.66 | 1.57 | NS |
| Creager et al (submitted) (N = 289) | Adenoviral HIF-1α | 1.34 | 1.77[c] | NS |

*Abbreviations:* HIF-1, hypoxia-inducible factor 1; PU, plaque forming units; VEGF; vascular endothelial growth factor; vp, viral particles.
[a] Combined analysis of single dose and double dose of intra-arterial bFGF.
[b] $4 \times 10^{10}$ PU (highest dose of AdVEGF).
[c] $2 \times 10^{11}$ vp (highest dose of Ad-HIF).

placebo by Beecher's classic article,[20] wherein a decided improvement was seen with placebo in 35% of cases. In a seminal article published 10 years ago, Hrobjartsson and Gotzsche[21] conducted a systematic review of clinical trials where patients were randomly assigned to no treatment or placebo. The trials were not blinded for obvious reasons and included a total of 130 studies, of which 32 included binary outcomes. The review was remarkable because there were trials designed just a few decades ago that compared placebo with no treatment, a design that would be preposterous to current institutional review boards. These trials included an array of 40 diverse clinical and psychological conditions that varied from hypertension and pain in Raynaud syndrome to orgasmic difficulties and marital discord. Trials with simple binary outcomes of improvement were included along with trials that had continuous scales of improvement. Placebos had no effect compared with no treatment when binary outcomes were used, regardless of whether these were subjective or objective. Alternatively, for continuous outcomes, placebos demonstrated a significant effect when assessing subjective but not objective outcomes. In 27 of the 130 trials involving the treatment of pain, there was a significant improvement with the placebo. The overall interpretation of the study was that there was little evidence for the placebo effect in clinical studies. An important conclusion of the study, however, was the effect of the placebo in improvement in trials involving pain and other subjective outcomes.[21] What implications may the results of this review have for intermittent claudication (IC) trials? First, IC in the classic definition of the disease is a painful condition. Clinical trials by definition only recruit the minority of patients who manifest classic IC. Thus, IC in the clinical trial context represents a condition in which a clinically significant placebo effect may be operative. Second, the interpretation of pain may vary significantly within patients and may be dependent on several poorly understood factors. As many a clinical trialist studying IC readily attests, the outcome of claudication onset time or PWT is known to vary considerably. In wide recognition of this variability, measures are commonly instituted with the intent of reducing variability of the exercise test.

### *Measures to Mitigate Variability in Baseline Treadmill Performance. Standardized Definitions*

The most important attribute of a standardized test measurement is its ability to discriminate an intervention when compared with the placebo group. By ensuring consistency in the baseline measurement, the estimate of treatment effect is robust. It is easy to see how varying baseline treadmill performance can result in attenuation of the change in response to an intervention, thereby reducing the ability to resolve true differences between treatment and placebo groups. For instance, in some studies the CV in the placebo group with repeat treadmill measures at baseline has been as high as 95%.[18] The change in placebo response at the end of 24 weeks, using the highest PWT of the 3 consecutively performed treadmills at baseline, was 2700%.[18] The rationale for including methods to identify such marked variability, and perhaps limit or even eliminate these outlier values, serves as the basis for such definitions. This degree of variation undoubtedly reduces any ability to resolve differences between placebo and active intervention. **Table 3** summarizes various approaches that have been used to limit this potential variability. As can be seen the repeat measures are typically instituted at baseline but not at exit. The assumption has been that by the time a patient exits a study, any of the variability is no longer operative. This, however, has not been put to formal test. What is the evidence that the use of any of the measures (see **Table 3**) can improve the effect estimate? Irrespective of the definition used, similar estimates of effect size are obtained, when formally tested at least in 1 trial over a 24-week duration.[18] The exception to the rule was the use of the highest measure of baseline PWT that yielded a much smaller difference in performance at the end of 24 weeks with implications for a larger sample size requirement with this measure. The baseline assessment approach had little impact on the effect size. The implication of this analysis are that the performance of 3 treadmill tests at baseline and use of any 1 of different metrics (see **Table 3**) are as good as using the results of the first treadmill test.

## *The Case for Alternate Surrogate Endpoints*

There is a need for newer endpoints that can provide a measure of efficacy that is better than existing exercise-derived endpoints. Although it is unlikely that such surrogates in the near future would result in regulatory FDA approval, they could provide important information on proof of concept and mechanism and serve as the basis for larger clinical trials. The surrogate markers of efficacy of most interest in PAD are those that involve assessment of changes at the level of perfusion and metabolism. The former could provide proof of concept for drugs that work by regulating lower-extremity flow. Alternatively, metabolic markers of effect would be attractive in studies that involve compounds that ameliorate metabolic defects associated with PAD. In some cases, both flow and metabolic markers would be helpful. What surrogates markers of efficacy should be considered and which measures are best suited for clinical trials in PAD? Surrogate markers that are noninvasive, sensitive to changes with an intervention, and easy to execute are ideal. Imaging-based surrogates fulfill these criteria well and there are many that may be attractive in PAD. Imaging has long had a role in the drug development process.[22–24] The number of image-derived endpoints that have been used as primary justification for preliminary or final drug approval is small, and of that list, tumor burden in cancer trials,[25] and changes in numbers of enhancing multiple sclerosis lesions are perhaps good examples.[26] Changes in atheroma volume is an example of additional language in the labeling of the drug but

**Table 3**
**Trials in angiogenesis involving patients with claudication and exercise endpoints**

| | | |
|---|---|---|
| First only | PWT of the first baseline treadmill test | Only 1 test required if test highly reproducible |
| Last only | PWT of the third baseline treadmill test | Most accurate if learning effect substantial over 3 tests |
| Highest | Highest PWT of the 3 baseline treadmill tests | Most reflective of true pathophysiologic limitations |
| Mean of 2 | Mean PWT of the first and second baseline treadmill tests | Removes requirement of third test if test reproducible |
| Mean of 3 | Mean PWT of all 3 baseline treadmill tests | Uses data from all 3 tests as the best point estimate |
| Median of 3 | Median value of 3 baseline treadmill tests | Removes the influence of outlier test |
| Reproducible | If ([treadmill 1 – treadmill 2]/([treadmill 1 + treadmill 2]/2) <0.25, then the means of the first and second baseline treadmills are used. If this is not the case, then third treadmill test performed.<br>If ([treadmill 2 – treadmill 3]/([treadmill 2 + treadmill 3]/2) <0.25, then mean of the second and third baseline treadmills is used.<br>If neither, then patient is not reproducible and excluded. | Decreases impact of an extreme value but subselects patients |

did not serve as primary justification for approval (rosuvastatin).[27] These situations are exclusively those where the change in imaging surrogate matches well with disease progression and regression, an important attribute of the Austin Bradford Hill criteria for surrogate competence.[28] Thus, the scarcity of quantitative imaging endpoints in medicine in general is related to the fact that few endpoints definitively fulfill the criteria of consistency (association in all circumstances), plausibility, specificity, and dose responsiveness. For several image-based endpoints, relating changes in any particular biomarker to endpoints that matter, such as exercise performance or perception of pain, has not been established. The majority of situations where imaging has played a role typically involves small numbers of patients, often performed in single centers (suggesting regional expertise that cannot be readily translated in the context of a clinical trial). In many instances, the interpretation of endpoints is subjective (eg, thallium). Thus, the clinical application of imaging-based surrogates will involve the simultaneous development of methodologies that are executable within the context of a clinical trial and fulfill the criteria of a surrogate for endpoints that matter to patients. An example of this situation is the relationship of exercise performance to exercise-induced depletion of phosphocreatine (PCr). Although changes in the latter in response to drug is indication of specific modulation of a pathway and hence proof of concept, for the surrogate to be viewed as such, it also needs to satisfy the criterion of clinical relevance. In other words, it must correlate with patient symptoms. Several emerging endpoints that may eventually serve an important role in validation of drugs and perhaps in regulatory approval are discussed.

### *Optimizing Drug Development with Surrogates*

The traditional paradigm of drug development has come under scrutiny in recent years. In this model, at least for cardiovascular drugs, phase I clinical trials are intended for preliminary assessment of safety, typically across a range of doses. It is not uncommon to include a few surrogate markers of efficacy, especially where measures exist, such as blood glucose, cholesterol, or blood pressure, that change rapidly enough for this to be examined within the context of safety goals. Thus, the dose-response relationship can be at least explored to arrive at an appropriate dose in phase II trial. This is often not the case, however, and the question of an effective dose can only be addressed within the context of a longer phase II study. Hard endpoints, such as death, myocardial infarction, and stroke, involve thousands of years of patient exposure, which is prohibitively expensive and a high-risk strategy. This has represented the most persuasive argument for surrogate measures to provide some measure of efficacy as part of phase II development (and even dose selection) before a longer trial involving thousands of patients. Surrogates, such as intravascular ultrasound and carotid intima media thickness, are probably the best examples of such a strategy where results from phase II studies using these surrogates have served as an early warning system for eventual drug failure. Although dose response may still be difficult to accomplish with such surrogates, this minimizes the expenditure of a large phase III study, if used early on in drug development. Alternatively, for drugs that work via amelioration of exercise performance on a treadmill and symptoms, such as pain, dose-response assessment may be difficult within the constraints of a phase II strategy. This may be due to the prohibitively large number of patients needed to elucidate a signal and, moreover, it can become difficult if the endpoint in question has considerable variability and takes time to change. In this context, at best, a limited range of doses can be tested and even these doses are chosen based on a best guess scenario. Thus, there is a high risk of using an incorrect dose. Furthermore, intermediate functional endpoints may have a complex relationship to the mechanism of action of the drug. This situation is best exemplified by a drug that improves blood flow via proangiogenic mechanism. The eventual expectation of the drug is that it improves lower-extremity function, because blood flow is an important determinant of function. Merely improving flow may not be enough (at least in the short term), however, to improve lower-extremity muscle function. In designing dose-finding studies, it would helpful to know that the drug improves blood flow and to determine the exact dose at which this effect occurs (proof of concept) before proceeding with larger studies to evaluate the effect of this treatment on function.

## EMERGING IMAGING-BASED SURROGATES

When considering rational drug development and how imaging may add value, it is helpful to consider key questions.

1. Does the surrogate measure help shed light on the mechanisms of action?
2. Did the surrogate help in dose selection for phase II trial?

3. Can the surrogate help with identification of populations who may respond better to therapy?
4. Can the surrogate predict eventual clinical benefit to patients?

The last question is critical because linkage to eventual benefit is a key attribute of an effective surrogate. The past several years have seen a tremendous surge in interest in developing surrogates that ultimately may help address some or all of these questions. **Table 4** lists some of these surrogates that seem promising. For space reasons, only some of these relating to MRI/magnetic resonance spectroscopy (MRS) and positron emission tomography (PET) are discussed.

## *MRI-Based Indices*

MRI has persuasive attributes to serve as a surrogate in clinical trials of PAD. It is a versatile technique that is able to assess both structure and function and, aside from some concerns around gadolinium-based contrast toxicity, it is almost entirely noninvasive. Recently, MRI has played an important part in clinical trials in indications, such as advanced solid tumors,[29] Alzheimer disease,[30,31] heart failure,[32–34] and chronic kidney disease.[35] In these situations, MRI-based measures are firmly established to correlate with disease activity. In PAD, MRI has the potential to provide data on facets that are integrally related to disease symptomatology, related to alterations in flow and metabolism. Both MRI and MRS use biologic relevant elements with an unbalanced nucleus where either the number of protons or neutrons is odd, thus a net angular moment is present. This may include hydrogen (proton) imaging commonly used in MRI or use of elements, such as $^{31}P$ in MRS, to allow assessment of high-energy phosphate components of metabolic pathways.

## *Flow-Based Indices*

MRI-based determination of flow and tissue perfusion is established in multiple circulatory beds and has been validated as a useful technique in quantifying blood flow to a territory or organ.[36–39] The techniques that have been extensively validated for MRI detection are noncontrast techniques that rely on the inherent magnetic properties of flowing protons or the oxygenation state of hemoglobin.[39] These techniques include arterial spin labeling (ASL) and blood oxygen level detection (BOLD).[40,41] In addition, contrast-enhanced techniques that rely on the wash-in and the wash-out of magnetic resonance (MR) contrast agent in tissue through the use of T1-weighted or $T2^*$-weighted sequences, are also of use.[29] Usually a bolus of paramagnetic contrast agent is administered intravenously into a patient. This changes the local relaxation parameters of the tissue and makes perfusion MR visible. Applying the principles of tracer kinetics for nondiffusible tracers, quantitative results can be obtained.

In general, noncontrast techniques function well in circulatory beds that are well perfused, such as the brain, myocardium, or kidney, especially when there is no flow-limiting disease.[39,40] ASL methods that use rapid readout techniques, such as echo planar imaging, are widely used in functional MRI of the brain where rapid changes in regional perfusion of subcortical areas are used to discern functional activation.[42,43] BOLD is also commonly used in functional MRI techniques to

**Table 4**
**Emerging surrogates to assess perfusion and metabolism in PAD**

| | MRI | MRS | PET | Contrast Ultrasound |
|---|---|---|---|---|
| Perfusion | Contrast agent–based DCE-MRI, $K^{trans}$<br>Noncontrast approaches<br>BOLD<br>ASL techniques | – | Flow measurements ($^{15}O$-$H_2O$ and $^{13}NH_3$) at rest and in response to exercise or pharmacologic vasodilation | Perfusion imaging with gas filled microbubbles of skeletal muscle at rest and exercise |
| Metabolism | – | $^{31}P$ spectroscopy<br>PCr/ATP Ratio<br>Rate of recovery of Pcreat<br>pH of tissue<br>ATP content | FDG uptake in skeletal muscle as index of metabolic activity | – |

*Abbreviation:* Pcreat, phosphocreatine.

discern functional brain activation.[44] Microscopic field inhomogeneity measured with T2*-weighted MRI is used to assess variations in the oxygen level of hemoglobin. The susceptibility change caused by paramagnetic deoxyhemoglobin as compared with diamagnetic oxyhemoglobin results in signal attenuation in T2*-weighted imaging, because the paramagnetic deoxyhemoglobin induces microscopic field inhomogeneity and a subsequent loss in intravoxel phase coherence. The ratio of concentrations of oxyhemoglobin to deoxyhemoglobin is proportional to the $Po_2$ of blood, which is supposed to be in balance with the surrounding tissue. A rise in $Po_2$ of tissue, therefore, leads to a subsequent increase in the signal intensity in T2*-weighted imaging. Assessment of regional perfusion with MRI using approaches, such as BOLD or ASL, in the skeletal muscle in the context of extremity imaging and PAD poses special challenges. Of foremost importance is that although absolute perfusion rates to the skeletal muscle in healthy adults are large, accounting for up to 17% of the cardiac output (900 mL/min), the specific perfusion rate averaged over the entire organ is a mere 3 mL/100 g/min. This contrasts with the brain and the liver, which receive 56 mL/100 g/min and 100 mL/100 g/min.[39] The skeletal muscle lower perfusion rate presents a major problem in generating adequate signal for detection. Augmentation of flow in response to an intervention is often leveraged as a tool to exaggerate perfusion as a way to obviate the low levels of rest perfusion.[45] The increase in perfusion with exercise or pharmacologic vasodilation is often dramatic in the skeletal muscle with a 20-fold to 50-fold increase in flow. Even with these measures, the relative increase in signal intensity seen with BOLD, at least in the upper extremity, is a 1% to 4% increase at best.[45] In PAD patients, the presence of a critical stenosis may impair both resting and exercise flow with implications for detecting changes. The inadequate dynamic range may impede the ability to detect differences across patient subsets that are meaningful.

Dynamic contrast-enhanced (DCE)-MRI involves the serial acquisition of MRIs of a tissue of before, during, and after an intravenous injection of contrast agent. As the agent perfuses into the tissue, the T1 and T2 values of tissue water decrease to an extent that is determined by the concentration of the agent. By considering a set of images acquired before, during, and after infusion, individual pixel/voxel elements in the region display a characteristic signal intensity time course that can be related to contrast concentration. This time course can be analyzed with an appropriate mathematical pharmacokinetic model. A 2-compartment model is used to model the distribution and transport of gadolinium across the blood vessel. A third (intracellular) compartment is assumed to exhibit no uptake of contrast agent. By fitting the DCE-MRI data to such a model, physiologic parameters can be extracted that relate to, for example, tissue perfusion, microvascular vessel wall permeability ($K^{trans}$) and extracellular volume fraction. Analysis of DCE-MRI data for perfusion requires knowledge of the concentration of the contrast in the blood plasma, the so-called arterial input function (AIF). This is a difficult problem and 3 main approaches have been developed to estimate input function. One approach involves introducing an arterial catheter into the subject and sampling blood during the imaging process for later analysis. This is impractical owing to its invasive nature, poor temporal resolution, and the nonavailability and expense of the technique required to measure contrast agents. A second method assumes that the arterial input is similar for all subjects and uses the calculation from a small cohort of subjects, which is then assumed to be valid for subsequent studies. The disadvantages include the influence of both intersubject and intrasubject variation and extrapolation to a diseased population who most certainly have variations in AIF, introducing large errors in analysis. A third method obtains the input function from the MRI data sets themselves. Methods have been developed that simultaneously measure signal intensity changes in both the blood and tissue. A calibration is then used to convert the blood signal intensity to the intravascular concentration of contrast agent. Such a method has the potential advantage of measuring the input function accurately on an individual basis and, because it does not require any further measurements, is completely noninvasive. It requires, however, the presence of a large vessel within the field of view. Additionally, the images must be acquired such that the lumen signal is devoid of partial volume or flow effects. Specialized pulse sequences can be used that selectively saturate spins to avoid inflow effects, allowing acquisition of a set of slices containing a feeding vessel without inflow effects. In general, accurate AIF measurements require (significantly) higher temporal resolution than tissue measurements, so the temporal resolution is dictated by the arterial inflow measurements process, and the spatial resolution and signal-to-noise ratio are compromised. The temporal resolution is potentially an important drawback to assessing perfusion accurately and the fact that an inflow vessel may not be available in the vicinity of imaged tissue is a challenge to consider. In a feasibility study involving 11 patients with PAD subjected to exercise in the MRI scanner, a dual-contrast sequence allowed measurement of arterial input (saturation recovery) and muscle perfusion (inversion recovery). The slope of the muscle perfusion time intensity curve was expressed as a ratio of the AIF to derive a perfusion index.[46]

In a another recent study, in a small sample of patients with PAD, DCE-MRI to determine the influx constant and area under the curve as well as dynamic BOLD imaging in calf muscle to measure maximal relative T2* changes and time to peak were quantified. The reproducibility of DCE-MRI and BOLD imaging was poor in patients with a CV up to 50.9%, suggesting that at least at 1.5 T these measures may not be practical in patients with PAD.[47] In the largest study that tested the usefulness of DCE-MRI and metabolic determinants of PAD, such as the PCr recovery time constants, Anderson and colleagues[48] evaluated 86 patients with PAD with a comprehensive protocol that included superficial femoral artery plaque volume, first-pass contrast-enhanced muscle perfusion, and $^{31}$P-MRS PCr recovery time constant measured at peak exercise in calf muscle. All patients underwent magnetic resonance angiography, treadmill testing with maximal oxygen consumption measurement, and a 6-minute walk test. The results demonstrated a disconnect (uncoupling) between metabolic measures and perfusion measures. PCr recovery time constant was the best correlate of treadmill exercise time, whereas calf muscle perfusion was the best correlate of 6-minute walk distance.

The availability of better instrumentation, including multichannel coil arrays and higher acceleration factors, may allow more coverage at acceptable spatial and temporal resolution. This may be important with this technique because previous studies have also shown striking differences in regional perfusion between muscle groups (eg, gastrochemius and soleus muscle groups).[46]

## *Metabolic Indices*

There is no doubt that PAD has a significant hemodynamic contribution. Hemodynamic abnormalities, however, do not adequately explain the degree of functional impairment. Several lines of evidence suggest that abnormalities of skeletal muscle metabolism may contribute to functional limitations in PAD patients. MRS has been used for more than 2 decades to assess metabolic function in vivo in organs, such as the skeletal muscle and heart.[49–53] $^{31}$P-MRS is performed using standard clinical MRI systems (usually 1.5 T) in humans. The premise of this technique is to measure indices of energy substrate and its use, such as ATP and PCr. $^{31}$P-MR spectra yield peaks for PCr and the 3 phosphorus atoms of ATP ($\gamma$-ATP, $\alpha$-ATP, and $\beta$-ATP) that are proportional to the concentrations of these metabolites. In PAD, cardiac mitochondria have structural abnormalities and may suffer from multiple functional alterations.[54] These may include alterations in mitochondrial electron transport–chain, resulting in reduced generation of ATP, reduced creatine kinase activity in both mitochondria and myofibrillar space, and inadequate creatine transfer into the mitochondria. In the muscle, the PCr shuttle plays a key role in ATP transfer and use. Mitochondrial creatine kinase plays an important role in the transfer of the high-energy phosphate bond in ATP to creatine to form PCr and ADP. The latter diffuses freely from the mitochondria to the myofibrils where myofibrillar creatine kinase recatalyzes the formation of ATP from PCr, releasing creatine. In general, the creatine kinase shuttle favors ATP synthesis over PCr synthesis; thus, ATP levels are maintained even though PCr levels may be depleted.[49] An early study to evaluate this hypothesis, tested the correlation of some of these measures in PAD. PCr and ADP recovery time constants and ATP production were determined during 3 exercise sessions and the results averaged and compared with known values obtained from a control population. ATP production was no different in PAD patients than in control subjects whereas PCr and ADP recovery time constants were significantly slower than normal. There was no correlation between these measures of mitochondrial function and any treadmill parameter.[55] The validity of PCr recovery was confirmed by another study using an incremental exercise design.[56]

The PCr/ATP ratio provides a global estimate of energy balance and has been used to differentiate normal subjects from PAD patients. PCr or PCr/ATP levels at rest and with exercise alone are poor discriminators of disease severity. PCr kinetics in response to exercise are commonly quantified by fitting the PCr changes over time with the help of a monoexponential model. In PAD, PCr levels show marked reduction in the anaerobic phase of exercise with a characteristic delayed response to normalization after a period of exercise. This time variable may be a better discriminator. Prior studies have provided conflicting data on the relationship between PCr recovery and exercise parameters. In an earlier study, Pipinos and colleagues[55] did not find a correlation between treadmill performance and PCr or ADP recovery. In contrast to this finding, a more recent study showed that the best correlate of treadmill exercise time was PCr recovery whereas calf muscle perfusion was the best correlate of 6-minute walk distance.[48] No correlation was noted between PCr and tissue perfusion, suggesting a mismatch between flow and metabolism parameters.

Can measures, such as PCr recovery and DCE-MRI, be integrated into clinical trials and can they serve as a robust surrogate for metabolic dysfunction in PAD? Although MRS techniques are sensitive, they are difficult to implement in a multicenter clinical trial context and have several considerations that affect performance. MRS techniques in general (such as chemical shift imaging) require homogenous magnetic fields. Even small field inhomogeneity can cause artifacts. The technique also is somewhat limited by sampling considerations and in general can assess metabolism in small regions and may not provide an estimate across large areas of muscle. This is important because there is tremendous heterogeneity in metabolism in the skeletal muscle of the lower extremity. Alterations of PCr recovery with exercise and its recovery generally demonstrate a limited dynamic range. Thus, although it may be possible to distinguish PAD from normal subjects, or even critical limb ischemia from IC, it may be more difficult to differentiate across patients with IC with varying degrees of impairment. Another technical consideration is that intracellular compartmentalization of high-energy substrates is not provided by MRS. In other words, the average cellular levels of ATP, PCr, or ADP are inferior discriminators compared with concentrations in the perimyofibrillar space and near the sarcoplasmic reticulum and sarcolemmal ion pumps. No method is currently available to make such measurements and, therefore, these have to be extrapolated from global measurements. In addition, they can be exceptionally helpful for assessment of specific mechanisms of drug action in the PAD context. The use of DCE-MRI and changes in the vascular parameter $K^{trans}$ before and after antitumor treatments has been performed successfully for many years.[29] The demonstration of an effect on $K^{trans}$ in tumor tissue has provided a good indication of tumor efficacy and provides a pharmacodynamic readout of clinical efficacy and could be adapted for use in atherosclerosis and PAD. This adaptation, however, would require re-engineering the approach in a way to allow such techniques to overcome the challenges (discussed previously) unique to PAD. Moreover, translation into the multicenter trial context will require careful attention to cross-platform protocol design, site training, equipment assessment (including periodic phantom scanning), and ongoing site monitoring—all vital to achieve reliable results in a multicenter trial involving quantitative MRI approaches.

### *Positron Emission Tomography-Based Indices of Flow*

PET is based on the use of chemically inert positron emitting radioisotopes, such as $^{11}C$, $^{15}O$, $^{18}F$, and the cationic potassium analog, $^{82}Rb$. These elements are used to tag naturally occurring compounds, such as ammonia ($^{13}NH_3$), water ($^{15}O\text{-}H_2O$), or glucose ($^{18}F$-fluorodeoxyglucose [FDG]). The tracer of choice is injected into circulation, and its concentration in the tissue over time is recorded using a detector. Based on the kinetics of the tracer, quantitative blood flow measurements can be derived. PET imaging is based on the detection of 2 photons created in an annihilation reaction between a positron and a tissue electron. The advantages over other isotope methods are the ability to measure tracer concentrations in tissue quantitatively, better spatial (2–6 mm) and temporal (seconds) resolution, and superior sensitivity as a result of multiple detectors. $^{15}O\text{-}H_2O$ is an ideal tracer for the muscle blood flow because it has a short half-life ($t_{1/2} = 123$ s) besides being freely diffusible. Relatively easy modeling of blood flow from tracer kinetics using single-compartment models enables accurate measurements of blood flow. In PET images, voxels (volume elements) that represent tiny regions of the muscle are used to quantify flow after coregistration with CT images that are also used for attenuation correction. An AIF to calculate arterial concentrations is needed and this is often provided by arterial cannulation. Within standard doses of $^{15}O\text{-}H_2O$, the accuracy has been comparable to microsphere-based approaches. PET has been used widely to quantify both skeletal muscle flow and metabolism using FDG, an $^{18}F$-labeled glucose analog, which is transported into the cells and phosphorylated but not further metabolized. Quantitative assessment of glucose uptake by FDG requires stable metabolic conditions during the measurement, which is usually accomplished by clamping glucose concentrations. PET flow measurements have been validated in PAD and as such may represent an attractive modality to assess therapeutic responses and to evaluate changes in flow and metabolism.[57,58] The major disadvantages of using PET in PAD are the need for an AIF, because image-based methods for assessment of input function may not be feasible, especially in patients with severe PAD, and multiple occlusions. Resting flow in PAD, although preserved except in advanced limb ischemia, is often insufficient to provide adequate signal in muscles, with provocative maneuvers, such as exercise and pharmacologic vasodilation, often required. The incorporation of PET as part of a rigorous phase Ib or even a phase IIa trial in a small group of patients may allow reaching the level of confidence necessary to proceed with additional studies, perhaps even incorporating traditional endpoints. The widespread availability of this technology and instrumentation (PET/CT) also renders the use of this approach feasible in clinical trials.

## RISK ASSESSMENT IN IC TRIALS

Risk assessment in trials involving drugs that alter surrogates have to fulfill additional expectations of safety, especially in the light of recent concerns raised in trials approved initially on the basis of surrogate outcome measures. This has forced a shift from the traditional approach of pooling adverse events, such as hard cardiovascular outcomes (death, MI, and stroke) and comparing the event rates between the treatment and the placebo groups. In IC trials involving small numbers of patients, the events, even after accruing those in multiple studies, are insufficient to exclude with certainty excess risk associated with the therapy. In trials involving drugs that alter symptoms or quality of life, there is the additional expectation that this does not come at the premium of safety. An alternate approach that has already gained favor in recent trials testing diabetic therapy is based on defining what constitutes unacceptable risk with an intended treatment and prospectively designing a phase II/III development program by focusing on the upper bound of the CI of the risk estimate rather than on the point estimate itself. Prespecification of this boundary allows for a clinical development plan to be designed prospectively to accrue sufficient patient exposure that rules out this risk with adequate certainty. This type of approach is similar to noninferiority studies, where the conclusion of noninferiority is made based on the CI boundaries, which allow rejecting the null hypothesis of no difference or noninferiority (treatments are comparable), if there is substantial chance that it is worse than the comparator by a preset amount.

## FINAL PERSPECTIVES

Moving forward in the PAD arena with new therapeutics is going to require some new thinking as to how best to evaluate efficacy and safety of drug therapies. This would spur confidence in pharmaceutical developers and renew enthusiasm in new approaches for treatment of this disorder. Currently, there is the widespread perception that PAD is the graveyard of pharmaceuticals. The availability of noninvasive imaging approaches that provide a handle on the fundamental processes of flow and metabolism and their changes in response to therapies may reinvigorate interest in development of new treatment modalities that target these pathways. For instance, the efficacy of newer angiogenic or cellular therapies on flow-based and metabolism-based indices may provide the necessary signal to design a larger study using more traditional endpoints. The way forward may be to consider incorporation of a meaningful (for the drug, based on the mechanism of action) surrogate endpoint that provides a measure of efficacy and has immediate implications for patient benefit.

## REFERENCES


1. Thompson PD, Zimet R, Forbes WP, et al. Meta-analysis of results from eight randomized, placebo-controlled trials on the effect of cilostazol on patients with intermittent claudication. Am J Cardiol 2002; 90(12):1314–9.
2. Brevetti G, Diehm C, Lambert D. European multicenter study on propionyl-L-carnitine in intermittent claudication. J Am Coll Cardiol 1999;34(5):1618–24.
3. Lievre M, Morand S, Besse B, et al. Oral Beraprost sodium, a prostaglandin I(2) analogue, for intermittent claudication: a double-blind, randomized, multicenter controlled trial. Beraprost et Claudication Intermittente (BERCI) research group. Circulation 2000;102(4):426–31.
4. Mohler ER 3rd, Hiatt WR, Olin JW, et al. Treatment of intermittent claudication with beraprost sodium, an orally active prostaglandin I2 analogue: a double-blinded, randomized, controlled trial. J Am Coll Cardiol 2003;41(10):1679–86.
5. Mohler ER 3rd, Klugherz B, Goldman R, et al. Trial of a novel prostacyclin analog, UT-15, in patients with severe intermittent claudication. Vasc Med 2000; 5(4):231–7.
6. Hiatt WR, Hirsch AT, Cooke JP, et al. Randomized trial of AT-1015 for treatment of intermittent claudication. A novel 5-hydroxytryptamine antagonist with no evidence of efficacy. Vasc Med 2004;9(1):18–25.
7. Hiatt WR, Klepack E, Nehler M, et al. The effect of inhibition of acyl coenzyme A-cholesterol acyltransferase (ACAT) on exercise performance in patients with peripheral arterial disease. Vasc Med 2004; 9(4):271–7.
8. Hiatt WR, Regensteiner JG, Creager MA, et al. Propionyl-L-carnitine improves exercise performance and functional status in patients with claudication. Am J Med 2001;110(8):616–22.
9. Brass EP, Anthony R, Cobb FR, et al. The novel phosphodiesterase inhibitor NM-702 improves claudication-limited exercise performance in patients with peripheral arterial disease. J Am Coll Cardiol 2006;48(12):2539–45.
10. Jaff MR, Dale RA, Creager MA, et al. Anti-chlamydial antibiotic therapy for symptom improvement in

peripheral artery disease: prospective evaluation of rifalazil effect on vascular symptoms of intermittent claudication and other endpoints in Chlamydia pneumoniae seropositive patients (PROVIDENCE-1). Circulation 2009;119(3):452–8.
11. Lederman RJ, Mendelsohn FO, Anderson RD, et al. Therapeutic angiogenesis with recombinant fibroblast growth factor-2 for intermittent claudication: the TRAFFIC study. Lancet 2002;359(9323):2053–8.
12. Rajagopalan S, Mohler ER 3rd, Lederman RJ, et al. Regional angiogenesis with vascular endothelial growth factor in peripheral arterial disease: a phase II randomized, double-blind, controlled study of adenoviral delivery of vascular endothelial growth factor 121 in patients with disabling intermittent claudication. Circulation 2003;108(16):1933–8.
13. Grossman PM, Mendelsohn F, Henry TD, et al. Results from a phase II multicenter, double-blind placebo-controlled study of Del-1 (VLTS-589) for intermittent claudication in subjects with peripheral arterial disease. Am Heart J 2007;153(5):874–80.
14. Mohler ER 3rd, Hiatt WR, Creager MA. Cholesterol reduction with atorvastatin improves walking distance in patients with peripheral arterial disease. Circulation 2003;108(12):1481–6.
15. Barter PJ, Caulfield M, Eriksson M, et al. Effects of torcetrapib in patients at high risk for coronary events. N Engl J Med 2007;357(21):2109–22.
16. Labs KH, Dormandy JA, Jaeger KA, et al. Transatlantic conference on clinical trial guidelines in peripheral arterial disease: clinical trial methodology. Basel PAD clinical trial methodology group. Circulation 1999;100(17):e75–81.
17. McDermott M, Greenland P, Liu K, et al. Leg symptoms in peripheral arterial disease: associated clinical characteristics and functional impairment. JAMA 2001;286(13):1599–606.
18. Brass EP, Jiao J, Hiatt W. Optimal assessment of baseline treadmill walking performance in claudication clinical trials. Vasc Med 2007;12(2):97–103.
19. Labs KH, Nehler MR, Roessner M, et al. Reliability of treadmill testing in peripheral arterial disease: a comparison of a constant load with a graded load treadmill protocol. Vasc Med 1999;4(4):239–46.
20. Beecher HK. The powerful placebo. JAMA 1955; 159(17):1602–6.
21. Hrobjartsson A, Gotzsche PC. Is the placebo powerless? An analysis of clinical trials comparing placebo with no treatment. N Engl J Med 2001;344(21):1594–602.
22. Bots ML, Visseren FL, Evans GW, et al. Torcetrapib and carotid intima-media thickness in mixed dyslipidaemia (RADIANCE 2 study): a randomised, double-blind trial. Lancet 2007;370(9582):153–60.
23. de Groot E, Hovingh GK, Wiegman A, et al. Measurement of arterial wall thickness as a surrogate marker for atherosclerosis. Circulation 2004;109(23 Suppl 1): III33–8.
24. Nissen SE, Nicholls SJ, Wolski K, et al. Effect of rimonabant on progression of atherosclerosis in patients with abdominal obesity and coronary artery disease: the STRADIVARIUS randomized controlled trial. JAMA 2008;299(13):1547–60.
25. Karrison TG, Maitland ML, Stadler WM, et al. Design of phase II cancer trials using a continuous endpoint of change in tumor size: application to a study of sorafenib and erlotinib in non small-cell lung cancer. J Natl Cancer Inst 2007;99(19):1455–61.
26. Anonymous FD. Approves fingolimod. Available at: http://www.fda.gov/NewsEvents/Newsroom/PressAnnouncements/ucm226755.htm. Last updated September 22, 2010.
27. Nissen SE, Nicholls SJ, Sipahi I, et al. Effect of very high-intensity statin therapy on regression of coronary atherosclerosis: the ASTEROID trial. JAMA 2006;295(13):1556–65.
28. Hill AB. The environment and disease: association or causation? Proc R Soc Med 1965;58:295–300.
29. Zweifel M, Padhani AR. Perfusion MRI in the early clinical development of antivascular drugs: decorations or decision making tools? Eur J Nucl Med Mol Imaging 2010;37(Suppl 1):S164–82.
30. Gilman S, Koller M, Black RS, et al. Clinical effects of Abeta immunization (AN1792) in patients with AD in an interrupted trial. Neurology 2005;64(9):1553–62.
31. Krishnan KR, Charles HC, Doraiswamy PM, et al. Randomized, placebo-controlled trial of the effects of donepezil on neuronal markers and hippocampal volumes in Alzheimer's disease. Am J Psychiatry 2003;160(11):2003–11.
32. Anand I, McMurray J, Cohn JN, et al. Long-term effects of darusentan on left-ventricular remodelling and clinical outcomes in the EndothelinA Receptor Antagonist Trial in Heart Failure (EARTH): randomised, double-blind, placebo-controlled trial. Lancet 2004;364(9431):347–54.
33. Bellenger NG, Rajappan K, Rahman SL, et al. Effects of carvedilol on left ventricular remodelling in chronic stable heart failure: a cardiovascular magnetic resonance study. Heart 2004;90(7):760–4.
34. Groenning BA, Nilsson JC, Sondergaard L, et al. Antiremodeling effects on the left ventricle during beta-blockade with metoprolol in the treatment of chronic heart failure. J Am Coll Cardiol 2000;36(7): 2072–80.
35. Chertow GM, Levin NW, Beck GJ, et al. In-center hemodialysis six times per week versus three times per week. N Engl J Med 2010;363(24):2287–300.
36. Martirosian P, Boss A, Fenchel M, et al. Quantitative lung perfusion mapping at 0.2 T using FAIR True-FISP MRI. Magn Reson Med 2006;55(5):1065–74.
37. Fenchel M, Martirosian P, Langanke J, et al. Perfusion MR imaging with FAIR true FISP spin labeling in patients with and without renal artery stenosis: initial experience. Radiology 2006;238(3):1013–21.

38. Boss A, Martirosian P, Claussen CD, et al. Quantitative ASL muscle perfusion imaging using a FAIR-TrueFISP technique at 3.0 T. NMR Biomed 2006; 19(1):125–32.
39. Martirosian P, Boss A, Schraml C, et al. Magnetic resonance perfusion imaging without contrast media. Eur J Nucl Med Mol Imaging 2010;37(Suppl 1):S52–64.
40. Iannetti GD, Wise RG. BOLD functional MRI in disease and pharmacological studies: room for improvement? Magn Reson Imaging 2007;25(6):978–88.
41. Prasad PV, Edelman RR, Epstein FH. Noninvasive evaluation of intrarenal oxygenation with BOLD MRI. Circulation 1996;94(12):3271–5.
42. Williams DS, Detre JA, Leigh JS, et al. Magnetic resonance imaging of perfusion using spin inversion of arterial water. Proc Natl Acad Sci U S A 1992; 89(1):212–6.
43. van Laar PJ, van der Grond J, Hendrikse J. Brain perfusion territory imaging: methods and clinical applications of selective arterial spin-labeling MR imaging. Radiology 2008;246(2):354–64.
44. Perthen JE, Bydder M, Restom K, et al. SNR and functional sensitivity of BOLD and perfusion-based fMRI using arterial spin labeling with spiral SENSE at 3 T. Magn Reson Imaging 2008;26(4):513–22.
45. Utz W, Jordan J, Niendorf T, et al. Blood oxygen level-dependent MRI of tissue oxygenation: relation to endothelium-dependent and endothelium-independent blood flow changes. Arterioscler Thromb Vasc Biol 2005;25(7):1408–13.
46. Isbell DC, Epstein FH, Zhong X, et al. Calf muscle perfusion at peak exercise in peripheral arterial disease: measurement by first-pass contrast-enhanced magnetic resonance imaging. J Magn Reson Imaging 2007;25(5):1013–20.
47. Versluis B, Backes WH, van Eupen MG, et al. Magnetic resonance imaging in peripheral arterial disease: reproducibility of the assessment of morphological and functional vascular status. Invest Radiol 2011;46(1):11–24.
48. Anderson JD, Epstein FH, Meyer CH, et al. Multifactorial determinants of functional capacity in peripheral arterial disease: uncoupling of calf muscle perfusion and metabolism. J Am Coll Cardiol 2009;54(7):628–35.
49. van der Grond J, Crolla RM, Ten Hove W, et al. Phosphorus magnetic resonance spectroscopy of the calf muscle in patients with peripheral arterial occlusive disease. Invest Radiol 1993;28(2):104–8.
50. Hardy CJ, Weiss RG, Bottomley PA, et al. Altered myocardial high-energy phosphate metabolites in patients with dilated cardiomyopathy. Am Heart J 1991;122(3 Pt 1):795–801.
51. Bottomley PA, Weiss RG, Hardy CJ, et al. Myocardial high-energy phosphate metabolism and allograft rejection in patients with heart transplants. Radiology 1991;181(1):67–75.
52. Neubauer S. The failing heart–an engine out of fuel. N Engl J Med 2007;356(11):1140–51.
53. Schocke M, Esterhammer R, Greiner A. High-energy phosphate metabolism in the exercising muscle of patients with peripheral arterial disease. Vasa 2008;37(3):199–210.
54. Pipinos II, Judge AR, Selsby JT, et al. The myopathy of peripheral arterial occlusive disease: part 1. Functional and histomorphological changes and evidence for mitochondrial dysfunction. Vasc Endovascular Surg 2007;41(6):481–9.
55. Pipinos II, Shepard AD, Anagnostopoulos PV, et al. Phosphorus 31 nuclear magnetic resonance spectroscopy suggests a mitochondrial defect in claudicating skeletal muscle. J Vasc Surg 2000;31(5):944–52.
56. Esterhammer R, Schocke M, Gorny O, et al. Phosphocreatine kinetics in the calf muscle of patients with bilateral symptomatic peripheral arterial disease during exhaustive incremental exercise. Mol Imaging Biol 2008;10(1):30–9.
57. Schmidt MA, Chakrabarti A, Shamim-Uzzaman Q, et al. Calf flow reserve with H(2)(15)O PET as a quantifiable index of lower extremity flow. J Nucl Med 2003;44(6):915–9.
58. Pande RL, Park MA, Perlstein TS, et al. Impaired skeletal muscle glucose uptake by [18F]fluorodeoxyglucose-positron emission tomography in patients with peripheral artery disease and intermittent claudication. Arterioscler Thromb Vasc Biol 2011;31(1):190–6.
59. Dawson DL, Cutler BS, Meissner MH, et al. Cilostazol has beneficial effects in treatment of intermittent claudication: results from a multicenter, randomized, prospective, double-blind trial. Circulation 1998; 98(7):678–86.
60. Beebe HG, Dawson DL, Cutler BS, et al. A new pharmacological treatment for intermittent claudication: results of a randomized, multicenter trial. Arch Intern Med 1999;159(17):2041–50.
61. Strandness DE Jr, Dalman RL, Panian S, et al. Effect of cilostazol in patients with intermittent claudication: a randomized, double-blind, placebo-controlled study. Vasc Endovascular Surg 2002;36(2):83–91.
62. Money SR, Herd JA, Isaacsohn JL, et al. Effect of cilostazol on walking distances in patients with intermittent claudication caused by peripheral vascular disease. J Vasc Surg 1998;27(2):267–74 [discussion: 274–5].
63. Dawson DL, Cutler BS, Hiatt WR, et al. A comparison of cilostazol and pentoxifylline for treating intermittent claudication. Am J Med 2000;109(7):523–30.
64. Lindgarde F, Jelnes R, Bjorkman H, et al. Conservative drug treatment in patients with moderately severe chronic occlusive peripheral arterial disease. Scandinavian Study Group. Circulation 1989;80(6): 1549–56.
65. Ernst E, Kollar L, Resch KL. Does pentoxifylline prolong the walking distance in exercised claudicants? A placebo-controlled double-blind trial. Angiology 1992;43(2):121–5.

# Management of Heart Failure with Renal Artery Ischemia

Madhav V. Rao, MD[a,*], Patrick Murray, MD[a],
Clyde W. Yancy, MD[b]

**KEYWORDS**

- Chronic kidney disease • Congestive heart failure
- Hypertension • Renal artery stenosis
- Renovascular disease

With improved treatment of coronary artery disease (CAD), valvular heart disease, and arrhythmias, more patients are surviving longer with impaired ventricular function. Similarly, hypertension results in ventricular remodeling in many affected patients. The resultant presence of an increasing number of persons who have impaired ventricular function creates the impetus to realize the natural history of altered ventricular function, which is the eventual development of heart failure (HF). Recent estimates indicate that 5.2 million people are living with HF in the United States with an additional 550,000 cases diagnosed each year.[1] Furthermore, these patients are older, living longer with HF, and likely to have one or more coexistent diseases also associated with aging. One such disease process that increases with age is chronic kidney disease (CKD). In a recent study of 3618 patients 70 years or older who did not have congestive heart failure (CHF) at the onset of the study period, a serum creatinine of greater than or equal to 1.5 mg/dL in men and 1.3 mg/dL in women was associated with increased CHF risk (multivariate hazard ratio [HR] 1.43; 95% CI, 1.17 to 1.74).[2] The combination of CHF and CKD has profound implications on patient mortality and morbidity. Smith and colleagues performed a meta-analysis of 16 studies that included 80,098 hospital admissions in patients who had HF. Sixty-three percent of these patients had any compromised renal function defined as an estimated glomerular filtration rate (GFR) defined as less than 90 mL per minute. Those patients who had decreased GFR had a HR of 1.56 (95% CI, 1.53 to 1.60) for all-cause mortality. Furthermore, with greater impairment of GFR (defined as estimated GFR less than 53) the risk for death increased (HR 2.31; 95% CI, 2.18 to 2.44).[3] This study showed that for every 10 mL per minute decrease in GFR, risk for mortality due to HF increased by 7%. Likewise, in 1002 patients hospitalized for CHF, worsening renal function (rise in serum creatinine greater than or equal to 0.3 mg/dL) predicted greater in-hospital mortality (sensitivity 81% and specificity 62%) and hospital length of stay greater than 10 days (sensitivity 64% and specificity 65%).[4] When using cystatin C, a novel biomarker of kidney injury, Shlipak and colleagues[5] found that this measurement was an even stronger predictor of mortality. These data were derived from a cohort of 279 patients in the Cardiovascular Health Study followed for a median of 6.5 years. They found that for every standard deviation rise in cystatin C (0.35 mg/L) was carried a 31% greater adjusted mortality risk (95% CI, 20% to 43%; *P*<.001) versus a 17% greater adjusted mortality risk (95% CI, 1% to 36%; *P* = .04) for each standard deviation rise in serum creatinine. In sum, with the aging population of the United

This article originally appeared in *Heart Failure Clinics, volume 4, number 4*.
[a] University of Chicago, Chicago, IL, USA
[b] Baylor University Medical Center, Dallas, TX, USA
* Corresponding author. Section of Nephrology, Department of Internal Medicine, University of Chicago, 5801 South Ellis, Chicago, IL 60637, USA.
*E-mail address:* madhav.rao@uchospitals.edu

Cardiol Clin 29 (2011) 433–445
doi:10.1016/j.ccl.2011.06.003

States, CHF and CKD prevalence will continue to rise and the coexistence of both conditions lends to poorer outcomes.

The relationship of CKD and HF implicates certain mechanistic considerations. Several consequences of CKD promote ventricular remodeling and the development of left ventricular hypertrophy (LVH). Because of progressive loss of renal mass in CKD leading to erythropoeitin deficiency, most patients who have CKD stage III (GFR less than 60 mL per minute) or greater are at risk for anemia of chronic disease. Anemia is a known risk factor for poorer outcomes in HF and for LVH development. In the aforementioned Canadian cohort study that prospectively enrolled 446 patients who had CKD (defined as Cockroft-Gault creatinine clearance between 25 and 75 mL per minute, chronicity on renal biopsy or clinical course, or small kidneys on renal ultrasound) the odds ratio (OR) for LVH was 1.32 for every 0.5 mg/dL ($P$ = .004) decrease in hemoglobin[6] Furthermore, the results also showed a step-wise increase in percentage of patients who had LVH for every 25 mL per minute loss of creatinine clearance with nearly 70% of patients having LVH at the time of dialysis initiation. In a subsequent study also examining the interaction of anemia and LVH, pooled data on 2423 patients who had CKD from the Atherosclerosis Risk in Communities study, Cardiovascular Health Study, Framingham Heart Study, and Framingham Offspring Study showed that LVH was associated with a HR of 1.67 (95% CI, 1.34–2.07) for the composite cardiac outcomes of myocardial infarction, stroke, or death. Anemia and LVH together heightened the HR to 4.15 (95% CI, 2.62 to 6.56; $P$ = .02).[7] In addition to anemia, the interaction of hypertension and end-stage renal disease (ESRD) also demonstrates worse cardiac outcomes. In a study of 432 patients who had ESRD and an average mean arterial pressure (MAP) of 101 $\pm$ 11 mm Hg, a 10–mm Hg rise in MAP was associated with increased presence of concentric LVH (OR 1.48; $P$ = .002) and in left ventricular (LV) mass ($P$ = .027) on serial echocardiography. These changes correlated with increased rates of HF (relative risk [RR] 1.44; $P$ = .007) and ischemic heart disease (RR 1.39; $P$ = .05). These results were adjusted for anemia, serum albumin, age, diabetes status, and ischemic heart disease and show that even modest elevations in blood pressure heighten the risk for poorer cardiovascular outcomes in the ESRD population.[8] In sum, risk factors that lead to CKD and its resultant side effects of the disease are shown to lead to the development of LVH and HF.

Another area of growing interest that may have an impact on the interplay between CKD and cardiac diseases, such as CHF, is vitamin D deficiency. Data from the Third National Health and Nutrition Examination Survey found that those patients who had a serum 25-hydroxyvitamin D level less than 21 ng/mL had a higher risk for hypertension (OR 1.30), diabetes mellitus (OR 1.98), obesity (OR 2.29), and high serum triglyceride levels (OR 1.47) compared with counterparts who had 25-hydroxvitamin D levels greater than or equal to 37 ng/mL.[9] Estimated GFR less than 30 mL per minute was a risk factor for lower vitamin D levels. Frequently, patients who have class III CKD or greater develop this condition because of decreased renal mass and 1$\alpha$-hydroxylase activity that leads to decreased levels of active vitamin D or calcitriol. It also is known, however, that patients who have CKD tend to have lower levels of inactive vitamin D or calcidiol. In the past, these deficiencies were studied to determine the effect on bone density and turnover, but with data from newer studies more focus has been placed on the effect on heart disease. In a recent study of 123 patients who had HF and vitamin D deficiency followed for 15 months, 50 $\mu$g of vitamin D3 per day oral supplementation was shown to decrease parathyroid hormone (PTH) level ($P$ = .007), tumor necrosis factor alpha ($P$ = .006), and interleukin 10 ($P$ = .042) and correlated with increase levels of serum 25-hydroxyvitamin D levels.[10] Beneficial results were seen in with the use of intravenous calcitriol in a cohort of 15 hemodialysis patients who had secondary hyperparathyroidism versus 10 dialysis patients not given supplementation. The use of calcitriol twice a week was associated with improved LV mass index (178 $\pm$ 73 vs 155 $\pm$ 61 g/m$^2$; $P$<.01) and correlated strongly with percent change in intact PTH levels (r = 0.52; $P$<.05). Furthermore, neurohormonal activation was down regulated as levels of plasma renin (18.5 $\pm$ 12.7 vs 12.3 $\pm$ 11.0 pg/mL; $P$ = .007), angiotensin II (79.7 $\pm$ 48.6 vs 47.2 $\pm$ 45.7 pg/mL; $P$ = .001), and atrial natriuretic peptide (16.6 $\pm$ 9.7 vs 12.2 $\pm$ 4.4 pg/mL) decreased.[11] More studies are evaluating the role of vitamin D supplementation. In particular, the paracalcitol capsules benefit renal failure induced cardiac morbidity in chronic kidney disease (PRIMO) study will be evaluating the use of paracalcitol levels in 220 patients who have an estimated GFR between 15 and 50 mL per minute and its effects on cardiac LV mass index as measured by serial cardiac MRI over the course of 48 weeks.[12] In addition, the Effect of Calcium and Vitamin D in Patients With Heart Failure (KarViDII) study will study vitamin D supplementation in 40 patients who have a known ejection fraction less than 40% to see if there is any improvement in the ejection fraction over the course of the follow-up period.[13] At present, there are no data to suggest that supplemental vitamin D is indicated in HF with CKD but this is a promising area of investigation.

Several causes of CKD exist, including chronic conditions, such as diabetes mellitus and hypertension, and more acute causes, such as the broad spectrum of glomerulonephritidies in younger patient populations. One such cause of CKD is renovascular disease. Although the magnitude of the effect of renovascular disease–induced CKD is not well characterized, studies show that it is likely a significant contributor to ESRD in the United States (**Fig. 1**). In a study that reviewed the United States Renal Data System database between 1996 and 2001, the prevalence of renovascular disease in patients older than age 67 ranged from 7.1% to 11.2% (adjusted OR for ESRD 1.68). One problem in this study was that the rise in renovascular disease was not reflected in the coding on the Medicare Evidence Report before starting dialysis, highlighting potential evidence of underestimation of frequency.[14]

Renovascular disease, specifically renal artery stenosis (RAS), is an area of medical interest fraught with varying opinions by physicians. This entity is further divided into RAS that is asymptomatic and RAS leading to ischemia. Nephrologists, cardiologists, and interventional radiologists all manage these diseases but often with different management strategies. The remainder of this article outlines renovascular disease as it relates to CKD; the pathophysiology of development of renovascular disease and subsequent effects leading to CHF; treatment modalities, especially when CHF develops; and outcomes of different treatment regimens.

A main cause for such heterogeneity in the approach to RAS is that it is not always diagnosed or that advances in technologies have made identification and stenting the renal arteries easy enough to intervene regardless of true medical benefit.[15] RAS should be investigated when long-term hypertension is refractory to medical therapy, hypertension occurs in a person before age 30, or for recurrent episodes of pulmonary edema. Often, renal function is not compromised as alternate routes of blood flow can develop in the extra- and intrarenal circulation, especially when this is a chronic process.[16] The causes of RAS that have garnered the most attention are atherosclerosis and fibromuscular dysplasia (FMD) because these are the most common causes in Western populations; however, in Southeast Asia, South America, and the Mediterranean, Takayasu's arteritis is attributed to cause up to 60% of cases.[17] FMD involves the entire width of the

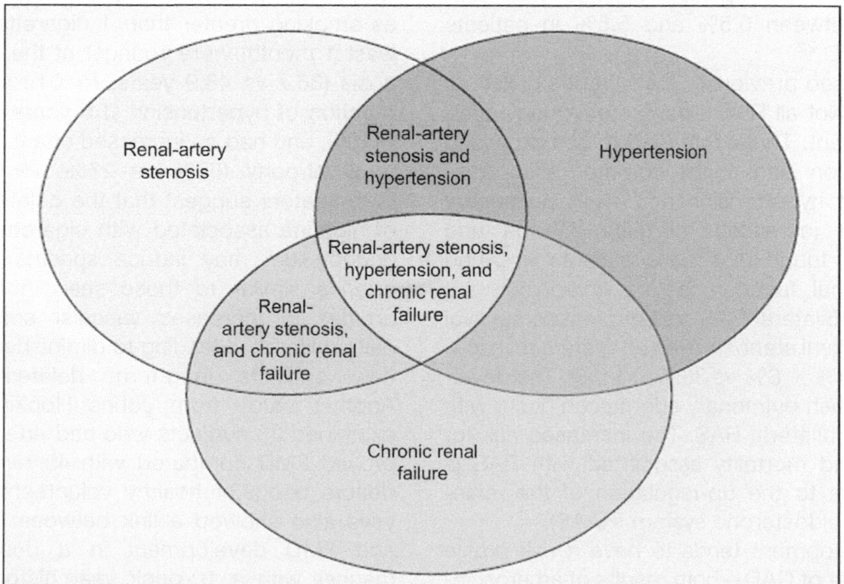


**Fig. 1.** Interrelation among RAS, hypertension, and chronic renal failure. RAS may occur alone (isolated anatomic RAS) or in combination with hypertension (renovascular or essential hypertension), renal insufficiency (ischemic nephropathy), or both. Patients who have RAS alone may benefit from revascularization to prevent loss of renal mass. In patients who have RAS and hypertension, hypertension seldom is cured by revascularization, except in those who have FMD. In patients who have RAS and chronic renal failure, renal revascularization may improve or stabilize renal function. (*From* Safian RD, Textor SC. Renal-artery stenosis. N Engl J Med 2001;344(6):431–42; with permission. Copyright © 2001, Massachusetts Medical Society.)

affected blood vessels. It tends to occur more often in women between ages 15 and 50, particularly in the distal two thirds of the renal arteries, and accounts for less than 10% of all cases of RAS.[18] Some have suggested that because of the limitations of different imaging modalities used to diagnosis RAS, the true prevalence of FMD is underestimated in the elderly.[19] FMD is not an isolated phenomenon to the renal arteries as it can occur in any area of the vascular bed. Much more common is the development of RAS resulting from atherosclerosis. In a recent study evaluating 1302 aortograms, the prevalence of significant RAS in patients referred for coronary angiography was 15% with 11% unilateral and 4% bilateral.[20] This was not a true sample of the general population as several these patients had significant comorbid conditions, such as diabetes mellitus or peripheral vascular disease, and were smokers. More recently, in an analysis of 324 patients referred for renal duplex ultrasound, unilateral RAS was found in 14% with occlusion occurring in 1.5% whereas 7% were diagnosed with bilateral RAS with 0.6% having complete occlusion. This was a retrospective, single-center study in a population with selection bias as they were referred specifically to rule out RAS.[21] Finally, in a retrospective analysis of 5% of the United States Medicare claims data, the prevalence of atherosclerotic renovascular disease was estimated at between 0.5% and 5.5% in patients who had CKD.[22]

As discussed previously, RAS can be unilateral or bilateral. Not all RAS lesions are hemodynamically significant. Those that lead to compromised renal perfusion lead to the common associated morbidity of hypertension and flash pulmonary edema and increased mortality. Dorros and colleagues[23] found that those patients who had impaired renal function (serum creatinine >2.0 mg/dL) and bilateral RAS had decreased survival versus unilateral stenosis even after stent revascularization (55% $\pm$ 6% vs 36% $\pm$ 11%). The development of flash pulmonary edema can occur with unilateral or bilateral RAS. The increased risk for morbidity and mortality associated with RAS is primarily due to the up-regulation of the renin-angiotensin-aldosterone system (RAAS).

RAS development tends to have a risk profile similar to that of CAD—both results of atherosclerotic disease (**Fig. 2**). In a recent study, the presence of vascular disease in the abdominal aorta or lower extremities (OR 2.06) or carotid arteries (OR 3.128) was associated with a greater risk for severe RAS (>70%) due to atherosclerosis.[24] Likewise, a multicenter study using renal duplex to diagnose renal vascular disease found that older age ($P$ = .028; OR 1.34; 95% CI, 1.03–1.73), high-density lipoprotein cholesterol levels less than 40 mg/dL ($P$ = .003; OR 2.63; 95% CI, 1.40–4.93), and higher systolic blood pressure ($P$ = .007; OR 1.44; 95% CI, 1.10–1.87) all were associated with increased risk. In addition, no difference in incidence was found between African Americans and Caucasians (6.7% vs 6.9%, $P$ = .933) or between men and women (9.1% vs 5.5%, $P$ = .053).[25]

The risks for development of FMD associated RAS are less defined. FMD can affect any vascular bed of the body. FMD is divided into three categories based on the location of pathology. They are intimal, medial, and perimedial lesions with 85% of all FMD-associated RAS resulting from the medial form of FMD, 5% from the intimal, and 10% from the perimedial lesions.[26] It is not uncommon for FMD-mediated RAS to have a combination of these lesions. As a result, the appearance of FMD angiographically has required its own classification first proposed by Kincaid and colleagues[27] in 1968. The four types are the classic string-of-beads appearance and tubular, focal, and solitary lesions with the classic form the most common iteration of FMD (**Fig. 3**).[28] A group from the University of Queensland reported that in a group of 50 subjects who had angiographically defined multifocal FMD with RAS, those who smoked cigarettes (defined as smoking greater than 1 cigarette daily for at least 1 month) were younger at the time of diagnosis (38.7 vs 48.9 years, $P$<.01), had a shorter duration of hypertension (1.5 years vs 8.5 years, $P$<.05), and had an increased chance of unilateral renal atrophy (67% vs 27%, $P$<.01).[29] These investigators suggest that the deleterious effects of nicotine associated with cigarette use on the endothelium may induce spasms in the renal arteries similar to those seen in the coronary arteries or increased vascular smooth muscle cell proliferation leading to diminished renal blood flow and its long-term deleterious effects. Another study from Johns Hopkins University examined 33 subjects who had arteriographically proved FMD compared with 45 renal transplant donors and 934 healthy volunteers. Their analyses also showed a link between cigarette use and FMD development in a dose-dependent manner with a 10-pack year history or greater of smoking having the highest risk for FMD formation. Furthermore, in this series all patients who had classically appearing FMD were Caucasian women. All patients were screened for HLA and HLA-DRw6 was more common in the FMD cohort versus transplant patients or healthy volunteers suggesting a genetic predisposition

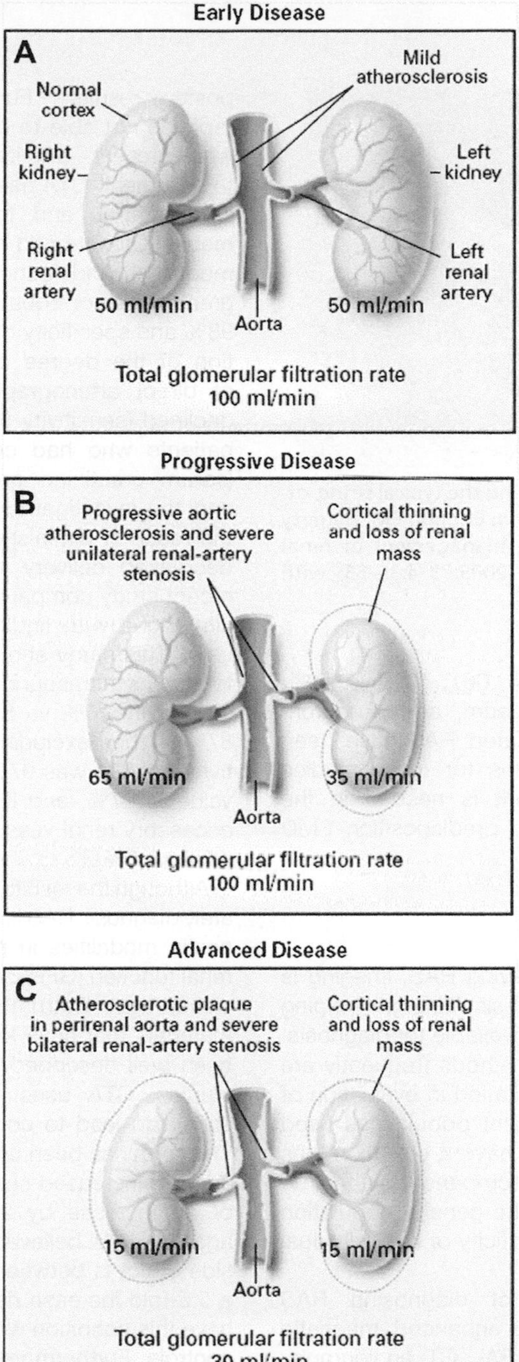


**Fig. 2.** Progressive atherosclerosis, RAS, and ischemic nephropathy. In the early phase (*A*), there is mild atherosclerosis of the perirenal abdominal aorta and normal renal function. Renal blood flow, renal mass, and the serum creatinine concentration are normal. The dimensions of the kidneys are normal, and there is no cortical atrophy. The total GFR (100 mL per minute) and the GFR in each kidney (50 mL per minute) are normal. As the disease progresses (*B*), there is progressive aortic atherosclerosis and severe unilateral RAS. The left kidney is smaller than the right kidney, and there may be cortical thinning and asymmetry in renal blood flow. The serum creatinine concentration remains normal as long as the right kidney is normal, despite the loss of renal mass. The total GFR may be normal (100 mL per minute) or only slightly depressed owing to compensatory changes in the right kidney, but renal blood flow is decreased in the left kidney (35 mL per minute). In advanced disease (*C*), there is bulky atherosclerotic plaque in the perirenal aorta and severe bilateral RAS. Both kidneys are small, and there is marked cortical thinning and irregularity. Loss of more than 50% of renal mass usually is associated with an elevation in the serum creatinine concentration (ischemic nephropathy), which may not be reversible. The total GFR (30 mL per minute) and the GFR in each kidney (15 mL per minute) are depressed. (*From* Safian RD, Textor SC. Renal-artery stenosis. N Engl J Med 2001;344(6):431–42; with permission. Copyright © 2001, Massachusetts Medical Society.)

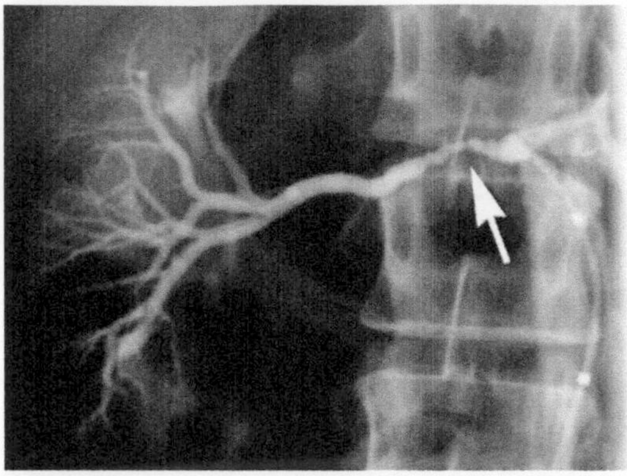

Fig. 3. Renal angiogram showing the typical string-of-beads appearance of FMD. (*From* Cheung CM, Hegarty J, Kalra PA. Dilemmas in the management of renal artery stenosis. Br Med Bull 2005;73–4:35–55; with permission.)

(43% vs 20%, OR 3.0, *P* = .067; 43% vs 23%, OR 2.51, *P* = .031).[30] In sum, certain factors associated with FMD-mediated RAS have been found, but the sample sizes for these studies were small and more work is needed in the area of a possible genetic predisposition FMD development.

## IMAGING

In patients suspected of having RAS, imaging is needed to confirm the diagnosis. Different imaging modalities and indices are available for diagnosis. Invasive and noninvasive methods frequently are used for diagnosis. The limitation in evaluation of these tools is that the patient populations used for these studies invariably have a selection bias and may lead to some discrepancy in the true prevalence of the RAS in the general population and the sensitivity and specificity of the individual modality used.

Noninvasive modalites of diagnosing RAS include duplex ultrasound, enhanced magnetic resonance angiography (MRA), CT angiography (CTA), and captopril renal scintigraphy. Captopril renal scintigraphy has been studied extensively in diagnosing RAS. When done, the captopril administration causes a fall in kidney function on the ipsilateral side where RAS is present. Maher and colleagues[31] evaluated this test in 44 patients who had hypertension, of whom 29 had renal impairment. They found that this test had a sensitivity of 85% and a specificity of 72%. Sensitivity and specificity decline further, however, when bilateral RAS is present.[16] In addition, the concomitant use of calcium channel blockers at the time of the captopril scan can lead to false-positive results.[32] Furthermore, captopril scintigraphy is not able to delineate the degree of RAS when present—a limitation in determining approach to treatment. CTA has been compared with direct arteriography and found to have comparable results. Olbricht and colleagues[33] compared both modalities and found that CTA for RAS lesions greater than or equal to 50% had a sensitivity of 98% and specificity of 94%. Furthermore, estimation of the degree of RAS was similar to that of direct arteriography. The accuracy of CTA declined (sensitivity 93% and specificity 81%) in patients who had compromised renal function (serum creatinine greater than 150 μmol/liter), and the investigators believe that this finding is the result of diminished renal blood flow causing decreased delivery of the contrast material. A recent study compared the use of MRA to duplex ultrasound with findings confirmed angiographically. This study showed that MRA was superior to duplex ultrasound in diagnosis of main RAS (sensitivity 90% vs 81% and specificity 86% vs 87%). When excluding cases of FMD, the sensitivity of MRA was 97% with a negative predictive value of 97%, and it was able to detect RAS in accessory renal vessels much better than duplex (96% vs 5%).[34]

Although the results of CTA and MRA in appropriately diagnosis RAS is impressive, using these diagnostic modalities in patients who have impaired renal function (GFR < 60 mL/min/1.73 m$^2$) must be discouraged. Both imaging techniques use contrast materials that have known side effects that have been well described subsequent to these earlier studies. CTA uses iodinated contrast material shown to lead to contrast-induced nephropathy. This term has been used to describe the phenomenon of increased serum creatinine by 0.5 mg/dL or an increase by 25% after exposure to this agent.[35] It is believed that the incidence of this side effect is between 7% and 15% and there is a 5.5-fold increase risk for death in patients who have this condition when compared with matched controls. Furthermore, known risks in addition to diminished renal function include, older age, diabetes, and HF.[36] A more recent iatrogenic condition, nephrogenic systemic fibrosis (NSF), is linked to the administration of gadolinium contrast, as used in MRA, to patients who have impaired renal function. The Food and Drug Administration (FDA) has published advisories regarding the use of gadolinium in patients who have moderate renal disease (eGRF less than 60 mL/min/1.73 m$^2$) and ESRD as of December 2006. According to this advisory, 90 patients had developed NSF within 2 days to 18 months of exposure.[37] Since that time, the FDA has placed a black box warning on all gadolinium-based contrast agents about the risk for NSF in any patient who has a GFR less than 30 mL/min/1.73 $m^2$, acute kidney injury, or hepatorenal syndrome or is in the perioperative phase of liver transplantation. It seems that this side effect occurs in a dose-dependent manner as detailed in a recent report that showed an OR of 12.1 for developing NSF when 0.2 mmol/kg of gadolinium versus 0.1 mmol/kg was administered. MRA uses 0.3 mmol/kg of gadolinium, which likely increases the risk further. To prevent NSF development, it is recommended that three hemodialysis treatments be performed to remove approximately 95% of the gadolinium from the circulation.[38] This is an additional drawback of MRA in addition to the issues associated with claustrophobia and the inability to perform this test in patients who have prior metallic implant.

As a result of these concerns, the most appropriate method to screen for RAS when suspected is duplex ultrasound. Ongoing advances in this modality of have led to improvements in its sensitivity and specificity. In a recent meta-analysis of 88 articles, including 8147 patient and 9974 arteries, duplex ultrasound using peak systolic velocity measurements had a sensitivity of 85% and specificity of 92%.[39] A retrospective analysis of 5950 patients referred for RAS evaluation via duplex ultrasound showed that a measure resistive index above 80 had the strongest association in univariate analysis of predicting renal function loss and lack of blood pressure improvement and vice versa before revascularization.[40] Furthermore, duplex ultrasound can be used to diagnose restenoses and evaluate both renal arteries concomitantly for RAS. In addition, duplex ultrasound is readily available compared with CTA and MRA and much less expensive to perform. The disadvantages that are associated with duplex ultrasound are that it takes 2 to 3 hours to complete an entire study and that there is an operator learning curve in performing a complete study.

## RENIN-ANGIOTENSIN-ALDOSTERONE SYSTEM

From a physiologic perspective, RAS leads to up-regulation of RAAS, prompted by an increase in rennin that can lead to the development or exacerbation of CHF. With RAS, renal blood flow frequently is diminished to varying extents. As the blood flow to the kidney decreases, the macula densa, located in the late thick ascending limb of the nephron, senses decreased luminal fluid. This occurs at a perfusion pressure of 70 to 80 mm Hg. As a result, the granular cells of the juxtaglomerular appartus secrete renin as a physiologic response to this diminished sodium chloride delivery. The renin that is secreted by these cells enters the blood stream where it activates angiotensin-converting enzyme. Mediated by the effects of angiotensin-converting enzyme in the pulmonary and renal vasculature, angiotensin I is transformed to angiotensin II. This substance is a direct vasoconstrictor and also promotes secretion of aldosterone from the adrenal glands. Aldosterone's effect is to cause the principal cells of the collecting duct to increase sodium absorption from the tubule fluid that enters the blood stream and increases effective circulating volume. As discussed later, newer data have come to light showing that aldosterone has potential to promote cardiac remodeling and renal fibrosis.

The effect of RAS on neurohormonal activation varies by duration of the lesion and the extent of the involvement. The presence of RAS has been shown to lead to up-regulation of prostaglandins E2 and I2 that leads to increased renin release.[41] When early unilateral RAS occurs, the elevated systemic pressure promotes blood flow to the contralateral kidney. This two-kidney, one-clip model, initially described by Goldblatt,[42] leads to increased medullary blood flow (**Fig. 4**). As a result, the hydrostatic forces are elevated and less luminal fluid is reabsorbed due to a diminished osmotic gradient leading to diuresis—also known as a pressure natriuresis. This escape phenomenon is not present in the two-kidney, two-clip model whereby bilateral RAS is present (**Fig. 5**). Without this compensatory pressure natriuresis, an elevated systemic blood pressure may occur. This elevated blood pressure is independent of the RAAS system. If renal ischemia is chronic in nature, RAAS is no longer up-regulated. With the chronicity, diminished kidney mass and nephrosclerosis occurs with resultant CKD and hypertension.[43]

The activation of the RAAS system also has detrimental effects on kidney volume and cardiac myocytes. Angiotensin II has been shown to increase transforming growth factor-beta (TGF-β) expression that is known to up-regulate fibrosis and extracellular matrix deposition in the interstitium of the kidney.[44] Similar findings of fibrosis have been found in cardiac myocytes under the influence of TGF-β. Such a pattern of extracellular matrix deposition seems to be more severe in hypertensive patients. In a recent study comparing hypertensive patients to nonhypertensive patients, those patients who had greater LV mass index and urinary albumin excretion were less likely to have suppression of TGF-β when treated with an angiotensin receptor blocker (ARB) compared with responder irrespective of blood pressure control.[45]

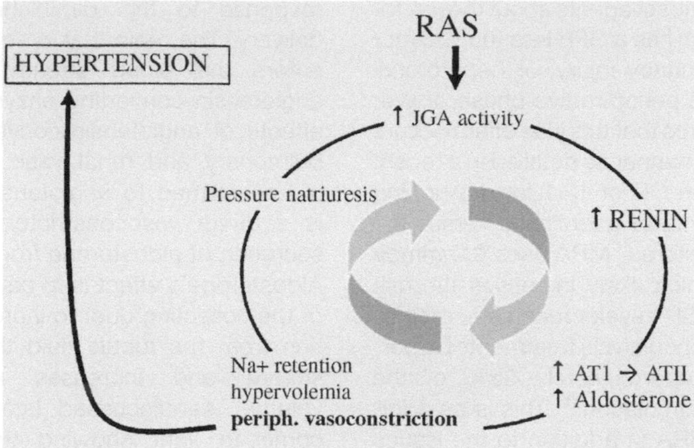


**Fig. 4.** Two-kidney, one-clip model of renovascular hypertension. ATI, angiotensin I; AT1I, angiotensin II; JGA, juxtaglomerular apparatus. (*From* Rundback JH, Murphy TP, Cooper C, et al. Chronic renal ischemia: pathophysiologic mechanisms of cardiovascular and renal disease. J Vasc Interv Radiol 2002;13(11):1085–92; with permission.)

These processes lead to end-organ damage in the form of nephrosclerosis and CHF.

The activation of the RAAS and the cascade of events outlined can have a detrimental effect at various levels in patients who have underlying HF. In mild forms of HF, GFR is preserved, but as HF worsens, it results in compromised renal blood flow leading to RAAS activation to maintain circulatory volume and preserve GFR.[46] Angiotensin II is implicated in having detrimental effects as a product of RAAS activation and angiotensin II is implicated in cardiac hypertrophy, remodeling, atherosclerosis, nephrosclerosis, and the earlier stages of HF.[47] Furthermore, some investigators suggest that neuroendocrine activation is higher in patients who have overt HF. It seems that activation of RAAS occurs in patients who have LV dysfunction before the onset of CHF. Angiotensin II is linked to abnormal collagen deposition in the heart after myocardial infarction. In addition to angiotensin II, studies have implicated renin release with detrimental effects—particularly in patients who have CHF. In the Studies of Left Ventricular Dysfunction (SOLVD), a multicenter study of patients who had ejection fraction less than 35%, patients who had overt CHF had increased median levels of plasma renin activity ($P = .03$) than patients who did not have overt HF or healthy subjects. In addition, those patients on diuretics also had elevated plasma renin levels compared with counterparts not on diuretics. In a recent study that compared 25 patients who had angiographically confirmed RAS to 25 patients who had hypertension and 25 healthy subjects, RAS patients had higher indices of oxidative stress and platelet activation that correlated with renal vein renin and angiotensin II levels.[48] Furthermore, aldosterone release in animal studies has shown

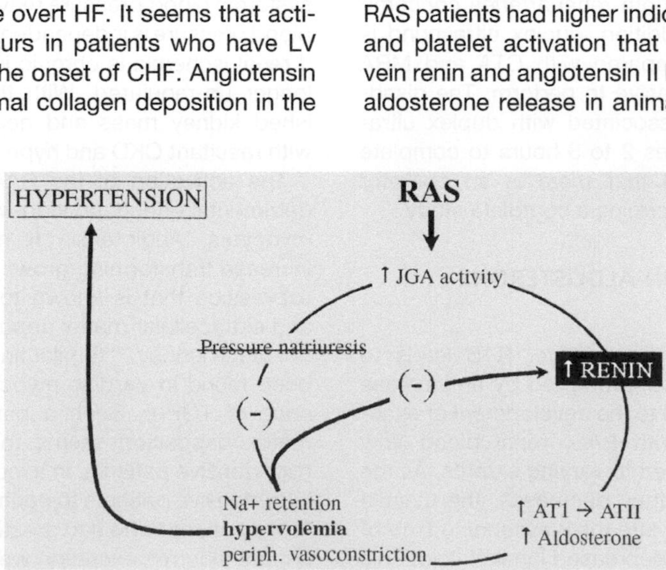


**Fig. 5.** Two-kidney, two-clip model of renovascular hypertension. AT, angiotensin; JGA, juxtaglomerular apparatus. (*From* Rundback JH, Murphy TP, Cooper C, et al. Chronic renal ischemia: pathophysiologic mechanisms of cardiovascular and renal disease. J Vasc Interv Radiol 2002;13(11):1085–92; with permission.)

the potential to inhibit nitric oxide synthesis by induction of interlukin-1β leading to endothelial dysfunction.[49] These animal studies have implicated that aldosterone promotes inflammation and fibrosis in vascular and nonvascular areas of cardiac injury that is caused by increased NADPH oxidase. This increase in fibrosis leads to cardiac remodeling and the development of ventricular hypertrophy and CHF.

Prolonged hypertension induced by chronic RAS may lead to hypertensive heart disease and diastolic dysfunction. These changes promote the formation of pulmonary edema. With the lack of pressure natriuresis, the systemic circulating volume increases. Bloch and colleagues[50] studied 90 patients who had bilateral RAS or unilateral RAS and found that patients who had bilateral RAS were much more likely to develop acute pulmonary edema of CHF than the unilateral RAS cohorts (77% vs 33%, $P = .004$). Likewise, a study of 38 patients who had acute pulmonary edema and systolic blood pressure greater than 160 mm Hg found that patients who had intact LV function likely had diastolic dysfunction.[51] None of these patients were evaluated for RAS. Pickering and colleagues[52] found that a risk for recurrent episodes of pulmonary edema in patients was bilateral RAS whereas diminished renal function and elevated blood pressure were not. Coronary heart disease also was an independent risk factor for pulmonary edema development. The lack of blood pressure as a risk factor for recurrent pulmonary edema is consistent with the normalization of renin and angiotensin levels seen in chronic RAS. As a result of such findings, it is recommended that in patients who have recurrent pulmonary edema and who do not have underlying coronary or valvular heart disease, a diagnosis of RAS must be excluded.[53]

## SCREENING CRITERIA

The American Heart Association (AHA) and the National Kidney Foundation have put forth guidelines addressing the timing and need for RAS screening.[54,55] Most of the suggestions outlined by these societies relate to blood pressure, in particular, early age of onset, malignant hypertension, or refractory hypertension. Furthermore, the onset of flash pulmonary edema or asymmetric kidney sizes on imaging are other factors to help clinicians in RAS diagnosis and evaluation (**Box 1**).

**Box 1**
**Clinical clues suggesting the presence of renal artery disease as the cause of hypertension and chronic kidney disease**

- Age at onset of hypertension <30 years or >55 years
- Abrupt onset of hypertension
- Acceleration of previously well-controlled hypertension
- Hypertension refractory to an appropriate three-drug regimen
- Accelerated hypertensive retinopathy
- Malignant hypertension
- History of tobacco use
- Systolic-diastolic abdominal bruit
- Flash pulmonary edema
- Evidence of generalized atherosclerosis obliterans
- Asymmetry in kidney size on imaging studies
- Acute kidney failure with treatment with an angiotensin-converting enzyme inhibitor (ACEI) or ARB

*Adapted from* American Journal of Kidney Diseases. Guideline 1: goals of antihypertensive therapy in CKD. Am J Kidney Dis 2004;43:S102; with permission.

## TREATMENT

The physiology of the RAS lesion determines the ideal method of treatment. Often lesions are angioplastied with or without stenting but it is difficult to determine before the procedure whether or not these interventions will have any clinical benefit. Furthermore, RAS due to FMD versus atherosclerosis can have an impact on the indication for and efficacy of medical versus interventional treatment.

The approach to treating RAS varies and controversy exists as to the most effective method to use. In 2005, the American College of Cardiology and the AHA formulated guidelines for treatment of RAS. The three strategies are medical therapy, angioplasty with or without stenting, and surgery.[54] Only lesions that have proved clinical significance, such as hypertension, should be treated. The first line treatment of unilateral RAS should be the use of ACEIs or ARBs. Tullis and colleagues[56] found that in patients who had greater than 60% RAS as a result of atherosclerosis, ACEIs were the only class of antihypertensive medications associated with significant improvement in systolic blood pressure (169 ± 22 mm Hg vs 157 ± 27 mm Hg; $P = .03$) and diastolic blood pressure (85 ± 9 mm Hg vs 79 ± mm Hg; $P = .001$). β-blockers and calcium channel blockers did not show significant benefit, with diuretic use showing a worsening systolic blood pressure (161 ± 24 mm Hg vs 168 ± 24 mm

Hg; $P = .05$). Another study with a 5-year follow-up compared 136 patients treated with revascularization technique to 54 counterparts treated medically. Either arm may or may not have been treated with ACEIs.[57] The use of ACEIs in either arm showed a positive effect on mortality with a greater effect seen in those treated only medically compared with the invasive cohort. Furthermore, a decreased rate of progressive renal impairment was seen with ACEI use (HR 0.29, 95% CI 0.09–0.92; $P = .036$). The difficulty with use of ACEIs in RAS is when to discontinue use in the event of rising serum creatinine. In a study of 108 patients considered at high risk for bilateral atherosclerotic RAS, ACEIs were given for a 2-week period where 69 patients developed significant increase in serum creatinine defined as greater than a 20% rise from baseline. Of these 69 patients, 52 had confirmed bilateral RAS, 17 less severe RAS, and 2 normal renal arteries. Twenty-six of these occurrences occurred within 4 days of initiation. When ACEIs were discontinued in all patients, the serum creatinine returned to baseline.[58] The rise in serum creatinine is believed the result of reduced poststenotic perfusion and disruption of the autoregulation of the GFR; this reduction in perfusion may lead to further loss of kidney mass.[59] Thus, using a threshold of 20% rise in serum creatinine as a cutoff to discontinue ACEIs after initiation is appropriate. Because of this potential side effect of ACEIs and the fact that atherosclerotic RAS can worsen, serial imaging has been considered and evaluated as part of a monitoring strategy to assess loss of renal function. In a study of 122 patients who had atherosclerotic RAS who underwent renal duplex every 6 months, those who had RAS greater than 60% had a 2-year cumulative incidence of renal atrophy of 20.8%. Risks for atrophy were systolic blood pressure above 180 mm Hg, a renal artery peak systolic of 400 cm per second, and a renal end diastolic velocity of greater than or equal to 5 cm per second. Use of ACEIs was not shown to have increased risk.[60] It is presumed that tight blood pressure control would be of benefit for RAS but this is not yet proved either.

The approach to the treatment of FMD is similar to that of athersclerotic RAS but with some caveats. Given that FMD occurs more often in younger patients, the threshold for invasive therapy should be lower. Medical therapy with the use of ACEIs is still a reasonable approach to control blood pressure, but FMD-associated RAS is shown to be responsive to angioplasty. In a study of 66 patients who had 85 lesions as a result of FMD, the angioplasty success rate was 100% with a 10-year patency rate of 87.07%.[61] All but one of the patients was cured of hypertension or had improvement of blood pressure. Recurrence of FMD lesions did occur in approximately 10% of the patients. Subsequent to this study, a prediction model of successful angioplasty of FMD associated RAS showed that the duration of hypertension, level of systolic blood pressure, and age were the key determinants.[62] In this series of 23 patients, age was an independent predictor of cure, which is believed the result of less intrarenal vascular disease and nephrosclerosis. As discussed previously, as RAS-induced hypertension persists over time, the neuroendocrine activation no longer continues and the secondary effects of RAAS activation exacerbate the elevated blood pressure making hypertension even less responsive to angioplasty.

Angioplasty with and without stenting should be used for treatment of atherosclerotic RAS but in limited circumstances. A known morbidity of bilateral RAS or unilateral RAS with one functioning kidney is pulmonary edema. In these circumstances the usefulness of stent placement has been studied. In a study of 90 patients who had renovascular disease, 56 patients had bilateral RAS with 23 having a history of pulmonary edema whereas 34 patients had unilateral RAS with one functioning kidney and four had a history of pulmonary edema.[50] Unilateral or bilateral stenting of the renal arteries prevented recurrence of pulmonary edema in 17 of 23 patients who had bilateral RAS and history of pulmonary edema but only one of three who had unilateral RAS. Five patients who had bilateral RAS and recurrent episodes of pulmonary edema had evidence of stent thrombosis or restenosis. In another study, Gray and colleagues[63] found that in a cohort of 39 patients who underwent renal artery stenting for recurrent or refractory pulmonary edema or CHF, mean blood pressure decreased (174/85 $\pm$ 32/23 mm Hg to 148/72 $\pm$ 24/14 mm Hg; $P<.001$), number of hospitalizations resulting from CHF in the year prior versus the year after declined (presenting 2.4 $\pm$ 1.4 hospitalizations vs 0.3 $\pm$ 0.7 hospitalizations; $P<.001$), and the New York Heart Association function class improved (2.9 $\pm$ 0.9 vs 1.6 $\pm$ 0.9 post stent). Angioplasty with and without stenting has not been demonstrated as effective in patient populations free of pulmonary edema or CHF. In a study of 106 patients who did not have HF or pulmonary edema but who had RAS greater than 50%, hypertension, and a mean serum creatinine of 2.3 mg/dL, no improvement in systolic or diastolic blood pressure, antihypertensive medication use, or renal function at 1 year was found.[64]

The role of surgery in the treatment of RAS has become more limited as successful treatment with ACEIs and angioplasty with and without stenting has improved. Surgery is associated with higher rates of morbidity and mortality with similar rates of improvement in blood pressure and renal function—2.1% to 6.1% perioperative mortality for bypass and 1% to 4.7% for endarterectomy.[18] The role for surgical correction usually is reserved for failed cases of angioplasty or in patients where the vascular anatomy is not amenable to correction with angioplasty. In a recent study of 92 patients status post surgical revascularization for RAS, worsening serum creatinine at discharge (OR 28.9; 95% CI, 5.0–165.4; $P$ = .0002), revascularization for unilateral RAS (OR 3.8; 95% CI, 0.8–16.6; $P$ = .05), and baseline serum above 1.5 mg/dL (OR 1.81; 95% CI, 1.15–2.85; $P$ = .011) all were associated with poor outcomes for preservation of renal function during the follow-up period (38.5 months).[65] Dialysis was started in 16 patients during the follow-up with dialysis-free survival at 5 years of 50%.

In sum, the combination of CKD and heart disease has profound ramifications for treatment, medical costs, and most importantly patient morbidity and mortality. Certain forms of renovascular disease, especially RAS, are associated with episodes of pulmonary edema and with HF and intact ejection fraction (diastolic dysfunction). Renovascular disease is not the culprit renal lesion in all cases where HF and chronic renal disease co-exist. Frequently, CAD is the cause of HF. Aside from FMD-induced RAS, the same risk factors for CAD lead to the development of atherosclerotic RAS. Early intervention for established atherosclerotic disease changes the natural history of CAD and may have an impact on RAS. Treatment of clinically important or symptomatic RAS begins with suppression of the RAAS with the use of ACEIs. Angioplasty with and without stenting is demonstrated to have clinical benefit in specific situations and should be used when medical therapy fails to control symptoms or cannot be tolerated because of side effects. Surgical revascularization should be used in limited situations. Although the concomitant presence of chronic renal disease and HF represents a worrisome clinical profile, certain forms of chronic renal disease are amenable to treatment interventions that may change the natural history and burden of HF.

## REFERENCES


1. Fonarow GC, Heywood JT, Heidenreich PA, et al. Temporal trends in clinical characteristics, treatments, and outcomes for heart failure hospitalizations, 2002 to 2004: findings from Acute Decompensated Heart Failure National Registry (ADHERE). Am Heart J 2007;153(6):1021–8.
2. Chae CU, Albert CM, Glynn RJ, et al. Mild renal insufficiency and risk of congestive heart failure in men and women > or = 70 years of age. Am J Cardiol 2003;92(6):682–6.
3. Smith GL, Lichtman JH, Bracken MB, et al. Renal impairment and outcomes in heart failure: systematic review and meta-analysis. J Am Coll Cardiol 2006;47(10):1987–96.
4. Gottlieb SS, Abraham W, Butler J, et al. The prognostic importance of different definitions of worsening renal function in congestive heart failure. J Card Fail 2002;8(3):136–41.
5. Shlipak MG, Katz R, Fried LF, et al. Cystatin-C and mortality in elderly persons with heart failure. J Am Coll Cardiol 2005;45(2):268–71.
6. Levin A, Thompson CR, Ethier J, et al. Left ventricular mass index increase in early renal disease: impact of decline in hemoglobin. Am J Kidney Dis 1999;34(1):125–34.
7. Weiner DE, Tighiouart H, Vlagopoulos PT, et al. Effects of anemia and left ventricular hypertrophy on cardiovascular disease in patients with chronic kidney disease. J Am Soc Nephrol 2005;16(6): 1803–10.
8. Foley RN, Parfrey PS, Harnett JD, et al. Impact of hypertension on cardiomyopathy, morbidity and mortality in end-stage renal disease. Kidney Int 1996;49(5):1379–85.
9. Martins D, Wolf M, Pan D, et al. Prevalence of cardiovascular risk factors and the serum levels of 25-hydroxyvitamin D in the United States: data from the Third National Health and Nutrition Examination Survey. Arch Intern Med 2007;167(11): 1159–65.
10. Schleithoff SS, Zittermann A, Tenderich G, et al. Vitamin D supplementation improves cytokine profiles in patients with congestive heart failure: a double-blind, randomized, placebo-controlled trial. Am J Clin Nutr 2006;83(4):754–9.
11. Park CW, Oh YS, Shin YS, et al. Intravenous calcitriol regresses myocardial hypertrophy in hemodialysis patients with secondary hyperparathyroidism. AJKD 1999;33(1):73–81.
12. Zittermann A, Schleithoff SS, Koerfer R. Vitamin D insufficiency in congestive heart failure: why and what to do about it? Heart Fail Rev 2006;11(1): 25–33.
13. National Institutes of Health. The effect of calcium and vitamin D in patients with heart failure [clinical trial]. Available at: http://www.clinicaltrials.gov/ct2/show/NCT00497900. Accessed August 6, 2008.
14. Guo H, Kalra PA, Gilbertson DT, et al. Atherosclerotic renovascular disease in older US patients starting dialysis, 1996 to 2001. Circulation 2007;115(1): 50–8.

15. Textor SC. Ischemic nephropathy: where are we now? J Am Soc Nephrol 2004;15(8):1974–82.
16. Alcazar JM, Rodicio JL. Ischemic nephropathy: clinical characteristics and treatment. Am J Kidney Dis 2000;36(5):883–93.
17. Cheung CM, Hegarty J, Kalra PA. Dilemmas in the management of renal artery stenosis. Br Med Bull 2005;73–74:35–55.
18. Safian RD, Textor SC. Renal-artery stenosis. N Engl J Med 2001;344(6):431–42.
19. Pascual A, Bush HS, Copley JB. Renal fibromuscular dysplasia in elderly persons. Am J Kidney Dis 2005;45(4):e63–6.
20. Harding MB, Smith LR, Himmelstein SI, et al. Renal artery stenosis: prevalence and associated risk factors in patients undergoing routine cardiac catheterization. J Am Soc Nephrol 1992;2(11):1608–16.
21. Labropoulos N, Ayuste B, Leon LR Jr. Renovascular disease among patients referred for renal duplex ultrasonography. J Vasc Surg 2007;46(4):731–7.
22. Kalra PA, Guo H, Kausz AT, et al. Atherosclerotic renovascular disease in United States patients aged 67 years or older: risk factors, revascularization, and prognosis. Kidney Int 2005;68(1):293–301.
23. Dorros G, Jaff M, Mathiak L, et al. Multicenter Palmaz stent renal artery stenosis revascularization registry report: four-year follow-up of 1,058 successful patients. Catheter Cardiovasc Interv 2002;55(2):182–8.
24. Buller CE, Nogareda JG, Ramanathan K, et al. The profile of cardiac patients with renal artery stenosis. J Am Coll Cardiol 2004;43(9):1606–13.
25. Hansen KJ, Edwards MS, Craven TE, et al. Prevalence of renovascular disease in the elderly: a population-based study. J Vasc Surg 2002; 36(3):443–51.
26. Plouin PF, Perdu J, La Batide-Alanore A, et al. Fibromuscular dysplasia. Orphanet J Rare Dis 2007;2–28.
27. Kincaid OW, Davis GD, Hallermann FJ, et al. Fibromuscular dysplasia of the renal arteries. Arteriographic features, classification, and observations on natural history of the disease. Am J Roentgenol Radium Ther Nucl Med 1968;104(2):271–82.
28. Lassiter FD. The string-of-beads sign. Radiology 1998;206(2):437–8.
29. Bofinger A, Hawley C, Fisher P, et al. Increased severity of multifocal renal arterial fibromuscular dysplasia in smokers. J Hum Hypertens 1999; 13(8):517–20.
30. Sang CN, Whelton PK, Hamper UM, et al. Etiologic factors in renovascular fibromuscular dysplasia. A case-control study. Hypertension 1989;14(5):472–9.
31. Maher ER, Othman S, Frankel AH, et al. Captopril-enhanced 99mTc DTPA scintigraphy in the detection of renal-artery stenosis. Nephrol Dial Transplant 1988;3(5):608–11.
32. Ludwig V, Martin WH, Delbeke D. Calcium channel blockers: a potential cause of false-positive captopril renography. Clin Nucl Med 2003;28(2):108–12.
33. Olbricht CJ, Paul K, Prokop M, et al. Minimally invasive diagnosis of renal artery stenosis by spiral computed tomography angiography. Kidney Int 1995;48(4):1332–7.
34. Leung DA, Hoffmann U, Pfammatter T, et al. Magnetic resonance angiography versus duplex sonography for diagnosing renovascular disease. Hypertension 1999;33(2):726–31.
35. Barrett BJ, Parfrey PS. Clinical practice. Preventing nephropathy induced by contrast medium. N Engl J Med 2006;354(4):379–86.
36. McCullough PA, Adam A, Becker CR, et al. Risk prediction of contrast-induced nephropathy. Am J Cardiol 2006;98(6A):27K–36K.
37. Food and Drug Administration. FDA public health advisory: gadolinium-containing contrast agents for magnetic resonance imaging (MRI). Available at: http://www.fda.gov/cder/drug/advisory/gadolinium_agents_20061222.htm. Accessed August 6, 2008.
38. Perazella MA, Rodby RA. Gadolinium-induced nephrogenic systemic fibrosis in patients with kidney disease. Am J Med 2007;120(7):561–2.
39. Williams GJ, Macaskill P, Chan SF, et al. Comparative accuracy of renal duplex sonographic parameters in the diagnosis of renal artery stenosis: paired and unpaired analysis. AJR Am J Roentgenol 2007;188(3):798–811.
40. Radermacher J, Chavan A, Bleck J, et al. Use of Doppler ultrasonography to predict the outcome of therapy for renal-artery stenosis. N Engl J Med 2001;344(6):410–7.
41. Imanishi M, Abe Y, Okahara T, et al. Effects of prostaglandin I2 and E2 on renal hemodynamics and function and renin release. Jpn Circ J 1980;44(11): 875–82.
42. Goldblatt HL, Hanzal RF, Summerville WW. Studies on experimental hypertension I: the production of persistent elevation of systolic blood pressure by means of renal artery ischemia. J Exp Med 1934; 59:347–80.
43. Rundback JH, Murphy TP, Cooper C, et al. Chronic renal ischemia: pathophysiologic mechanisms of cardiovascular and renal disease. J Vasc Interv Radiol 2002;13(11):1085–92.
44. Maschio G, Alberti D, Janin G, et al. Effect of the angiotensin-converting-enzyme inhibitor benazepril on the progression of chronic renal insufficiency. The Angiotensin-Converting-Enzyme Inhibition in Progressive Renal Insufficiency Study Group. N Engl J Med 1996;334(15):939–45.
45. Laviades C, Varo N, Diez J. Transforming growth factor beta in hypertensives with cardiorenal damage. Hypertension 2000;36(4):517–22.

46. Hillege HL, Girbes AR, de Kam PJ, et al. Renal function, neurohormonal activation, and survival in patients with chronic heart failure. Circulation 2000; 102(2):203–10.
47. Shokei K, Iwao H. Molecular and cellular mechanisms in angiotensin II-mediated cardiovascular and renal disease. Pharmacol Rev 2000;52:11–34.
48. Minuz P, Patrignani P, Gaino S, et al. Increased oxidative stress and platelet activation in patients with hypertension and renovascular disease. Circulation 2002;106(22):2800–5.
49. Ikeda U, Kanbe T, Nakayama I, et al. Aldosterone inhibits nitric oxide synthesis in rat vascular smooth muscle cells induced by interleukin-1 beta. Eur J Pharmacol 1995;290(2):69–73.
50. Bloch MJ, Trost DW, Pickering TG, et al. Prevention of recurrent pulmonary edema in patients with bilateral renovascular disease through renal artery stent placement. Am J Hypertens 1999;12(1 Pt 1):1–7.
51. Gandhi SK, Powers JC, Nomeir AM, et al. The pathogenesis of acute pulmonary edema associated with hypertension. N Engl J Med 2001; 344(1):17–22.
52. Pickering TG, Herman L, Devereux RB, et al. Recurrent pulmonary oedema in hypertension due to bilateral renal artery stenosis: treatment by angioplasty or surgical revascularisation. Lancet 1988; 2(8610):551–2.
53. Missouris CG, Belli AM, MacGregor GA. "Apparent" heart failure: a syndrome caused by renal artery stenoses. Heart 2000;83(2):152–5.
54. Hirsch AT, Haskal ZJ, Hertzer NR, et al. ACC/AHA 2005 Practice Guidelines for the management of patients with peripheral arterial disease (lower extremity, renal, mesenteric, and abdominal aortic): a collaborative report from the American Association for Vascular Surgery/Society for Vascular Surgery, Society for Cardiovascular Angiography and Interventions, Society for Vascular Medicine and Biology, Society of Interventional Radiology, and the ACC/AHA Task Force on Practice Guidelines (Writing Committee to Develop Guidelines for the Management of Patients With Peripheral Arterial Disease): endorsed by the American Association of Cardiovascular and Pulmonary Rehabilitation; National Heart, Lung, and Blood Institute; Society for Vascular Nursing; TransAtlantic Inter-Society Consensus; and Vascular Disease Foundation. Circulation 2006; 113(11):1474–547.
55. K/DOQI clinical practice guidelines on hypertension and antihypertensive agents in chronic kidney disease. Am J Kidney Dis 2004;43(5 Suppl 1):S1–290.
56. Tullis MJ, Caps MT, Zierler RE, et al. Blood pressure, antihypertensive medication, and atherosclerotic renal artery stenosis. Am J Kidney Dis 1999;33(4):675–81.
57. Losito A, Errico R, Santirosi P, et al. Long-term follow-up of atherosclerotic renovascular disease. Beneficial effect of ACE inhibition. Nephrol Dial Transplant 2005;20(8):1604–9.
58. van d V, Beutler JJ, Kaatee R, et al. Angiotensin converting enzyme inhibitor-induced renal dysfunction in atherosclerotic renovascular disease. Kidney Int 1998;53(4):986–93.
59. Hricik DE, Dunn MJ. Angiotensin-converting enzyme inhibitor-induced renal failure: causes, consequences, and diagnostic uses. J Am Soc Nephrol 1990;1(6):845–58.
60. Caps MT, Zierler RE, Polissar NL, et al. Risk of atrophy in kidneys with atherosclerotic renal artery stenosis. Kidney Int 1998;53(3):735–42.
61. Tegtmeyer CJ, Selby JB, Hartwell GD, et al. Results and complications of angioplasty in fibromuscular disease. Circulation 1991;83(Suppl 2):I155–61.
62. Davidson RA, Barri Y, Wilcox CS. Predictors of cure of hypertension in fibromuscular renovascular disease. Am J Kidney Dis 1996;28(3):334–8.
63. Gray BH, Olin JW, Childs MB, et al. Clinical benefit of renal artery angioplasty with stenting for the control of recurrent and refractory congestive heart failure. Vasc Med 2002;7(4):275–9.
64. van Jaarsveld BC, Krijnen P, Pieterman H, et al. The effect of balloon angioplasty on hypertension in atherosclerotic renal-artery stenosis. Dutch Renal Artery Stenosis Intervention Cooperative Study Group. N Engl J Med 2000;342(14): 1007–14.
65. Marone LK, Clouse WD, Dorer DJ, et al. Preservation of renal function with surgical revascularization in patients with atherosclerotic renovascular disease. J Vasc Surg 2004;39(2):322–9.

# Ventricular–Vascular Interaction in Heart Failure

Barry A. Borlaug, MD[a,*], David A. Kass, MD[b]

**KEYWORDS**

- Ventriculorterial stiffening
- Preserved ejection fraction
- Verapamil

The cardiovascular system is designed to provide ample pressure and flow to the body at rest and over broad ranges of stress. Because blood flow is pulsatile, changes in cardiac output are accompanied by alterations in the arterial pulse wave amplitude and pressure. In health, the heart–artery system is compliant to prevent wide swings in pressure that otherwise can lead to vascular and end-organ damage. For the vasculature, this compliance is largely contained within the proximal conduit vessels, and the stiffness (elastance) achieved during contraction by the left ventricle is closely matched or coupled to this arterial elastance to optimize mechanical efficiency and maintain a normal ejection fraction. Perhaps more important than the coupling ratio of ventricular and vascular stiffness are their absolute values. Indeed, maintaining low ventricular and arterial elastances in the normal human allows a dynamic range of volume transfer to be achieved during ejection with minimal change in pressure.

With advancing age, ventricular and arterial stiffness increase, changes that are further amplified by comorbidities, such as hypertension, diabetes, and kidney disease. This stiffening greatly augments systolic and pulse pressure swings during ejection, increasing arterial pressure decay during diastole and ventricular afterload. When incident (ejected) pressure waves encounter zones of impedance mismatch (eg, arterial bifurcations), part of the wave is reflected backward, interfering with flow but augmenting pressure. Pressure and flow wave transmission is enhanced in stiff blood vessels; thus the principal reflected wave returns to the heart in late systole, exacerbating systolic load. This increase in net and late-systolic afterload importantly alters ventricular systolic and diastolic function, increasing the amount of hydraulic work (and myocardial oxygen consumption) needed to provide the body with a given amount of blood flow. This increase in work in turn leads to impaired cardiovascular reserve function, labile systemic blood pressures, diminished coronary flow reserve, and increased diastolic filling pressures. Greater pulse perfusion in a stiff arterial system is a risk factor for vascular disease, and may compromise endothelial-dependent vasorelaxation. One can consider this adverse interaction between stiff heart and arteries as a form of coupling disease that ultimately limits the ability of the integrated cardiovascular system to respond to stress.

Ventricular–arterial stiffening is common in patients who have heart failure and apparent preservation of systolic function. Such patients are typically older, female, hypertensive, and display a high prevalence of diabetes, obesity, and renal dysfunction. They often develop marked systolic hypertension under conditions of stress, and their arterial and ventricular systolic pressures are sensitive to blood volume status. Although abnormal diastolic function is believed to contribute to failure symptoms by increasing congestion, it cannot explain the observed increases in systemic

This article originally appeared in *Heart Failure Clinics, volume 4, number 1.*
[a] Mayo Clinic and Foundation, Rochester, MN, USA
[b] Johns Hopkins Medical Institutions, Baltimore, MD, USA
* Corresponding author. Division of Cardiovascular Diseases, Mayo Clinic and Foundation, Gonda 5-455, 200 First Street SW, Rochester, MN 55905.
*E-mail address:* borlaug.barry@mayo.edu

Cardiol Clin 29 (2011) 447–459
doi:10.1016/j.ccl.2011.06.004
0733-8651/11/$ – see front matter 

pressures nor does it fully underlie limitations of cardiac reserve. Recent animal and human data have refocused attention on the impact of arterial afterload on ventricular diastolic relaxation and compliance. Here we review the pathophysiology of ventricular–arterial stiffening and its role in the syndrome of heart failure with a preserved ejection fraction (HFpEF).

## VENTRICULAR–ARTERIAL COUPLING

The influence of ventricular and vascular stiffness on net cardiovascular function is most easily appreciated in the pressure–volume plane. Ventricular systolic stiffness (contractility) is expressed as end-systolic elastance (Ees; **Fig. 1**), the slope of the end-systolic pressure–volume relationship.[1] Cardiac afterload is often conceived of as being equivalent to systolic blood pressure—a practice that can lead to erroneous conclusions and interpretations. Systemic blood pressures are determined by the complex and dynamic interaction of ventricle and vasculature,[2] and vary with preload, contractility, and heart rate also. An alternative is to assess the vascular load that opposes ejection independent of ventricular function. The traditional gold standard is aortic input impedance, derived from Fourier analysis of aortic pressure and flow waves.[3,4] Input impedance is expressed in the frequency domain, making it difficult to match with typical measures of ventricular systolic function, which exist in the time domain. Sunagawa and colleagues[5,6] conceived of a "net" vascular stiffness, effective arterial elastance (Ea), which shares the same units as Ees and is more easily calculated to study ventricular–arterial interaction. Ea is not a measure of a specific vascular property, but combines mean and pulsatile loading, providing a lumped parameter that reflects the net impact of this load on the heart. Kelly and colleagues[7] showed that the simple ratio of end-systolic pressure to stroke volume (Pes/SV) accurately estimates Ea in hypertensive and normal humans. Graphically, Ea is the negative slope of a line through the end-systolic and end-diastolic volume ($P = 0$) points (see **Fig. 1**) Coupling of heart and artery is often then depicted by the interaction of these two relations, and expressed as a ratio of Ea/Ees.[2,8,9] The intersection of these lines at a given preload value determines the end-systolic pressure and volume (see **Fig. 1**) The Ea/Ees ratio is preserved with normal aging to maintain optimal efficiency in men, but declines somewhat in women, because the denominator (ventricular stiffness) increases out of proportion to the increase in the numerator (vascular load).[10]

Effective coupling of heart to artery can be defined in several ways. One is the optimal transfer of blood from heart to periphery without excessive changes in blood pressure. Another is to provide optimal cardiovascular flow reserve without compromising arterial pressures. One can mathematically express optimal coupling as the interaction that best enhances the work performed by the heart on the body (ie, optimal external work). Last, one must consider the efficiency of the heart in performing this work—the energy consumption required by the heart to affect external work. Experimental and clinical studies have tended to focus on the latter two definitions (ie, optimizing external work or efficiency). For this, one can both predict[5] and observe experimentally[9] that an Ea/Ees coupling ratio of 0.6 to 1.2 achieves near-optimal work and efficiency. This range is normally

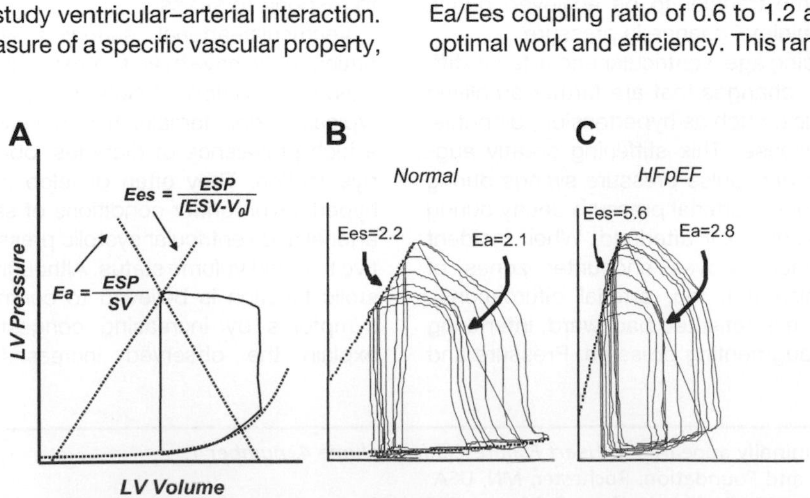


**Fig. 1.** (*A*) Left ventricular end-systolic elastance (Ees) is described by the slope and intercept of the end-systolic pressure–volume relationship, whereas arterial elastance (Ea) is defined by the negative slope between the end-systolic pressure–volume point and end-diastolic volume. (*B*) A normal adult has relatively low Ees and Ea, with a coupling ratio around unity, whereas older aged, hypertensive and HFpEF subjects (*C*) display marked increases in ventricular and arterial elastance.

maintained under various physiologic stresses. It can become very high, so-called "afterload mismatch," as in systolic heart failure, whereby depressed systolic function (low Ees) is coupled to a high arterial impedance (high Ea).[8] The coupling ratio is inversely related to ejection fraction (EF = 1/[1 + Ea/Ees]), and normally drops with exercise, as the increase in Ees (contractility) exceeds the increase in afterload (Ea) to augment cardiac output and blood pressure.[11] With aging, the exercise drop in Ea/Ees becomes compromised, partly explaining the age-dependent reduction in aerobic capacity.[11]

## DECONSTRUCTING AFTERLOAD

Ea is dominated by nonpulsatile load—systemic vascular resistance (SVR)—but it is also altered by artery stiffening to increase pulsatile load. Blood pressure pulsatility increases with aging and this is reflected in the pressure–volume diagram in the elderly individual (**Fig. 1**C) by the greater increase in systolic pressure throughout ejection.[10,12–16] Because Ea is determined by Pes/SV, the greater the disparity between Pes and mean arterial pressure (ie, the more pulsatile or stiff the arterial system), the higher Ea will be relative to mean resistance load.[7] Ea varies directly with SVR and heart rate and inversely with arterial compliance.[17,18] Different combinations of resistive and compliance loading alterations can lead to dramatic fluctuations in cardiac stroke work and peak power, despite stable Ea and Ea/Ees ratios, so it is worth considering the individual components of total arterial afterload (Ea).

A commonly used system to model the behavior of the vasculature is that of the three-element Windkessel, which deconstructs arterial load into a proximal resistance to pulsatile flow in the ascending aorta (characteristic impedance, Zc) proximal to a distal arteriolar resistance (mean SVR) and large vessel compliance (total arterial compliance, Ca) arranged in parallel (**Fig. 2**A).[7,17] An increase in steady load is manifest as an increase in SVR, whereas a change in pulsatile load would alter Zc and/or Ca. The Windkessel does not incorporate the effects of wave reflections, which become much more relevant with aging and vascular stiffening, often leading to dramatic increases in late-systolic load.[19] Wave reflections and late-systolic load are most readily quantified by examining the amplitude of the reflected pressure wave relative to total pulse pressure. This ratio, usually expressed as a percentage, is known as the augmentation index (**Fig. 2**B). Increases in late-systolic load may be particularly deleterious in their effects on diastolic relaxation.[20]

## VENTRICULAR–ARTERIAL STIFFENING IN HEART FAILURE WITH A PRESERVED EJECTION FRACTION

In patients who have HFpEF, the Ea/Ees ratio decreases compared with younger individuals, but is similar to that of asymptomatic hypertensive elderly patients.[13,15,21,22] Importantly, it still falls in a range where external work and efficiency are not likely compromised.[9] Although the ratio itself is reduced, the absolute value of both numerator and denominator are significantly elevated.

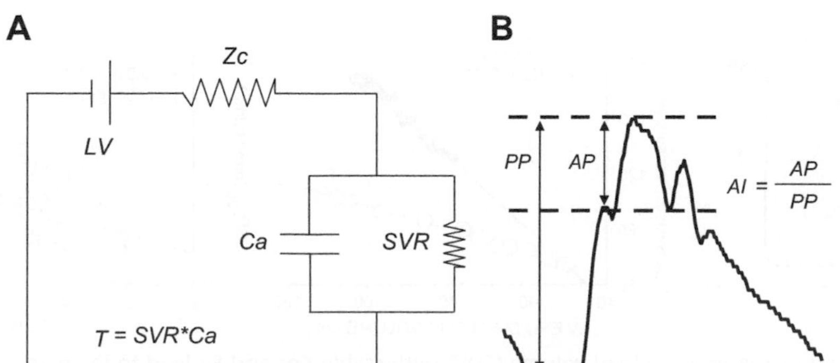


$$Ea = \frac{SVR + Zc}{t_s + T(1-e^{-td/T})} \sim \frac{ESP}{SV}$$

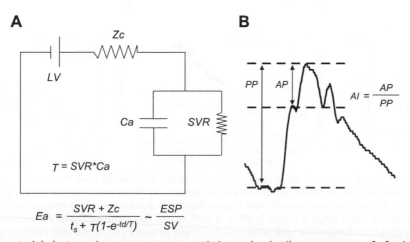

**Fig. 2.** Effective arterial elastance incorporates mean resistive and pulsatile components of afterload. (*A*) Electrical circuit analog of the three-element Windkessel model, which consists of a proximal characteristic impedance (Zc) upstream of total arterial compliance (Ca) and systemic vascular resistance (SVR) arranged in parallel. (*B*) With vascular stiffening, pulse wave velocity increases, such that reflected waves return to the ascending aorta in late systole rather than early diastole. The magnitude of late-systolic load can then be quantified by the augmentation index (AI), described by the ratio of augmented (AP) to pulse pressure (PP).

Patients who have HFpEF thus have elevated vascular stiffness and increased ventricular stiffness in systole and diastole.[15,21–23]

The net interaction between ventricular and arterial stiffness is important because it can significantly impact the first two components of optimal coupling: blood pressure homeostasis and preservation of adequate cardiovascular reserve. As displayed in **Fig. 3**A and B, an increase in both Ea and Ees means that systolic pressures are much more sensitive to changes in left ventricular (LV) end-diastolic volume, and thus central blood volume. Small changes in volume that might accompany dietary indiscretion or diuretic usage translate to more exaggerated changes in arterial pressure in a stiffer ventricle–artery system. The same can be said for changes in afterload: a given change in Ea in the setting of an increased Ees produces very large shifts in systemic blood pressures despite little change in stroke volume (**Fig. 3**C, D). These higher pressures during stress increase the amount of myocardial oxygen consumption required to deliver a given stroke volume, and can potently influence systolic and diastolic function.[15] Increased ventriculoarterial stiffening amplifies the systemic blood pressure response to acute preload alteration, as is seen with normal aging in humans (**Fig. 3**E, F).[13]

## MECHANISMS OF VENTRICULAR–VASCULAR STIFFENING

Ees is determined by active and passive muscle properties. Passive behavior is somewhat of a misnomer, because diastolic tone is regulated in part by calcium handling and also by qualitative (including posttranslational phosphorylation state) and quantitative changes in multiple sarcomeric proteins.[24] Diastolic stiffening is related to properties of myocyte size, chamber geometry, intrasarcomeric protein composition, cytosolic and membrane distensibility, and extracellular matrix composition, fibrillar crosslinking, and biophysical properties. Systolic ventricular elastance is related

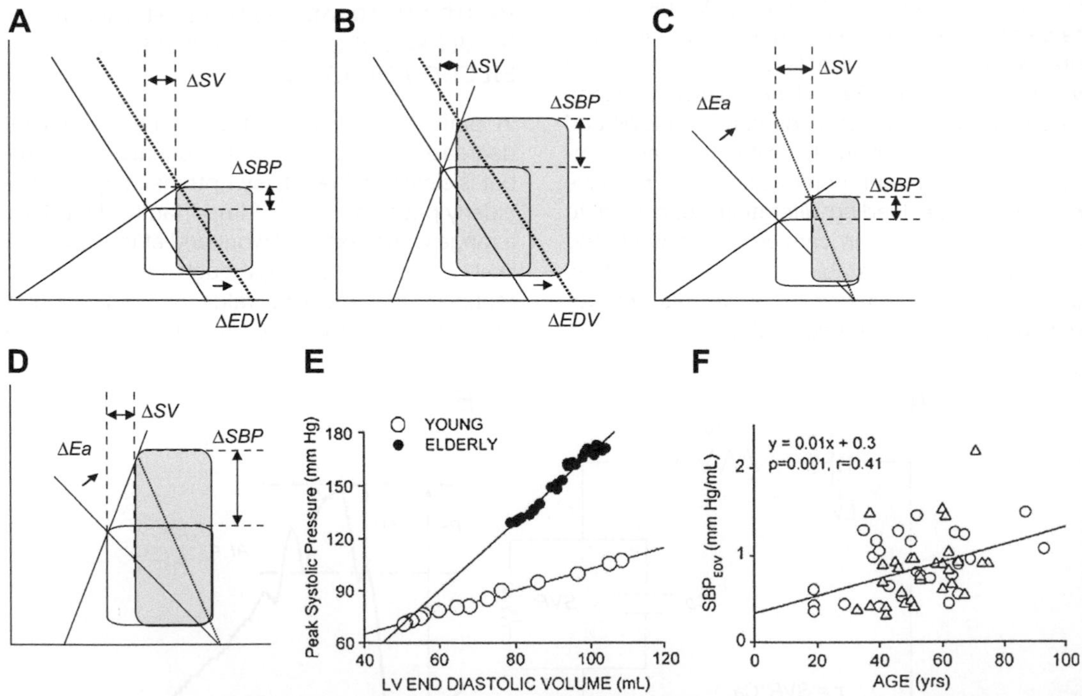


**Fig. 3.** (*A*) Isolated increases in preload volume (EDV) with stable Ees and Ea lead to increases in blood pressure (BP) and stroke volume, but in a stiff ventriculoarterial system. (*B*) The same increase in EDV produces a much larger increase in BP with proportionately less augmentation in stroke volume. Similarly, an isolated increase in afterload produces much more increase in BP in a stiff system (*D*) compared with normal or low elastances (*C*). Note again that the change in stroke volume is much less pronounced in the stiff heart–artery system, and the stroke work or pressure–volume area (*shaded*) is much greater, indicating higher myocardial oxygen demand to achieve the same net volume transfer. Increased stiffness explains why older adults show much greater dependence of BP on preload (*E*). The slope of the SBP–preload relation is higher in healthy older versus younger subjects (*F*). (*Panels E and F from* Chen CH, Nakayama M, Nevo E, et al. Coupled systolic-ventricular and vascular stiffening with age: implications for pressure regulation and cardiac reserve in the elderly. J Am Coll Cardiol 1998;32(5):1221–7; with permission. Copyright © 1998, American College of Cardiology.)

to the same determinants, and activated myofilament properties, changes in structural protein behavior shortened to smaller lengths, and interactions of the activated myocytes with the matrix. Vascular stiffening also stems from structural and muscle tone–dependent factors. Smooth muscle tone plays an important role, as does the geometry of the vessel (eg, dilation), elastin and collagen content, cross-linking of matrix components, and other factors. These topics have been reviewed extensively elsewhere.[25]

How does increased ventriculoarterial stiffness relate to patients who have HFpEF? Hypertension with left ventricular hypertrophy or concentric chamber remodeling is common in this disorder.[26,27] In a large observational study of consecutive patients presenting with HFpEF, the mean LV mass index was several standard deviations above normal cutoff partition values defining LV hypertrophy.[27] Myocyte hypertrophy has been documented, along with a modest increase in myofibrillar content, and increases in passive myocyte stiffness in triton-skinned cells.[28,29] Myocardial fibrosis is common, although this is not necessarily different than that observed in patients who have systolic heart failure.[29] Ventricular cellular passive stiffness has been found to correlate with estimates of diastolic chamber stiffness in HFpEF subjects,[28] consistent with clinical data.[22,23] Not all of the increase in diastolic stiffening is ascribable to ventricular properties, however, because external loading factors (including pericardial and right heart interaction) also contribute importantly to observed diastolic stiffening, as indicated by invasive pressure–volume analysis.[15,30]

Diastolic stiffening leads to fluid redistribution into the lungs and limits filling, but it cannot explain why patients who have HFpEF typically present with severe, uncontrolled hypertension when they develop pulmonary edema[31] and often display marked blood pressure sensitivity to vasodilator or diuretic therapy. The latter more directly relates to increased left ventricular systolic stiffening (Ees).[13,15] In addition to arterial systolic pulse pressure and stiffness, which are known to increase with age, Ees also increases in tandem.[7,10,12–14] In subjects who have hypertensive heart disease, and those who go on to develop HFpEF, this stiffening is more pronounced over age-matched controls (see **Figs. 1**C, **3**; **Fig. 4**). Because Ees has also been viewed as a measure of systolic contractile function, one might conclude that this reflects enhanced contractility. This seems unlikely, however, because other less chamber geometric–dependent parameters do not increase with aging. Early studies showed that Ees increased out of proportion to Ea in HFpEF,[15] but more recent studies indicate that many patients who have hypertensive heart disease may also have similar increases in ventricular–arterial stiffness.[21,22] The presence of ventriculoarterial stiffening in patients who do not have HF does not mean that it is not important in the pathophysiology of HF, just as the presence of diastolic dysfunction in patients who do not have HF does not indicate that the latter is not relevant in HFpEF. Rather, it underlines the highly integrated and multifaceted

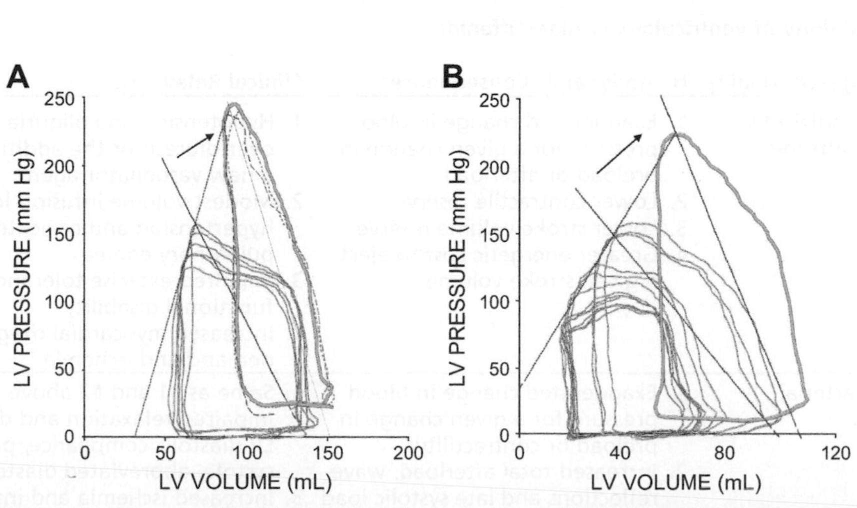


**Fig. 4.** (*A, B*) Example pressure–volume loops taken from patients who had HFpEF at baseline and with acute increases in Ea induced by isometric handgrip (*arrows*). Because of elevated baseline stiffness, the "gain" is much greater with further increases, leading to severe hypertension. Note the greatly increased end-diastolic LV pressures during handgrip. (*From* Kawaguchi M, Hay I, Fetics B, et al. Combined ventricular systolic and arterial stiffening in patients with heart failure and preserved ejection fraction: implications for systolic and diastolic reserve limitations. Circulation 2003;107(5):714–20; with permission.)

mechanisms that conspire to cause symptoms in patients who have HFpEF.

In addition to being older and hypertensive, most patients who have HFpEF are female,[26] and this factor may also influence abnormal ventricular–arterial stiffening. Women develop more concentric LV hypertrophy in the setting of pressure overload as compared with men.[10,32,33] A large population-based study showed that the age-dependent increases in ventricular systolic and arterial stiffness are much greater in women compared with men. With exercise, healthy older women display a greater increase in arterial elastance than younger women, whereas men do not show this interaction between age and acute stiffness changes.[11] These factors might provide clues to explain the increased prevalence of HFpEF in older women.[10] In contrast to vascular and ventricular systolic stiffening, mean peripheral vascular resistance does not show this age-dependent increase and is greater in men. Women are thus more likely to display accentuated increases in pulsatile loading with age, associated with greater coupled ventricular–arterial stiffening.[10]

## PATHOPHYSIOLOGY OF VENTRICULAR–ARTERIAL STIFFENING

### *Systolic Effects*

**Table 1** summarizes the effects of ventriculoarterial stiffening. One major consequence is increased blood pressure lability and sensitivity to volume and vascular loading.[13] In a normal heart–artery system, an increase in EDV results in a given increase in end-systolic pressure (see **Fig. 3**A). In a typical HFpEF patient, however, even if the coupling ratio is normal the same change in EDV leads to an exaggerated change in blood pressure (see **Fig. 3**B). The pressure–volume area or stroke work (shaded) to achieve this given stroke volume is therefore also higher in the patient who has HFpEF.[15] Similarly, decreases in preload lead to greater decreases in systolic pressure in this stiffly-coupled system, and changes in afterload (Ea) are also associated with enhanced changes in blood pressure because of an elevated baseline Ees (see **Figs. 3**C, D). The heart–artery system in HFpEF patients is thus "high gain" in pressure changes with small loading perturbations, and there is less change in stroke volume for a given alteration in blood pressure. **Fig. 4** shows marked increases in systemic and LV filling pressures during isometric handgrip in two patients who have HFpEF—changes that are much more dramatic because of the steep baseline Ees. This distinction is key in comparing HFpEF with systolic heart failure, in which large increases in stroke volume are often associated with minimal change in systemic blood pressure with vasodilators, because of greatly diminished Ees.[34]

In addition to enhanced load sensitivity, systolic reserve function also becomes limited with increased stiffening. A high basal Ees means there is less effective change in systolic performance for

**Table 1**
**Pathophysiology of ventricular-vascular stiffening**

| Underlying Abnormality | Hemodynamic Consequences | Clinical Relevance |
|---|---|---|
| Increased ventricular systolic stiffness | 1. Exaggerated change in blood pressure for a given change in preload or afterload<br>2. Lower contractile reserve<br>3. Lower stroke volume reserve<br>4. Greater energetic cost to eject a given stroke volume | 1. Hypotension and oliguria with slight over-diuresis or the addition of a new vasodilator agent<br>2. Modest volume infusion leads to hypertension and/or acute pulmonary edema<br>3. Impaired exercise tolerance and functional disability<br>4. Increased myocardial oxygen demand and ischemia |
| Increased arterial stiffness | 1. Exaggerated change in blood pressure for a given change in preload or contractility<br>2. Increased total afterload, wave reflections and late systolic load<br>3. Greater dependence upon systolic pressure for coronary flow<br>4. Abnormal endothelial mechanotransduction | 1. Same as #1 and #2 above<br>2. Impaired relaxation and decreased LV diastolic compliance, prolonged systole, abbreviated diastole<br>3. Increased ischemia and infarct size for a given drop in systolic blood pressure<br>4. Endothelial dysfunction, abnormal vasodilation response to stress |

a given percent increase in Ees during stress demands. Increases in Ees reflect contractility reserve, but the impact of a change in Ees on net cardiac output is nonlinear, being much greater when the starting value is low than when it increases (**Fig. 5**A). If you link a heart with a high Ees to a stiff arterial system, the net effect on systolic pressure is exacerbated,[13,15] and thus ejection is further compromised. Because exercise duration is predominately determined by cardiac output reserve,[35,36] combined systolic ventricular and vascular stiffening can be an important contributor to exertional incapacity.

A third consequence of combined arterial–ventricular systolic stiffening is that the cardiac work required to deliver a given cardiac output increases. **Fig. 5**B shows the estimated increase in cardiac work necessary to achieve a given change in stroke volume as a function of ventricular (Ees) and arterial (Ea) properties for four patient groups, including subjects who have HFpEF (who have double or more the energetic cost to the heart as compared with younger controls), and age-matched hypertensive subjects who do not have left ventricular hypertrophy.[15]

## *Diastolic Effects*

Cardiac interaction with a stiff arterial system amplifies late systolic pressure loading because of an increase in pulse wave velocity and the amplitude of reflected waves (ie, increased augmentation index [AI]), impacting systolic and diastolic processes.[16] Acute increases in afterload prolong relaxation in humans and animals.[24,37–39] Afterload dependence is more pronounced in heart failure,[37] possibly related to abnormal phosphorylation of troponin I (TnI). Our laboratory recently showed that constitutive activation of protein kinase A (PKA) phosphorylation sites attenuates afterload-induced impairment in early diastolic relaxation, suggesting that part of the response seen in heart failure might be related to downstream abnormalities in β-adrenergic signaling.[40] More recently, Bilchick and colleagues[41] examined a transgenic murine model expressing partially dephosphorylated PKA sites and constitutively active PKC sites. Transgenic animals displayed a doubling in isovolumic relaxation time with a given increase in afterload, an effect that could not be rescued with isoproterenol coadministration.

There is less abundant human data concerning the afterload-dependence of diastole, particularly in HFpEF patients. **Fig. 4** shows pressure–volume responses with acute isometric handgrip for two patients who have HFpEF.[15] Because of the steep end-systolic pressure–volume relationship (high Ees), there is a greatly exaggerated increase in systolic blood pressure, associated with acute increases in diastolic filling pressures and prolongation of early pressure decay. Increases in late-systolic load may be most deleterious in their effects on early relaxation,[39] possibly related to qualitative changes in thick–thin filament dissociation with altered loading sequence (late vs early peak load).[42] We recently showed that LV early

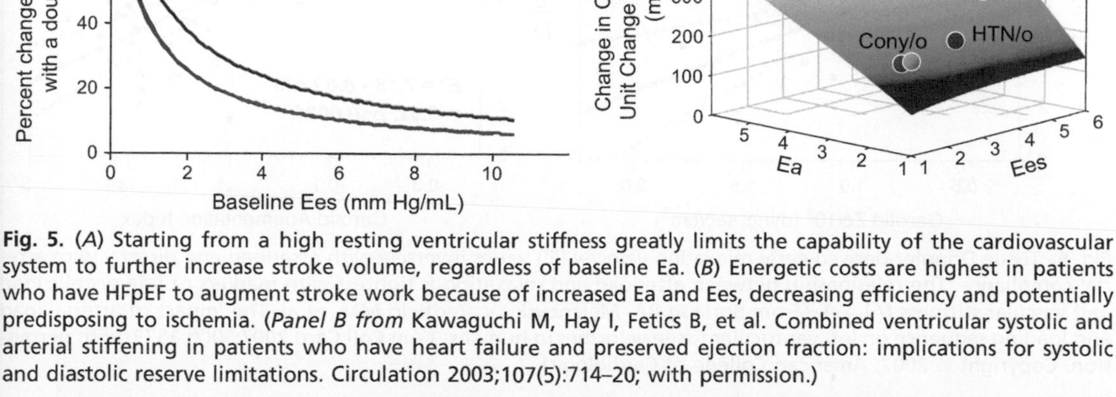

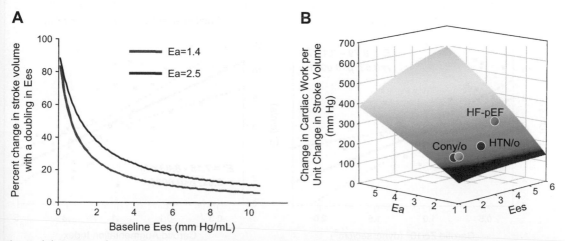


**Fig. 5.** (*A*) Starting from a high resting ventricular stiffness greatly limits the capability of the cardiovascular system to further increase stroke volume, regardless of baseline Ea. (*B*) Energetic costs are highest in patients who have HFpEF to augment stroke work because of increased Ea and Ees, decreasing efficiency and potentially predisposing to ischemia. (*Panel B from* Kawaguchi M, Hay I, Fetics B, et al. Combined ventricular systolic and arterial stiffening in patients who have heart failure and preserved ejection fraction: implications for systolic and diastolic reserve limitations. Circulation 2003;107(5):714–20; with permission.)

diastolic relaxation, as assessed with tissue Doppler echo, varies inversely with net afterload and vascular stiffness, and directly with total arterial compliance in patients who have and do not have hypertensive heart disease.[20] Intriguingly, relaxation was most strongly correlated with the pulsatile components, particularly late-systolic load (**Fig. 6**). These results suggest that therapies specifically targeting vascular stiffness and wave reflection may be beneficial to improve diastolic relaxation. These findings are consistent with a recent clinical trial demonstrating improved relaxation velocity with chronic vasodilator therapy.[43]

Rates of early pressure decay have traditionally been believed to have little effect on LV end diastolic pressure, because the latter is believed to be influenced primarily by passive chamber compliance.[44,45] Despite evidence for afterload modulation of early relaxation, there is little known about how afterload might modulate passive diastolic compliance.[46] Leite-Moreira and colleagues[39] showed that increases in afterload prolong relaxation and shift the pressure–dimension relationship upward in rabbits, although the single beat method used could not discount pericardial restraining effects, and the amount of increase required to elicit a change (80% of isovolumic contraction) may not be physiologically relevant in humans. More recently, Shapiro and colleagues[47] examined afterload dependence of diastolic compliance in an aged-hypertension canine model of HFpEF. Acute phenylephrine-induced increases in Ea reduced LV diastolic capacitance and increased filling pressures. At each level of load, stiffness was higher in the aged-hypertension dogs compared with young controls (consistent with more severe diastolic dysfunction), but intriguingly, there was no difference in the slope of the relationship between afterload and diastolic compliance between the groups. Even more intriguing is the observation that the variation in capacitance as a function of afterload

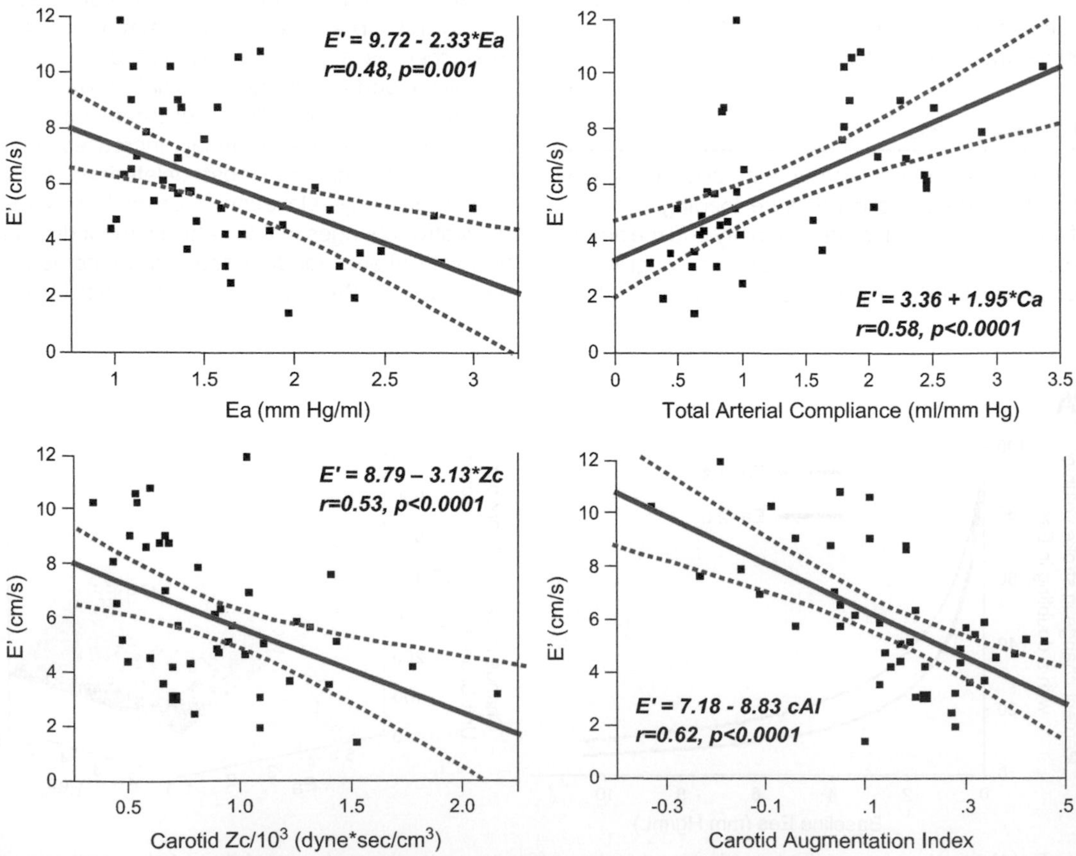


**Fig. 6.** Tissue Doppler-derived early relaxation velocity (E′) varies inversely with afterload and directly with arterial compliance. The relationship between afterload and relaxation is tightest with markers of late systolic load and vascular stiffness (AI, Zc). (*From* Borlaug BA, Melenovsky V, Redfield MM, et al. The impact of arterial load and loading sequence on left ventricular tissue velocities in humans. J Am Coll Card 2007;50(7):1573; with permission. Copyright © 2007, American College of Cardiology.)

was much more substantial than the absolute differences attributable to disease presence or absence alone. Further study is required to better define how afterload might dynamically modulate LV chamber compliance.

### *Vascular Effects*

The left ventricle normally depends on diastolic arterial pressure as the driving force for coronary artery perfusion, with more than 70% of left coronary flow occurring during diastole. When the heart ejects into a stiff vasculature, however, it becomes more dependent on systolic coronary flow.[48,49] This change in pulse perfusion pattern may render the heart more sensitive to acutely impaired systolic performance. When the heart ejects into a compliant arterial system, acute left coronary occlusion is well compensated for by moderate chamber dilation, and there is little decline in systolic pressure. When the same heart ejects into a stiff vascular system by means of an in vivo aortic bypass tube,[49] the results are markedly different, however: the heart dilates much more, and the magnitude of the ischemic bed size and resulting decline in function is exacerbated.

The endothelium is a major physical force transducer that senses local changes in shear stress (flow) and vessel distension (stretch), translating these signals to regulate endothelial function and vascular tone. Pulsatile perfusion combines both stimuli, and recent studies from our laboratory have revealed that these two signals combined provide additive stimulation for nitric oxide synthase, a primary upstream kinase activator (Akt), and cytoprotective effects against oxidant stress.[50] The latter seem to be primarily mediated by the augmented increase in Akt activation. Pulse perfusion in the relative absence of wall cyclic distension yields a different response, however. Here, Akt activation is blunted, there is correspondingly less increase in nitric oxide synthase activation, and a substantial blunting of the protection to oxidant stress. This signaling seems specifically coupled to the stretch stimulation (rather than shear), and although the exact cascade responsible remains to be elucidated, it has intriguing implications. One is that reduced arterial compliance can itself blunt the normal flow-mediated dilatory response that is a central component of vasodilator reserve under stress. Although this direct link has yet to be proved in vivo, it may indeed contribute to vasodilator reserve limitations in the elderly, and in particular individuals who have HFpEF, who need to recruit this reserve as a compensation for the loss of other cardiovascular mechanisms.[36]

## VENTRICULAR–ARTERIAL STIFFENING AND EXERCISE RESERVE

Increases in ventricular and vascular stiffness affect cardiovascular reserve function with exercise stress. Warner and colleagues[51] studied the effects of losartan on exercise performance in 20 asymptomatic subjects who had echo-Doppler diastolic dysfunction and a hypertensive response to exercise, suggesting increased ventricular–vascular stiffness. Although losartan had no effect on resting blood pressure, it blunted the peak systolic pressure during exercise, increased the time to blood pressure greater than 190 mm Hg, and was associated with an approximate 10% increase in peak oxygen consumption. More recently, the same group performed a separate, randomized exercise intervention study, in which subjects received either 6 months of losartan or hydrochlorothiazide. They found similar reductions in exercise-induced hypertension with each treatment, but only losartan improved exercise performance and quality of life measures, suggesting that direct ventricular or vascular effects, rather than blood pressure changes per se, are critical in determining cardiovascular reserve function.[52]

Hundley and colleagues[53] studied the relationship between MRI-derived proximal aortic distensibility and exercise performance in 10 young, 10 older, and 10 HFpEF subjects. Aortic distensibility is highest in the young and most compromised in patients who have HFpEF, even compared with healthy older subjects. The authors went on to show that aortic distensibility strongly predicts exercise performance (**Fig. 7**), even after adjusting for age and gender in multivariate regression analysis. Aortic wall thickness was significantly greater in subjects who had HFpEF compared with both other groups, supporting the notion that abnormal vascular remodeling contributes to increased arterial stiffening in these patients independent of, or in addition to, normal aging.

In a noninvasive hemodynamic study, we compared subjects who had HFpEF to matched controls who had hypertensive LVH, and found that patients who had HFpEF displayed a markedly impaired ability to augment cardiac output with exercise, despite similar increases in preload.[36] The inability to augment cardiac output with stress correlated with chronotropic incompetence and an inability to vasodilate and drop systemic vascular resistance during exercise. Baseline blood pressure and vascular stiffness were similarly elevated in both groups, and only by measuring changes with exercise was the deficit in vascular reserve function observed. More recently, we found that among subjects who had hypertensive heart

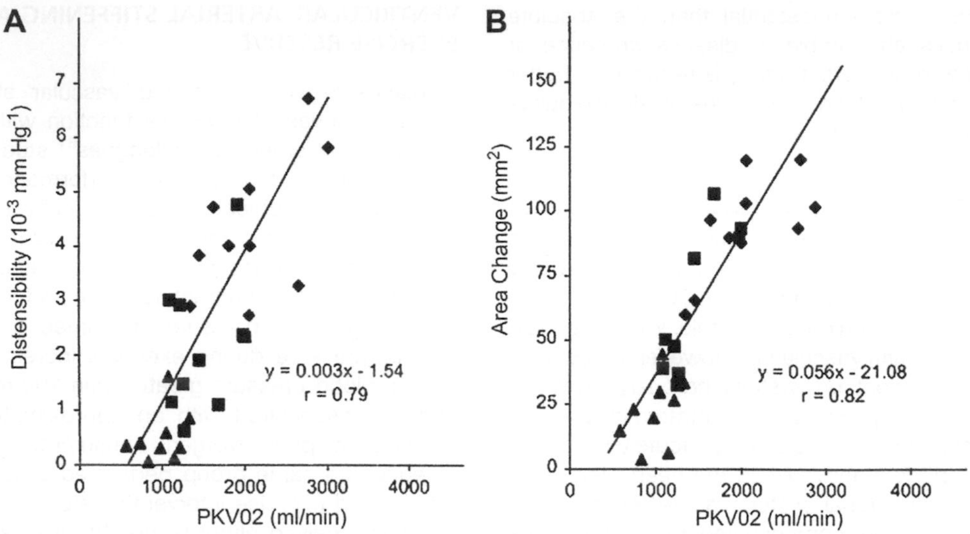


**Fig. 7.** Metabolic exercise performance is directly related to aortic distensibility (*A*) and cross-sectional area change (*B*) in patients who have HFpEF, older-aged controls, and young healthy controls. (*From* Hundley WG, Kitzman DW, Morgan TM, et al. Cardiac cycle-dependent changes in aortic area and distensibility are reduced in older patients with isolated diastolic heart failure and correlate with exercise intolerance. J Am Coll Cardiol 2001;38(3):796–802; with permission. Copyright © 2001, American College of Cardiology.)

disease referred to the catheterization laboratory for evaluation of dyspnea, acute exercise-induced increases in LV diastolic filling pressures were highest in subjects who had the greatest exercise-induced increase in Ea and Ees, highlighting the importance of resting and exercise-induced stiffening in affecting exercise reserve.[54]

## THERAPEUTIC STRATEGIES TARGETING STIFFNESS

Ventricular–vascular stiffening can be treated with agents that acutely modulate ventricular systolic and diastolic performance, vascular smooth muscle tone, and endothelial function. Verapamil, which acutely reduces ventricular and vascular stiffness, improves exercise capacity in patients who have HFpEF, hypertrophic cardiomyopathy, and elderly subjects who have hypertension and hypertrophy.[55–57] A recent trial in older hypertensive patients found that verapamil led to significant reductions in ventricular and vascular stiffness and these changes were in turn associated with a 50% improvement in aerobic exercise performance.[57] Short-term treatment with the angiotensin receptor antagonist losartan improves exercise performance in subjects who have a hypertensive response to exercise as described above,[51,52] whereas acute vasodilation with sodium nitroprusside did not share such beneficial effects.[58] Because isolated reduction in Ea results in greater decreases in blood pressure with less increase in stroke volume with a high baseline Ees (see **Fig. 3**), vasodilators that do not also treat ventricular stiffness tend to have less benefit. Propranolol, which does decrease Ees, but also increases Ea, does not improve exercise performance.[59] Given the extent of chronotropic incompetence in patients who have HFpEF,[36,60] drugs such as calcium channel antagonists and beta blockers require more study to compare offsetting effects on ventricular and arterial stiffness and heart rate, in addition to examining differences in acute versus chronic effects.

Many of the changes in ventricular–arterial stiffness in HFpEF are chronic, because of alterations in the material properties of the cardiovascular system.[25,61] In the largest randomized trial of HF with near-normal EF, there was a borderline-significant treatment effect driven by a reduction in hospitalizations for HF.[62] This trial enrolled subjects who had HF and EF greater than 40%, however, and many would consider those who have EF less than 50% to 55% to have some element of systolic dysfunction.[26,27] ACE inhibitors, which also reduce vascular stiffness, may be useful in HFpEF.[63] Other treatments under evaluation include aldosterone,[64,65] TGF-β,[66] and chymase antagonists.[67] A large-scale randomized trial funded by the National Institutes of Health (NIH) is currently underway testing the efficacy of the aldosterone antagonist spironolactone in HFpEF.

Ventricular hypertrophy is commonly seen in HFpEF, and the increase in stiffening and concentric remodeling seen with hypertensive heart disease commonly results in increased Ees; thus hypertrophy may be a novel therapeutic target in this disorder and those at risk. Controlling blood pressure and afterload is the most obvious way to ameliorate hypertrophy, but strategies specifically targeting concentric remodeling may be synergistically useful also. Among the panoply of candidate small molecules involved in hypertrophic signaling is Rho kinase, a key downstream effecter of $G_q$-protein coupled angiotensin-II signaling.[24,68] Rho kinase increases vascular smooth muscle cell tone, and the Rho kinase inhibitor fasudil is being evaluated as an anti-anginal drug. Fasudil also attenuates Ang-II–induced cardiac hypertrophy; thus therapies interfering with rho kinase may prove synergistically useful in relation to its vasodilatory and anti-hypertrophic properties.[69,70] HMG CoA-reductase inhibitors (statins) have recently been shown to be associated with improved survival in a retrospective analysis of patients who had HFpEF, and intriguingly, are known to also inhibit Rho kinase activation.[70,71] We recently demonstrated that the phosphodiesterase 5 inhibitor sildenafil prevents the hypertrophic response to pressure overload in mice.[72] In humans, sildenafil suppresses acute β-adrenergic stimulated contractility.[73] The NIH-sponsored RELAX trial will soon begin enrollment, studying whether chronic PDE5 inhibition with sildenafil can improve exercise performance and reduce ventricular hypertrophy and vascular stiffening in patients who have HFpEF.

As clinically based pathophysiologic research continues to identify mechanisms whereby ventricular–arterial stiffening impairs cardiovascular function, and basic research defines the key cellular players involved in promoting ventriculoarterial stiffness, remodeling, and hypertrophy, we will increasingly be able to better treat patients who have HFpEF by targeting these multiple complex coexisting and highly integrated pathways related to ventriculoarterial stiffening.

## REFERENCES


1. Suga H, Sagawa K. Instantaneous pressure-volume relationships and their ratio in the excised, supported canine left ventricle. Circ Res 1974;35(1):117–26.
2. Kass DA, Kelly RP. Ventriculo-arterial coupling: concepts, assumptions, and applications. Ann Biomed Eng 1992;20(1):41–62.
3. Milnor WR. Arterial impedance as ventricular afterload. Circ Res 1975;36(5):565–70.
4. Murgo JP, Westerhof N, Giolma JP, et al. Aortic input impedance in normal man: relationship to pressure wave forms. Circulation 1980;62(1):105–16.
5. Sunagawa K, Maughan WL, Burkhoff D, et al. Left ventricular interaction with arterial load studied in isolated canine ventricle. Am J Physiol 1983; 245(5 Pt 1):H773–80.
6. Sunagawa K, Maughan WL, Sagawa K. Optimal arterial resistance for the maximal stroke work studied in isolated canine left ventricle. Circ Res 1985;56(4):586–95.
7. Kelly RP, Ting CT, Yang TM, et al. Effective arterial elastance as index of arterial vascular load in humans. Circulation 1992;86(2):513–21.
8. Asanoi H, Sasayama S, Kameyama T. Ventriculoarterial coupling in normal and failing heart in humans. Circ Res 1989;65(2):483–93.
9. De Tombe PP, Jones S, Burkhoff D, et al. Ventricular stroke work and efficiency both remain nearly optimal despite altered vascular loading. Am J Physiol 1993; 264(6 Pt 2):H1817–24.
10. Redfield MM, Jacobsen SJ, Borlaug BA, et al. Age- and gender-related ventricular-vascular stiffening: a community-based study. Circulation 2005;112(15): 2254–62.
11. Najjar SS, Schulman SP, Gerstenblith G, et al. Age and gender affect ventricular-vascular coupling during aerobic exercise. J Am Coll Cardiol 2004; 44(3):611–7.
12. Avolio AP, Chen SG, Wang RP, et al. Effects of aging on changing arterial compliance and left ventricular load in a northern Chinese urban community. Circulation 1983;68(1):50–8.
13. Chen CH, Nakayama M, Nevo E, et al. Coupled systolic-ventricular and vascular stiffening with age: implications for pressure regulation and cardiac reserve in the elderly. J Am Coll Cardiol 1998;32(5):1221–7.
14. Nichols WW, O'Rourke MF, Avolio AP, et al. Effects of age on ventricular-vascular coupling. Am J Cardiol 1985;55(9):1179–84.
15. Kawaguchi M, Hay I, Fetics B, et al. Combined ventricular systolic and arterial stiffening in patients with heart failure and preserved ejection fraction: implications for systolic and diastolic reserve limitations. Circulation 2003;107(5):714–20.
16. Nichols WW, O'Rourke MF, Avolio AP, et al. Ventricular/vascular interaction in patients with mild systemic hypertension and normal peripheral resistance. Circulation 1986;74(3):455–62.
17. Segers P, Stergiopulos N, Westerhof N. Relation of effective arterial elastance to arterial system properties. Am J Physiol Heart Circ Physiol 2002;282(3): H1041–6.
18. Chemla D, Antony I, Lecarpentier Y, et al. Contribution of systemic vascular resistance and total arterial compliance to effective arterial elastance in humans. Am J Physiol Heart Circ Physiol 2003;285(2):H614–20.
19. Kelly R, Hayward C, Avolio A, et al. Noninvasive determination of age-related changes in the human arterial pulse. Circulation 1989;80(6):1652–9.

20. Borlaug BA, Melenovsky V, Redfield MM, et al. The impact of arterial load and loading sequence on left ventricular tissue velocities in humans. J Am Coll Card 2007;50(16):1570–7.
21. Melenovsky V, Borlaug BA, Rosen B, et al. Cardiovascular features of heart failure with preserved ejection fraction versus nonfailing hypertensive left ventricular hypertrophy in the urban Baltimore community: the role of atrial remodeling/dysfunction. J Am Coll Cardiol 2007;49(2):198–207.
22. Lam CS, Roger VL, Rodeheffer RJ, et al. Cardiac structure and ventricular-vascular function in persons with heart failure and preserved ejection fraction from Olmsted county, Minnesota. Circulation 2007;115(15):1982–90.
23. Zile MR, Baicu CF, Gaasch WH. Diastolic heart failure—abnormalities in active relaxation and passive stiffness of the left ventricle. N Engl J Med 2004;350(19):1953–9.
24. Borlaug BA, Kass DA. Mechanisms of diastolic dysfunction in heart failure. Trends Cardiovasc Med 2006;16(8):273–9.
25. Zieman SJ, Melenovsky V, Kass DA. Mechanisms, pathophysiology, and therapy of arterial stiffness. Arterioscler Thromb Vasc Biol 2005;25(5):932–43.
26. Owan TE, Redfield MM. Epidemiology of diastolic heart failure. Prog Cardiovasc Dis 2005;47(5):320–32.
27. Klapholz M, Maurer M, Lowe AM, et al. Hospitalization for heart failure in the presence of a normal left ventricular ejection fraction: results of the New York heart failure registry. J Am Coll Cardiol 2004;43(8):1432–8.
28. Borbely A, van der Velden J, Papp Z, et al. Cardiomyocyte stiffness in diastolic heart failure. Circulation 2005;111(6):774–81.
29. van Heerebeek L, Borbely A, Niessen HW, et al. Myocardial structure and function differ in systolic and diastolic heart failure. Circulation 2006;113(16):1966–73.
30. Dauterman K, Pak PH, Maughan WL, et al. Contribution of external forces to left ventricular diastolic pressure. Implications for the clinical use of the Starling law. Ann Intern Med 1995;122(10):737–42.
31. Gandhi SK, Powers JC, Nomeir AM, et al. The pathogenesis of acute pulmonary edema associated with hypertension. N Engl J Med 2001;344(1):17–22.
32. Carroll JD, Carroll EP, Feldman T, et al. Sex-associated differences in left ventricular function in aortic stenosis of the elderly. Circulation 1992;86(4):1099–107.
33. Villari B, Campbell SE, Schneider J, et al. Sex-dependent differences in left ventricular function and structure in chronic pressure overload. Eur Heart J 1995;16(10):1410–9.
34. Kass DA, Maughan WL. From "Emax" to pressure-volume relations: a broader view. Circulation 1988;77(6):1203–12.
35. Franciosa JA, Leddy CL, Wilen M, et al. Relation between hemodynamic and ventilatory responses in determining exercise capacity in severe congestive heart failure. Am J Cardiol 1984;53(1):127–34.
36. Borlaug BA, Melenovsky V, Russell SD, et al. Impaired chronotropic and vasodilator reserves limit exercise capacity in patients with heart failure and a preserved ejection fraction. Circulation 2006;114(20):2138–47.
37. Gillebert TC, Leite-Moreira AF, De Hert SG. Load dependent diastolic dysfunction in heart failure. Heart Fail Rev 2000;5(4):345–55.
38. Gillebert TC, Lew WY. Influence of systolic pressure profile on rate of left ventricular pressure fall. Am J Physiol 1991;261(3 Pt 2):H805–13.
39. Leite-Moreira AF, Correia-Pinto J, Gillebert TC. Afterload induced changes in myocardial relaxation: a mechanism for diastolic dysfunction. Cardiovasc Res 1999;43(2):344–53.
40. Takimoto E, Soergel DG, Janssen PM, et al. Frequency- and afterload-dependent cardiac modulation in vivo by troponin I with constitutively active protein kinase A phosphorylation sites. Circ Res 2004;94(4):496–504.
41. Bilchick KC, Duncan JG, Ravi R, et al. Heart failure-associated alterations in troponin I phosphorylation impair ventricular relaxation-afterload and force-frequency responses and systolic function. Am J Physiol Heart Circ Physiol 2007;292(1):H318–25.
42. Brutsaert DL, Sys SU. Relaxation and diastole of the heart. Physiol Rev 1989;69(4):1228–315.
43. Solomon SD, Janardhanan R, Verma A, et al. Effect of angiotensin receptor blockade and antihypertensive drugs on diastolic function in patients with hypertension and diastolic dysfunction: a randomised trial. Lancet 2007;369(9579):2079–87.
44. Gilbert JC, Glantz SA. Determinants of left ventricular filling and of the diastolic pressure-volume relation. Circ Res 1989;64(5):827–52.
45. Kass DA, Wolff MR, Ting CT, et al. Diastolic compliance of hypertrophied ventricle is not acutely altered by pharmacologic agents influencing active processes. Ann Intern Med 1993;119(6):466–73.
46. Leite-Moreira AF, Correia-Pinto J. Load as an acute determinant of end-diastolic pressure-volume relation. Am J Physiol Heart Circ Physiol 2001;280(1):H51–9.
47. Shapiro BP, Lam CS, Patel JB, et al. Acute and chronic ventricular-arterial coupling in systole and diastole. Insights from an elderly hypertensive model. Hypertension 2007;50(3):503–11.
48. Saeki A, Recchia F, Kass DA. Systolic flow augmentation in hearts ejecting into a model of stiff aging vasculature. Influence on myocardial perfusion-demand balance. Circ Res 1995;76(1):132–41.
49. Kass DA, Saeki A, Tunin RS, et al. Adverse influence of systemic vascular stiffening on cardiac

dysfunction and adaptation to acute coronary occlusion. Circulation 1996;93(8):1533–41.
50. Li M, Chiou KR, Bugayenko A, et al. Reduced wall compliance suppresses Akt-dependent apoptosis protection stimulated by pulse perfusion. Circ Res 2005;97(6):587–95.
51. Warner JG Jr, Metzger DC, Kitzman DW, et al. Losartan improves exercise tolerance in patients with diastolic dysfunction and a hypertensive response to exercise. J Am Coll Cardiol 1999;33(6):1567–72.
52. Little WC, Zile MR, Klein A, et al. Effect of losartan and hydrochlorothiazide on exercise tolerance in exertional hypertension and left ventricular diastolic dysfunction. Am J Cardiol 2006;98(3):383–5.
53. Hundley WG, Kitzman DW, Morgan TM, et al. Cardiac cycle-dependent changes in aortic area and distensibility are reduced in older patients with isolated diastolic heart failure and correlate with exercise intolerance. J Am Coll Cardiol 2001;38(3):796–802.
54. Jaber WA, Borlaug BA, Redfield MM, et al. Determination of the mechanism of elevated left ventricular filling pressures with exercise: a simultaneous echocardiographic-catheterization study [abstract 1756]. Circulation 2007;116:371.
55. Bonow RO, Dilsizian V, Rosing DR, et al. Verapamil-induced improvement in left ventricular diastolic filling and increased exercise tolerance in patients with hypertrophic cardiomyopathy: short- and long-term effects. Circulation 1985;72(4):853–64.
56. Setaro JF, Zaret BL, Schulman DS, et al. Usefulness of verapamil for congestive heart failure associated with abnormal left ventricular diastolic filling and normal left ventricular systolic performance. Am J Cardiol 1990;66(12):981–6.
57. Chen CH, Nakayama M, Talbot M, et al. Verapamil acutely reduces ventricular-vascular stiffening and improves aerobic exercise performance in elderly individuals. J Am Coll Cardiol 1999;33(6):1602–9.
58. Nussbacher A, Gerstenblith G, O'Connor FC, et al. Hemodynamic effects of unloading the old heart. Am J Physiol 1999;277(5 Pt 2):H1863–71.
59. Fleg JL, Schulman S, O'Connor F, et al. Effects of acute beta-adrenergic receptor blockade on age-associated changes in cardiovascular performance during dynamic exercise. Circulation 1994;90(5):2333–41.
60. Brubaker PH, Joo KC, Stewart KP, et al. Chronotropic incompetence and its contribution to exercise intolerance in older heart failure patients. J Cardiopulm Rehabil 2006;26(2):86–9.
61. Kass DA. Ventricular arterial stiffening: integrating the pathophysiology. Hypertension 2005;46(1):185–93.
62. Yusuf S, Pfeffer MA, Swedberg K, et al. Effects of candesartan in patients with chronic heart failure and preserved left-ventricular ejection fraction: the CHARM-Preserved Trial. Lancet 2003;362(9386):777–81.
63. Cleland JG, Tendera M, Adamus J, et al. The perindopril in elderly people with chronic heart failure (PEP-CHF) study. Eur Heart J 2006;27(19):2338–45.
64. Pitt B, Reichek N, Willenbrock R, et al. Effects of eplerenone, enalapril, and eplerenone/enalapril in patients with essential hypertension and left ventricular hypertrophy: the 4E-left ventricular hypertrophy study. Circulation 2003;108(15):1831–8.
65. Pitt B, Zannad F, Remme WJ, et al. The effect of spironolactone on morbidity and mortality in patients with severe heart failure. Randomized Aldactone Evaluation Study Investigators. N Engl J Med 1999;341(10):709–17.
66. Kuwahara F, Kai H, Tokuda K, et al. Transforming growth factor-beta function blocking prevents myocardial fibrosis and diastolic dysfunction in pressure-overloaded rats. Circulation 2002;106(1):130–5.
67. Matsumoto T, Wada A, Tsutamoto T, et al. Chymase inhibition prevents cardiac fibrosis and improves diastolic dysfunction in the progression of heart failure. Circulation 2003;107(20):2555–8.
68. Lai A, Frishman WH. Rho-kinase inhibition in the therapy of cardiovascular disease. Cardiol Rev 2005;13(6):285–92.
69. Higashi M, Shimokawa H, Hattori T, et al. Long-term inhibition of Rho-kinase suppresses angiotensin II-induced cardiovascular hypertrophy in rats in vivo: effect on endothelial NAD(P)H oxidase system. Circ Res 2003;93(8):767–75.
70. Morikawa-Futamatsu K, Adachi S, Maejima Y, et al. HMG-CoA reductase inhibitor fluvastatin prevents angiotensin II-induced cardiac hypertrophy via Rho kinase and inhibition of cyclin D1. Life Sci 2006;79(14):1380–90.
71. Fukuta H, Sane DC, Brucks S, et al. Statin therapy may be associated with lower mortality in patients with diastolic heart failure: a preliminary report. Circulation 2005;112(3):357–63.
72. Takimoto E, Champion HC, Li M, et al. Chronic inhibition of cyclic GMP phosphodiesterase 5A prevents and reverses cardiac hypertrophy. Nat Med 2005;11(2):214–22.
73. Borlaug BA, Melenovsky V, Marhin T, et al. Sildenafil inhibits beta-adrenergic-stimulated cardiac contractility in humans. Circulation 2005;112(17):2642–9.

# Exercise Intolerance

Dalane W. Kitzman, MD[a,*], Leanne Groban, MD[b]

**KEYWORDS**

- Diastolic heart failure • Heart rate
- Hypertrophic cardiomyopathy • Systolic heart failure

Exercise intolerance is the primary symptom of chronic diastolic heart failure (DHF). It is part of the definition of heart failure and is intimately linked to its pathophysiology. Further, exercise intolerance affects the diagnosis and prognosis of heart failure. In addition, understanding the mechanisms of exercise intolerance can lead to developing and testing rational treatments for heart failure. This article focuses on the fundamental principles of exercise physiology and on the assessment, pathophysiology, and potential treatment of exercise intolerance in DHF.

## IMPORTANCE OF EXERCISE INTOLERANCE

Heart failure is defined as a syndrome in which cardiac output is insufficient to meet metabolic demands. This definition implies that insufficient cardiac output will be expressed symptomatically. Heart failure often may manifest by occasional episodes of acute decompensation with overt systemic volume overload and pulmonary edema.[1,2] Exertional fatigue and dyspnea, however, are the primary chronic symptoms in outpatients, even when well compensated and non-edematous, and whether associated with reduced or normal ejection fraction (EF).[3] In addition, these symptoms and other consequences of exercise intolerance are potent determinants of health-related quality of life in patients who have heart failure. Several investigators have reported that objective measures and even subjective estimates of exercise tolerance are predictors of survival.[4,5]

Exercise intolerance can be quantified objectively using semiquantitative assessments, such as interview (New York Heart Association [NYHA] classification) and surveys (Minnesota Living with Heart Failure or Kansas City Cardiomyopathy questionnaires), and quantitative methods, including timed walking tests (6-minute walk distance) and graded exercise treadmill or bicycle exercise tests. Cardiopulmonary exercise testing on a treadmill or a bicycle ergometer provides the most accurate, reliable, and reproducible assessments of exercise tolerance and yields multiple important outcomes, including metabolic equivalents, exercise time, exercise workload, blood pressure and heart rate responses, and rate–pressure product. Using commercially available instruments that perform automated concentration and volume analyses of expired gas, one can assess simultaneously measures of oxygen consumption ($VO_2$), carbon dioxide generation, and ventilatory response both at rest and during exercise. Patient effort is an important modifier of data quality and can itself be assessed simultaneously, objectively by expired gas analysis (as the respiratory exchange ratio) and by the somewhat subjective but more easily obtained measures of perceived effort by the Borg scale and percent age-predicted maximal heart rate.

Submaximal exercise is in some ways a more important outcome variable than peak exercise capacity because it is more applicable to everyday life and is relatively independent of effort. Submaximal exercise capacity can be assessed as the

This article originally appeared in *Heart Failure Clinics, volume 4, number 1*.
This work was supported in part by National Institute on Aging Grants, R37-AG18915 (MERIT), Dennis Jahnigen Career Development and Paul Beeson Award (K08-AG026764) and Claude D. Pepper Older Americans Independence Center (P30 AG21332).
[a] Wake Forest University Health Sciences, Winston-Salem, NC, USA
[b] Wake Forest University Health Sciences Center, Winston-Salem, NC, USA
* Corresponding author. Section of Cardiology, Wake Forest University School of Medicine, Medical Center Boulevard, Winston-Salem, NC 27157.
*E-mail address:* dkitzman@wfubmc.edu

Cardiol Clin 29 (2011) 461–477
doi:10.1016/j.ccl.2011.06.002

ventilatory anaerobic threshold by expired gas analysis, using either the Wasserman-Whipp or the V-slope method. Cardiopulmonary exercise testing measurements and expired gas analysis with automated, commercially available instruments provides measures of both peak oxygen consumption and of ventilatory anaerobic threshold that are valid and highly reproducible in elderly patients who have DHF as well as in those who have systolic heart failure (SHF) (**Fig. 1**). Another variable provided by these methods, the ventilation/carbon dioxide production ($VE/VCO_2$) slope, is a strong predictor of survival, independent of $VO_2$.[6] The $VE/VCO_2$ slope is abnormal in patients who have DHF, although it is not as abnormal as it is in those who have SHF.[7]

Submaximal exercise performance also can be assessed by timed and distance walk tests. These tests are simple to perform and are widely available. The authors have shown that the 6-minute walk distance is decreased considerably in elderly patients who have DHF. In group data, the reduction is in proportion to both peak exercise oxygen consumption and ventilatory anaerobic threshold. The authors' published studies, however, suggest that 6-minute walk testing has only modest accuracy for predicting peak exercise capacity in individual patients compared with direct measurement with cardiopulmonary exercise testing with expired gas analyses and also is not as reproducible.[8]

## PATHOPHYSIOLOGY OF EXERCISE INTOLERANCE

To understand the pathophysiology of exercise intolerance in DHF, the authors performed a comparative study of maximal exercise testing with expired gas in 119 older subjects in three distinct, well-defined groups: persons who had heart failure with severe left ventricular (LV) systolic dysfunction (mean EF, 30%); persons who had isolated DHF (EF $\geq$50% and no significant coronary, valvular, pericardial, or pulmonary disease and no anemia); and age-matched controls.[3] In comparison with the controls, peak exercise $VO_2$ was severely reduced in the patients who had DHF, to a degree similar to the reduction in those with SHF (**Fig. 2**).[3] Submaximal exercise capacity, as measured by the ventilatory anaerobic threshold, was reduced in patients who had DHF versus those who had SHF, and this reduced exercise capacity was accompanied by reduced health-related quality of life.[3]

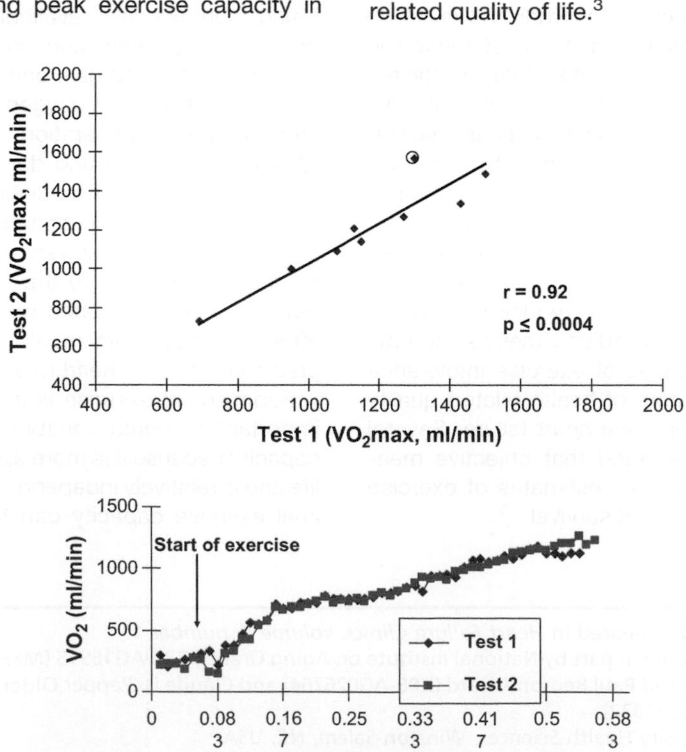


**Fig. 1.** Excellent reproducibility of peak exercise $VO_2$ in older patients who have heart failure, including those who have LVEF. (*Top panel*) Group data. (*Bottom panel*) 15-Second averaged data from a representative patient. (*From* Marburger CT, Brubaker PH, Pollock WE, et al. Reproducibility of cardiopulmonary exercise testing in elderly heart failure patients. Am J Cardiol 1998;82:905–9; with permission.)

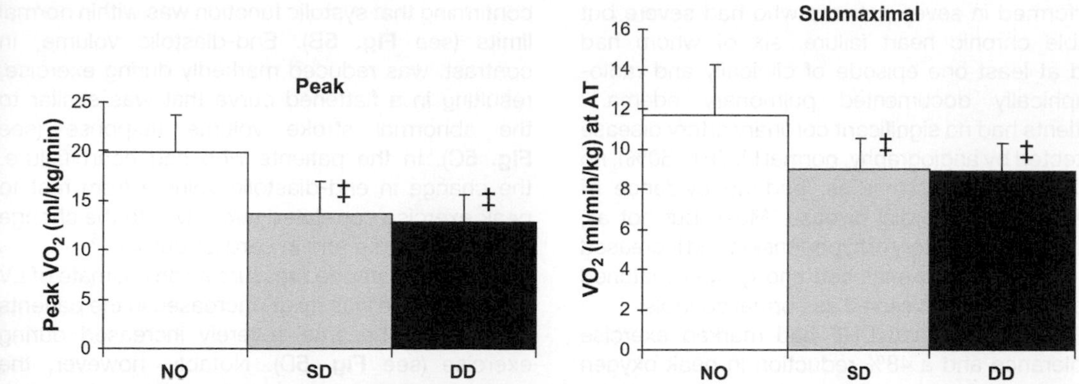


**Fig. 2.** $VO_2$ during peak exhaustive exercise (*left panel*) and during submaximal exercise at the ventilatory anaerobic threshold (*right panel*) in age-matched normal subjects (NO), elderly patients who have heart failure caused by systolic dysfunction (SD), and elderly patients who have heart failure with normal systolic function, that is, presumed diastolic dysfunction (DD). Exercise capacity is severely reduced in patients who have DHF compared with normal controls ($P<.001$), to a degree similar to the reduction in patients who have SHF. Overall, peak exercise $VO_2$ was 33% lower in the women than in the men (not shown). (*Data from* Kitzman DW, Little WC, Brubaker PH, et al. Pathophysiological characterization of isolated diastolic heart failure in comparison to systolic heart failure. JAMA 2002;288(17):2144–50.)

By the Fick equation, peak $VO_2$ during exercise is the product of cardiac output and arteriovenous oxygen (A-$VO_2$) difference, indicating that exercise intolerance is related to one or both of these factors and to the variables that influence them. Measurement of peak exercise $VO_2$ and at least one of these other two factors (cardiac output or A-$VO_2$ difference) allows one to calculate the remaining unknown factor and to begin to isolate specific factors that contribute to exercise intolerance in individual patients and within groups (**Fig. 3**).

## *Central Cardiac Response to Exercise*

These principles were used to examine the determinants of exercise performance in normal persons and in patients who had heart failure. A series of cardiopulmonary exercise studies was performed using symptom-limited upright bicycle exercise with indwelling pulmonary artery and brachial

**Potential Mechanisms of Exercise Intolerance from the Fick Equation**

**Heart Rate:**
**chronotropic incompetence**
**Stroke Volume:**
**↓contractility (systolic dysfunction: ESV)**
**↓LV filling (diastolic dysfunction: EDV)**
**Arteriovenous $O_2$ Difference:**
**↓peripheral vascular function**
**↓skeletal muscle bulk and function**
**↓hemoglobin (anemia)**

**Fig. 3.** Potential mechanisms of exercise intolerance from the factors of the Fick equation. EDV, end-diastolic volume; ESV, end-systolic volume.

artery catheters and simultaneous expired gas analysis and radionuclide ventriculography.[9–17] Cardiac output was determined by the Fick principle for oxygen, and LV end-diastolic volume and end-systolic volume were calculated from the Fick stroke volume and the radionuclide EF (LVEF).

In healthy young and middle-aged male and female volunteers, $VO_2$ increases 7.7-fold from rest to peak exercise during upright bicycle exercise,[9,14] and this increase is achieved by a 3.2-fold increase in cardiac output and a 2.5-fold increase in A-$VO_2$ difference. The increase in cardiac output results from a 2.5-fold increase in heart rate and a 1.4-fold increase in stroke volume. Stroke volume increases during low levels of exercise via the Frank-Starling mechanism; during higher levels of exercise, stroke volume increases predominantly because of increased contractility and even may decline slightly because of tachycardia and limited filling time.

Aging is accompanied by reduced peak exercise $VO_2$ caused by an age-related decline in peak exercise cardiac output, heart rate, stroke volume, and LVEF.[10,13] Thus, in normal subjects, stroke volume and end-diastolic volume response are important contributors to the increase in $VO_2$ and cardiac output during upright exercise and are altered by normal aging but not by gender.

This information regarding the physiology of exercise in normal persons and changes with aging provides background for a series of studies the authors performed to understand the cardiovascular and peripheral mechanisms of the reduced exercise capacity in patients who have DHF. Invasive cardiopulmonary exercise testing was performed in seven patients who had severe but stable chronic heart failure, six of whom had had at least one episode of clinically and radiographically documented pulmonary edema.[15] Patients had no significant coronary artery disease detected by angiography, normal LVEF ($\geq$50%), no wall motion abnormalities, and no evidence of valvular or pericardial disease. Most, but not all, patients had a history of hypertension and increased LV mass. Ten age-matched and gender-matched healthy volunteers served as normal controls.

Patients who had DHF had marked exercise intolerance and a 48% reduction in peak oxygen consumption. In patients and normal subjects, exercise was limited primarily by leg fatigue, and dyspnea also was reported frequently.[15] The peak respiratory exchange ratio was greater than 1.10 and was similar in patients who had DHF and normal subjects, suggesting good exercise effort in both groups. In both groups, arterial lactate concentration increased several fold from rest to peak exercise. During submaximal exercise at 50 watts, where oxygen consumption was similar in patients and controls, lactate concentration tended to be increased in the patients compared with the normal subjects ($2.2 \pm 1.1$ vs $1.4 \pm 0.7$ mmol/L).

At rest, there were no intergroup differences between the two groups in cardiac output, central A-$VO_2$ difference, stroke volume, or heart rate. Cardiac output was significantly reduced in the patients at submaximal workloads, however, and was severely reduced by 41% at peak exercise (**Fig. 4**A). Central A-$VO_2$ difference was increased by approximately 10% in the patients during the submaximal exercise, partially compensating for the reduced cardiac index (**Fig. 4**B). At peak exercise, however, this mechanism was outstripped, and the A-$VO_2$ difference was reduced by 13%. In the patients, the change in cardiac output from rest to peak exercise correlated closely with the increase in $VO_2$ during exercise ($r = 0.81$; $P<.03$).

Stroke volume was reduced in the patients during submaximal exercise and was markedly reduced (−26%) at peak exercise (**Fig. 4**C).[15] Likewise, heart rate was reduced by 18% in patients compared with controls at peak exercise (**Fig. 4**D). The change in stroke volume correlated well with the increase in cardiac output during exercise, suggesting that reduced stroke volume was the primary factor for reduced cardiac output and for the 48% reduction in peak $VO_2$ in the patients who had DHF.

A number of factors might contribute to the abnormal stroke volume response in the patients (**Fig. 5**A–D). The LVEF and end-systolic volume index during rest and exercise were not different from those in normal subjects (see **Fig. 5**A, B), confirming that systolic function was within normal limits (see **Fig. 5**B). End-diastolic volume, in contrast, was reduced markedly during exercise, resulting in a flattened curve that was similar to the abnormal stroke volume response (see **Fig. 5**C). In the patients who had heart failure, the change in end-diastolic volume from rest to peak exercise correlated strongly with the change in stroke volume and in cardiac output.[15]

Pulmonary wedge pressure as an estimate of LV filling pressure was mildly increased in the patients at rest and became severely increased during exercise (see **Fig. 5**D). Notably, however, the change in pulmonary wedge pressure from rest to peak exercise did not correlate significantly with the change in stroke volume or the increase in $VO_2$ during exercise. The LV end-diastolic pressure–volume ratio tended to be elevated in the patients at rest and became markedly increased during exercise. The upward, left-shifted LV diastolic pressure–volume relationship in the patients who had DHF (**Fig. 6**)[15] indicates that the patients did not use the Frank-Starling mechanism, probably primarily because of diastolic LV dysfunction. In contrast, patients who have heart failure and reduced systolic function have an operating pressure–volume relationship that is shifted upward and to the right during exercise.[18]

Although these invasively assessed LV filling pressures offers key insights into exercise intolerance, their invasive nature limits their overall utility. Noninvasive Doppler mitral filling indices, particularly the more recently developed tissue Doppler indices, can give insight into LV diastolic function. The time constant of isovolumic pressure decline ($\tau$) can be estimated noninvasively by measuring the early diastolic velocity of the mitral annulus ($E'$).[19] Furthermore, the ratio of early LV diastolic filling velocity (E) to $E'$ correlates well with invasively measured LV end-diastolic pressures.[20] Notably, an increased $E/E'$ ratio at rest has been correlated with maximal and submaximal exercise intolerance.[21,22] In addition, an increase in $E/E'$ during exercise correlates with exercise intolerance.[23]

Comparison of the exercise cardiovascular responses in the two different groups of patients who had heart failure (those who had normal EFs[15] and those who had reduced EFs[11,13,15]) can be instructive. Both had severe exertional symptoms and objective evidence of exercise intolerance, markedly reduced peak cardiac output and stroke volume, mildly reduced peak heart rate, and slightly reduced peak A-$VO_2$ difference (**Fig. 7**). Both groups also had mildly increased resting and markedly elevated exercise mean pulmonary capillary wedge pressures. The means by which LV stroke volume was reduced differed,

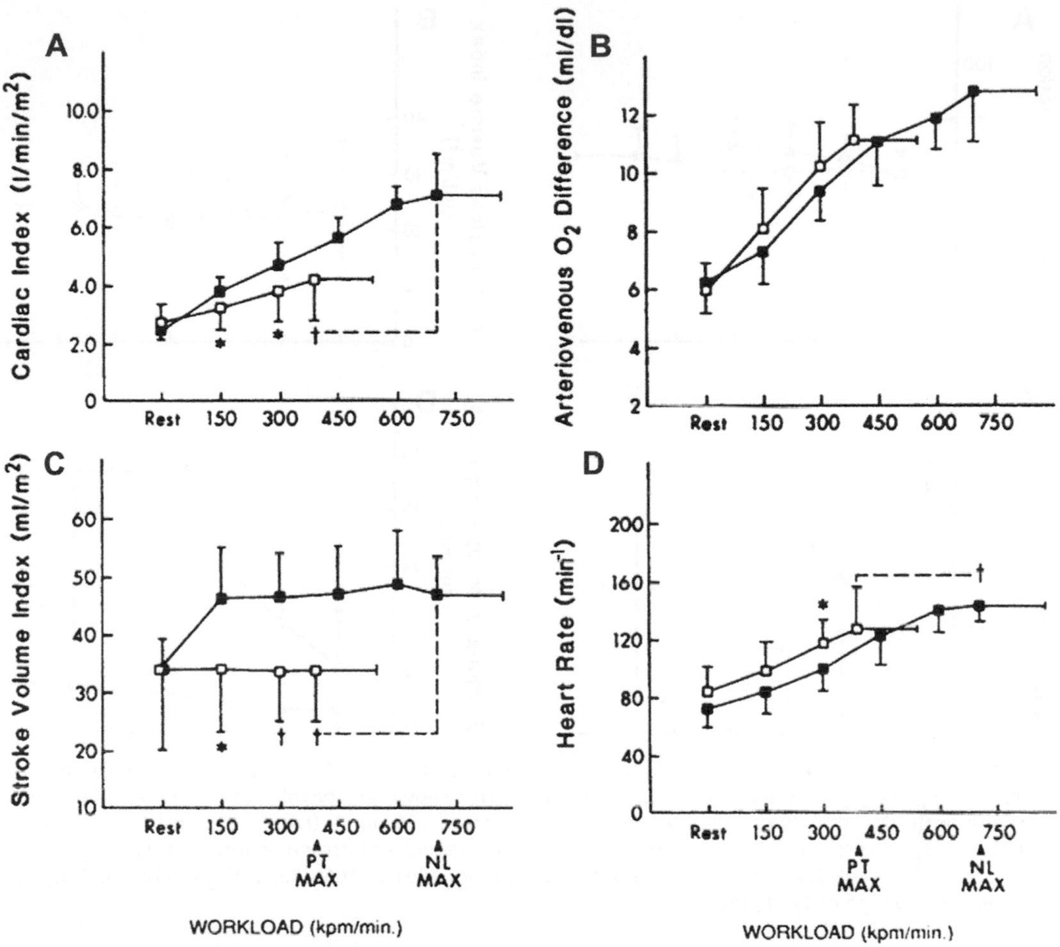


**Fig. 4.** Cardiovascular function assessed by invasive cardiopulmonary exercise testing in patients who have heart failure and normal systolic function (*open boxes*) and age-matched normal controls (*closed boxes*). The primary components of the Fick equation for $VO_2$, cardiac output, and A-$VO_2$ difference are shown in panels A and B, respectively. The components of cardiac output, stroke volume, and heart rate are shown in panels C and D. The X-axis is exercise workload in kilopounds/min (kpm); 150 kpm is equivalent to 25 W. (*From* Kitzman DW, Higginbotham MB, Cobb FR, et al. Exercise intolerance in patients with heart failure and preserved left ventricular systolic function: failure of the Frank-Starling mechanism. J Am Coll Cardiol 1991;17:1065–72; with permission. Copyright © 1991, American College of Cardiology.)

however. In one group patients had profound systolic contractile dysfunction and were able to use markedly increased LV filling pressure to produce greater-than-normal use of the Frank-Starling mechanism to compensate partially and maintain an increase in exercise stroke volume.[11,13] In the other group, despite normal systolic contractile function and markedly increased LV filling pressure,[15] patients were unable to use the Frank-Starling mechanism to increase stroke volume during exercise (see **Fig. 7**).[24]

## *Heart Rate Response to Exercise*

Decreased heart rate response also contributes to the reduced cardiac output at peak exercise and thus to reduced peak exercise $VO_2$. Indeed, chronotropic incompetence has been a frequent finding during cardiopulmonary exercise studies in SHF, but data were lacking for older patients and particularly for those who had normal EFs. Therefore, the authors compared heart rate and expired gas analyses responses in elderly patients who had DHF with those in a group of age- and gender-matched patients who had SHF and in healthy normal controls. Using the most standard definition of chronotropic incompetence, the authors found that chronotropic incompetence was present in 20% to 25% of older patients who had heart failure, that the prevalence was similar in patients who had DHF and those who had SHF, that the presence of chronotropic

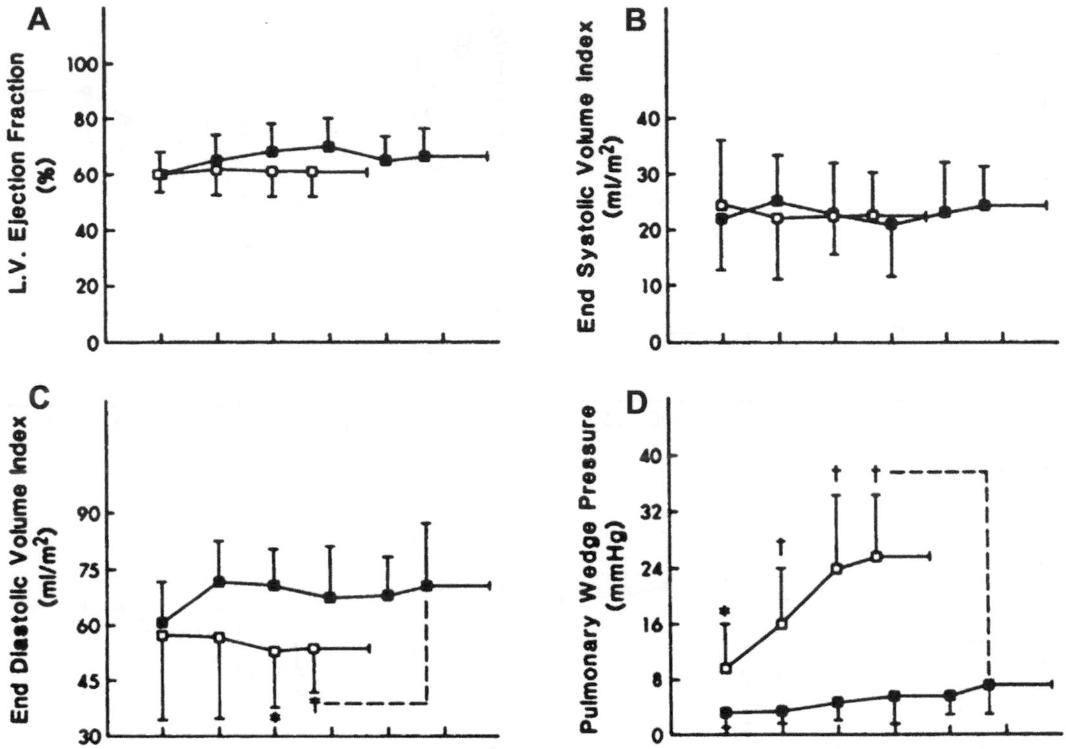


**Fig. 5.** The components of the LV stroke volume response during exercise, LVEF, end-systolic volume, end-diastolic volume, and LV filling pressure are shown in panels *A–D*. Not shown are systolic and mean arterial pressures, which were not different between groups. The key is the same as in **Fig. 4**. (*From* Kitzman DW, Higginbotham MB, Cobb FR, et al. Exercise intolerance in patients with heart failure and preserved left ventricular systolic function: failure of the Frank-Starling mechanism. J Am Coll Cardiol 1991;17:1065–72; with permission. Copyright © 1991, American College of Cardiology.)

incompetence contributed significantly to the degree of exercise intolerance, measured as maximal $VO_2$, and that this contribution was independent of medications, including beta-adrenergic antagonists (**Fig. 8**).[25] The important contribution of chronotropic incompetence to exercise intolerance in patients who had DHF was confirmed by Borlaug and colleagues,[26] who studied a cohort of primarily elderly, African American women who had hypertension and heart failure with a preserved EF. They reported that significant reductions in the rate of heart rate increase during exercise were primary contributors to reduced peak cardiac index and maximal exercise $VO_2$ (**Fig. 9**). The implication of this finding merits further investigation and has therapeutic implications.

## *Central and Peripheral Vascular Contributions to Exercise Intolerance*

Abnormal afterload and abnormal ventricular–vascular coupling may contribute to the abnormal Frank-Starling response seen in the patients who have DHF. Nearly all such patients (88%) have a history of chronic systemic hypertension.[27–29] In animal models, diastolic dysfunction develops early in systemic hypertension, and LV diastolic relaxation is sensitive to increased afterload,[30–35] which can impair relaxation, leading to increased LV filling pressures and decreased stroke volume and could lead to symptoms of dyspnea and congestion.[1,2,33]

In animal models and in humans, chronic systolic hypertension accelerates and magnifies the age-related increase in fibrotic thickening of the aortic wall and resultant increase in aortic stiffness, which is a major determinant of LV afterload and ventricular–vascular coupling.[36,37] To determine whether abnormally decreased aortic distensibility contributes to the severe exercise intolerance in heart failure with normal EF, the authors performed MRI and maximal exercise testing with expired gas analysis in a group of elderly patients who had isolated DHF, as defined earlier, with young healthy subjects and age-matched healthy subjects as normal controls. The patients who had DHF had severe exercise

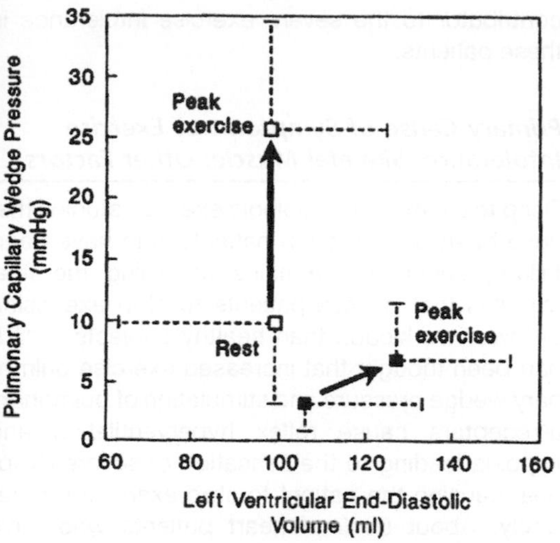


**Fig. 6.** LV diastolic function assessed by invasive cardiopulmonary exercise testing. The key is the same as in **Fig. 4**. The pressure–volume relationship was shifted upward and leftward at rest. In the patients undergoing exercise testing, LV diastolic volume did not increase despite the marked increase in diastolic (pulmonary wedge) pressure. Because of diastolic dysfunction, failure of the Frank-Starling mechanism resulted in severe exercise intolerance. (*From* Kitzman DW, Higginbotham MB, Cobb FR, et al. Exercise intolerance in patients with heart failure and preserved left ventricular systolic function: failure of the Frank-Starling mechanism. J Am Coll Cardiol 1991;17:1065–72; with permission. Copyright © 1991, American College of Cardiology.)

intolerance that was associated with increased pulse pressure and concentric hypertrophic LV remodeling. Thoracic aortic wall thickness was increased 50%, and there was markedly decreased aortic distensibility (**Fig. 10**). In univariate analysis, decreased aortic distensibility correlated closely with severely decreased peak exercise $VO_2$ (**Fig. 11**).[38] In multivariate analysis, decreased aortic distensibility was the strongest independent predictor of reduced exercise capacity. These data support a potentially important role of increased aortic stiffness, caused by underlying aging and amplified by chronic hypertension, in the pathophysiology of chronic heart failure symptoms.[39]

Peripheral arteries must dilate early during exercise to accommodate and facilitate the conveyance of increased nutritive blood flow to working skeletal muscle. Multiple lines of evidence suggest that in patients who have SHF this response is impaired and contributes to exercise intolerance and that this impairment is modifiable with exercise training and other interventions.[40–43] The authors examined the flow-mediated arterial dilation (FMAD) response to ischemia-induced by 3- to 5- minute cuff inflation in the femoral artery in elderly patients who had DHF, patients who had SHF, and normal age-matched controls using phase-contrast MRI. They also performed cardiopulmonary exercise testing with expired gas analysis.[44] Cardiopulmonary exercise testing again demonstrated severe exercise

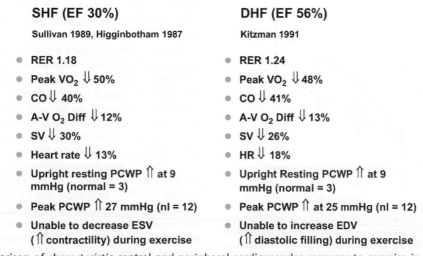

**Central Hemodynamic Response to Upright Bicycle Exercise in SHF vs. DHF Compared to Normals**

| **SHF (EF 30%)** | **DHF (EF 56%)** |
| --- | --- |
| **Sullivan 1989, Higginbotham 1987** | **Kitzman 1991** |
| • **RER 1.18** | • **RER 1.24** |
| • **Peak $VO_2$ ⇓ 50%** | • **Peak $VO_2$ ⇓ 48%** |
| • **CO ⇓ 40%** | • **CO ⇓ 41%** |
| • **A-V $O_2$ Diff ⇓ 12%** | • **A-V $O_2$ Diff ⇓ 13%** |
| • **SV ⇓ 30%** | • **SV ⇓ 26%** |
| • **Heart rate ⇓ 13%** | • **HR ⇓ 18%** |
| • **Upright resting PCWP ⇑ at 9 mmHg (normal = 3)** | • **Upright Resting PCWP ⇑ at 9 mmHg (normal = 3)** |
| • **Peak PCWP ⇑ 27 mmHg (nl = 12)** | • **Peak PCWP ⇑ at 25 mmHg (nl = 12)** |
| • **Unable to decrease ESV (⇑ contractility) during exercise** | • **Unable to increase EDV (⇑ diastolic filling) during exercise** |

**Fig. 7.** Comparison of characteristic central and peripheral cardiovascular response to exercise in patients who have heart failure associated with severe LV systolic dysfunction (HFpEF) versus normal LVEF. See text for discussion. CO, carbon dioxide; EDV, end-diastolic volume; ESV, end-systolic volume; PCWP, pulmonary capillary wedge pressure; RER, respiratory exchange ratio; SV, stroke volume. (*Data from* Refs.[11,12,15])

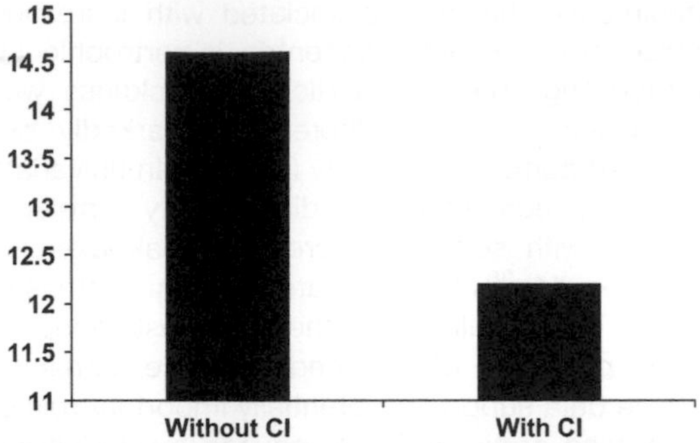


**Fig. 8.** Peak exercise $VO_2$ (y-axis, in mL/kg/min) in patients who have heart failure with and without chronotropic incompetence (CI). Patients who have chronotropic incompetence have more severe exercise intolerance, suggesting a contributory role for CI. (*Adapted from* Brubaker PH, Joo KC, Steward KP, et al. Chronotropic incompetence and its contribution to exercise intolerance in older heart failure patients. J Cardiopulm Rehab 2006;26:86–9; with permission.)

intolerance in the patients who had DHF that was similar in degree to that in patients who had SHF. The patients who had SHF had severely reduced femoral FMAD compared with normal subjects. In the patients who had DHF, however, the FMAD was relatively preserved and did not differ significantly from that in normal controls (**Fig. 12**). Thus, the authors concluded that abnormal FMAD was not present in DHF and was not a significant

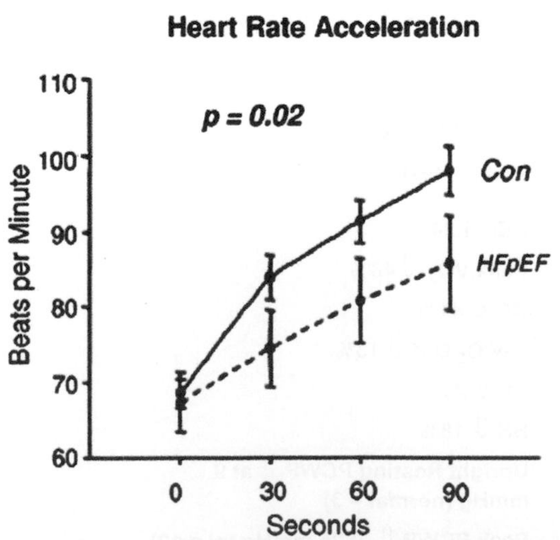


**Fig. 9.** Heart rate acceleration during exercise in controls (Con) and patients who have heart failure and preserved EF (HFpEF). (*From* Borlaug BA, Melenovsky V, Russell SD, et al. Impaired chronotropic and vasodilator reserves limit exercise capacity in patients with heart failure and a preserved ejection fraction. Circulation 2006;114:2144; with permission.)

contributor to the severe exercise intolerance in these patients.

### *Primary Cause of Symptoms of Exercise Intolerance; Skeletal Muscle; Other Factors*

Despite the many physiologic exercise studies that have been performed in patients who have heart failure, uncertainty remains regarding the final stimulus that causes patients to stop exercising at lower workloads than healthy subjects.[45–48] It had been thought that increased exercise pulmonary wedge pressure and stimulation of pulmonary J-receptors cause reflex hyperventilation and hypoxia leading to the sensation of severe dyspnea, causing the patient to stop exercise prematurely. About 50% of heart patients who have either SHF or DHF, however, discontinue exercise primarily because of general fatigue or leg fatigue rather than because of dyspnea. In addition, investigators have demonstrated that arterial hypoxia does not occur during exercise in patients who have heart failure and that excess ventilation is related to pulmonary hypoperfusion and reduced cardiac output rather than elevated LV filling pressures.[16,49] Furthermore, exercise intolerance, as measured objectively by peak $VO_2$, is unrelated to invasively measured pulmonary capillary wedge pressures, including in patients who have DHF.[15] The decreased exercise cardiac output probably causes skeletal muscle hypoperfusion, a potent stimulus for early anaerobic metabolism, and subsequent generation of muscle lactate and other metabolites that could produce the sensation of peripheral and central fatigue.[50,51] Indeed, in the studies that reported lactate production during exercise, the production of lactate in persons who had heart failure was abnormal compared with that in normal persons.[3,15]

Based on the extensive experience in seeking to understand exercise intolerance in patients who have SHF, it is likely that several factors in addition to those discussed previously may contribute to exercise intolerance in patients who have DHF. Such potential contributors include anemia (which is highly prevalent in DHF, as it is in SHF),[52] and skeletal muscle bulk, fiber type, and function.[11,42,53–61] There have been particularly compelling findings regarding skeletal muscle remodeling in SHF[11,56,62–73] but there are no data regarding skeletal muscle remodeling in DHF. Skeletal muscle could be an even more relevant factor in DHF than in SHF, given increasing data regarding the role of skeletal muscle atrophy and dysfunction in older patients who have a variety of disabling chronic syndromes. This area seems to be a particularly promising area for future investigation.[74–78] In

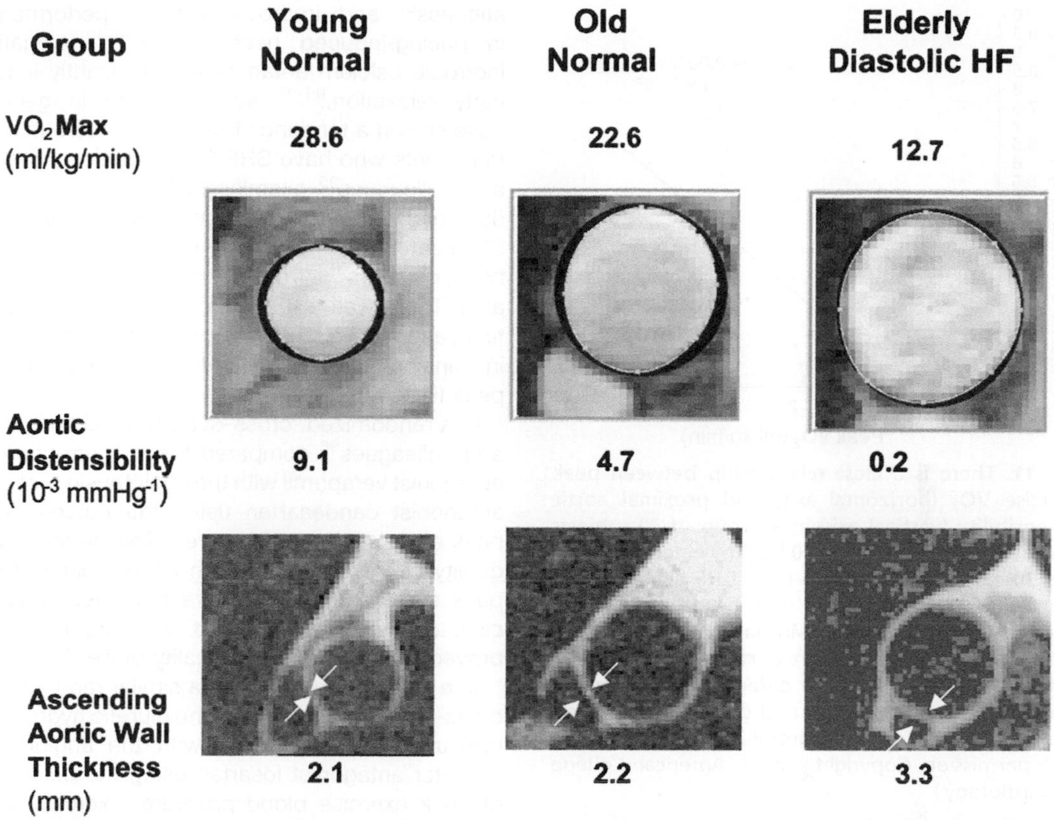


**Fig. 10.** Data and images from representative subjects from healthy young persons, healthy elderly persons, and elderly patients who have diastolic heart failure (HF). Maximal exercise oxygen consumption ($VO_2max$), aortic distensibility at rest, and the LV mass:volume ratio are shown. Patients who have DHF have severely reduced exercise tolerance ($VO_2max$) and aortic distensibility and increased aortic wall thickness (*arrows*). (*Adapted from* Hundley WG, Kitzman DW, Morgan TM, et al. Cardiac cycle dependent changes in aortic area and aortic distensibility are reduced in older patients with isolated diastolic heart failure and correlate with exercise intolerance. J Am Coll Cardiol 2001;38(3):796–802; with permission. Copyright © 2001, American College of Cardiology.)

addition, the amount of adipose tissue between skeletal muscle bundles seems to be a potential modifier of skeletal muscle function and of exercise capacity as well. This area probably will also be a fruitful area for future research, particularly because skeletal muscle bulk and function seem to be potentially modifiable through nutrition and exercise interventions.[79]

## INTERVENTIONS TO IMPROVE EXERCISE TOLERANCE

During exercise in normal subjects, systolic and pulse pressure increase substantially, and this response is magnified by increased arterial stiffness. Data from animal models suggest that the exercise-related increase in systolic blood pressure is mediated, in part, by exercise-induced increases in circulating angiotensin II. Indeed, in a randomized, double-blind, placebo-controlled cross-over trial, angiotensin receptor blockade reduced the exaggerated exercise increase in systolic and pulse pressures, resulting in significantly improved exercise treadmill time and quality of life (**Fig. 13**).[80]

In a group of patients who had NYHA class III heart failure and presumed diastolic dysfunction (EF >50%), Aronow and Kronzon[81] showed that the angiotensin-converting enzyme inhibitor enalapril significantly improved functional class, exercise duration, EF, diastolic filling, and LV mass.

In hypertrophic cardiomyopathy, a disorder in which diastolic dysfunction is common, verapamil seems to improve symptoms and objectively measured exercise capacity.[82–85] This agent also improves ventricular vascular coupling and exercise performance in aged individuals who have hypertension.[86] In laboratory animal models calcium antagonists, particularly dihydropyridines, prevent ischemia-induced increases in LV diastolic

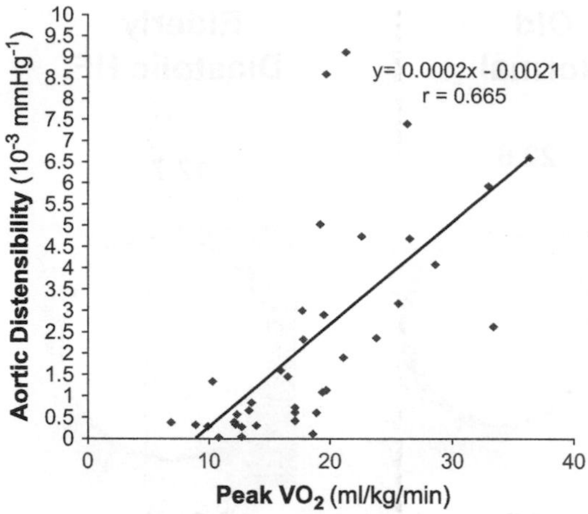


**Fig. 11.** There is a close relationship between peak exercise $VO_2$ (horizontal axis) and proximal aortic distensibility (vertical axis) in a group of 30 subjects (10 healthy young persons, 10 healthy elderly persons, and 10 elderly patients who have DHF). Each symbol represents the data from one participant. (*From* Hundley WG, Kitzman DW, Morgan TM, et al. Cardiac cycle dependent changes in aortic area and aortic distensibility are reduced in older patients with isolated diastolic heart failure and correlate with exercise intolerance. J Am Coll Cardiol 2001;38(3):796–802; with permission. Copyright © 2001, American College of Cardiology.)

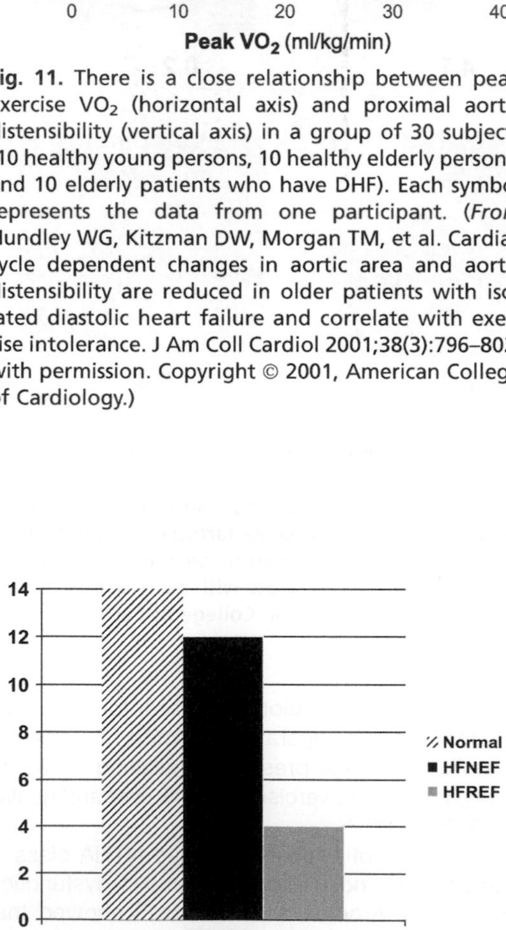


**Fig. 12.** Flow-mediated arterial dilation (FMAD) of the femoral artery by phase-contrast MRI in normal subjects, elderly patients who have heart failure and normal EF (HFNEF), and patients who have heart failure and reduced EF (HFREF). FMAD is severely reduced in HFREF but is relatively preserved in HFNEF compared with age-matched healthy normal subjects. (*From* Hundley WG, Bayram E, Hamilton CA, et al. Leg flow-mediated arterial dilation in elderly patients with heart failure and normal left ventricular EF. Am J Physiol Heart Circ Physiol 2007;292(3):H1427–34; with permission.)

stiffness[87] and improve diastolic performance in pacing-induced heart failure.[88–90] Negative inotropic calcium antagonists significantly impair early relaxation,[90–94] however, and in general have shown a tendency toward adverse outcome in patients who have SHF.[90] Nonetheless, Setaro and colleagues[95] examined 22 men (mean age, 65 years) who had clinical heart failure despite an EF greater than 45% in a randomized, double-blind, placebo-controlled cross-over trial of verapamil. There was a 33% improvement in exercise time, and there also were significant improvements in clinicoradiographic heart failure scoring and peak filling rate.

In a randomized, cross-over, blinded trial, Little and colleagues[96] compared the calcium-channel antagonist verapamil with the angiotensin receptor antagonist candesartan using the outcomes of peak exercise blood pressure, exercise time, and quality of life. Although both agents blunted the peak systolic blood pressure response to exercise, only candesartan, but not verapamil, improved exercise time and quality of life.[96]

In a subsequent trial with a similar randomized, cross-over, blinded design, the diuretic hydrochlorothiazide was compared with the angiotensin receptor antagonist losartan using the outcomes of peak exercise blood pressure, exercise time, and quality of life.[97] Although both agents blunted the peak systolic blood pressure response to exercise, only losartan, but not hydrochlorothiazide, improved exercise time and quality of life.[97]

The addition of low-dose spironolactone (12.5–50 mg daily) to standard therapy has been shown to improve exercise tolerance in patients who have severe SHF. Aldosterone antagonism has numerous potential benefits in patients who have DHF, including LV remodeling, reversal of myocardial fibrosis, and improved LV diastolic function and vascular function.[98–100] Few data, however, are presently available regarding aldosterone antagonism in DHF. In one small study, low-dose spironolactone was well tolerated and seemed to improve exercise capacity and quality of life in older women who had isolated DHF.[101] In another, spironolactone improved measures of myocardial function in hypertensive patients who had DHF.[102]

Glucose cross-links increase with aging and diabetes and cause increased vascular and myocardial stiffness. Alagebrium, a novel cross-link breaker, improved vascular and LV stiffness in dogs. In a small, open-label, 4-month trial of this agent in elderly patients, LV mass, quality of life, and tissue Doppler diastolic function indexes improved (**Fig. 14**), but there were no significant improvements in exercise capacity or aortic distensibility, the primary outcomes of the trial.[103]

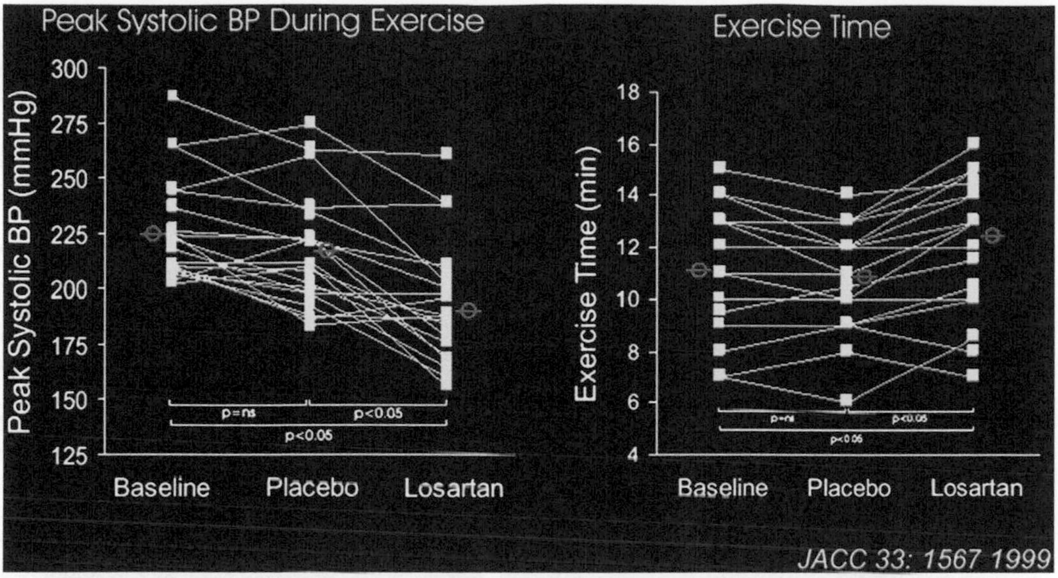


**Fig. 13.** Plots of peak systolic blood pressure (BP) and exercise duration during baseline, during placebo administration, and during losartan administration in a randomized, controlled, cross-over trial. Treatment with the angiotensin II antagonist losartan increased exercise time. (*From* Warner JG, Metzger C, Kitzman DW, et al. Losartan improves exercise tolerance in patients with diastolic dysfunction and a hypertensive response to exercise. J Am Coll Cardiol 1999;33:1567–72; with permission. Copyright © 1999, American College of Cardiology.)

A variety of other agents and strategies for this syndrome, including a selective endothelin antagonist, are being evaluated currently or are under consideration.

The substantial chronotropic incompetence seen in patients who have DHF and its correlation with reduced exercise capacity described earlier provides a rationale for electronic pacing interventions to improve exercise capacity. Indeed, one modest-sized single-center study using such a strategy demonstrated substantially improved exercise performance in selected patients who had hypertensive LV hypertrophy with supranormal systolic ejection and distal cavity obliteration and who experienced debilitating exertional fatigue and dyspnea.[104] These data merit confirmation in larger, multicenter, randomized, controlled trials.

Thus, a variety of pharmacologic and other interventions in small studies have shown improvements in exercise tolerance with verapamil,[95] enalapril,[81] angiotensin receptor antagonism,[80,96] and aldosterone antagonism.[101] It should be remembered that in patients who have SHF, some types of pharmacologic interventions that improve exercise tolerance have had paradoxical effects on long-term survival.[105,106] Therefore the VE/$VCO_2$ slope during exercise, which is a powerful predictor of survival independent of $VO_2$, should be included in future intervention trials of exercise tolerance.[6]

Aerobic exercise training has the potential to improve a variety of key abnormalities in patients who have heart failure and normal EF, including LV diastolic compliance, aortic distensibility, blood pressure, and skeletal muscle function.[72,107,108] Indeed, in SHF, aerobic exercise training has been shown to improve exercise tolerance, probably by favorable effects on multiple factors.[17,109,110] A recent report indicates that LV diastolic compliance is preserved in older masters athletes compared with their age-matched and young counterparts, suggesting that exercise training may be beneficial in DHF as well.[111] A preliminary report indicates that exercise training improves exercise tolerance and quality of life in older patients who have heart failure and normal EF.[112] A recent report from a clinical exercise rehabilitation program suggests that exercise training also may benefit patients who have DHF.[113] Although the role of exercise training in the clinical management of this syndrome remains to be defined, it would seem prudent to recommend regular, moderate physical activity as tolerated, as is the accepted practice in SHF. The effect of exercise training on survival in patients who have SHF is being examined in a large, multicenter, randomized, controlled trial sponsored by the National

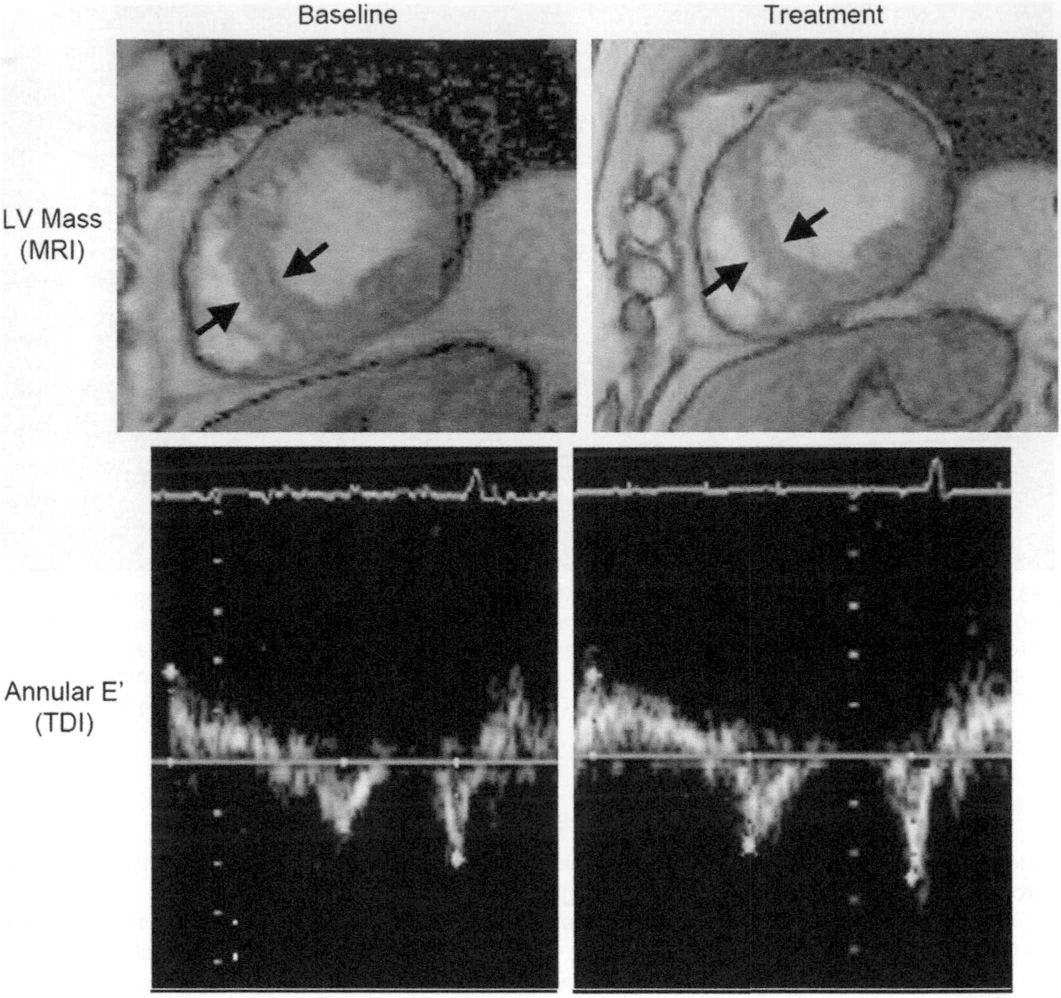


**Fig. 14.** Effect of alagebrium on LV mass seen by MRI (*top panel*) and E′ seen by tissue Doppler imaging (TDI) in older patients who have DHF. (*From* Little WC, Zile MR, Kitzman DW, et al. The effect of alagebrium chloride (ALT-711), a novel glucose cross-link breaker, in the treatment of elderly patients with diastolic heart failure. J Card Fail 2005;11(3):191–5; with permission.)

Institutes of Health (HF-ACTION). Presently, there is no trial examining mortality and exercise training in patients who have heart failure and normal EF.

## SUMMARY

Even when stable and non-edematous, patients who have heart failure and normal EF have severe, chronic exercise intolerance. The pathophysiology of exercise intolerance in this syndrome is incompletely understood but probably is multifactorial. Presently available data suggest that important contributors include decreased LV diastolic compliance, decreased aortic distensibility, exaggerated exercise systolic blood pressure, relative chronotropic incompetence, and possibly anemia and skeletal muscle remodeling. Because it is a primary determinant of quality of life, can be quantified objectively, is reproducible, and is modifiable, exercise intolerance is an attractive therapeutic target. A number of pharmacologic and other interventions seem to improve exercise intolerance in DHF. Although it is unknown whether these interventions will be accompanied by improved survival, the parallel outcome of improved quality of life supports the clinical relevance of exercise performance outcomes.

## REFERENCES

1. Gandhi SK, Powers JE, Fowle KM, et al. The pathogenesis of acute pulmonary edema associated with hypertension. N Engl J Med 2000;344(1):17–22.
2. Powers JE, Gandhi SK, Kramer RK, et al. Predictors of poor outcome in patients with hypertensive

pulmonary edema [abstract]. J Am Coll Cardiol 2004;43(5A):227A.
3. Kitzman DW, Little WC, Brubaker PH, et al. Pathophysiological characterization of isolated diastolic heart failure in comparison to systolic heart failure. JAMA 2002;288(17):2144–50.
4. Bol E, de Vries WR, Mosterd WL, et al. Cardiopulmonary exercise parameters in relation to all-cause mortality in patients with chronic heart failure. Int J Cardiol 2000;72:255–63.
5. Jones RC, Francis GS, Lauer MS. Predictors of mortality in patients with heart failure and preserved systolic function in the Digitalis Investigation Group trial. J Am Coll Cardiol 2004;44(5):1025–9.
6. Francis DP, Shamin W, Davies LC, et al. Cardiopulmonary exercise testing for prognosis in chronic heart failure: continuous and independent prognostic value from VE/VCO2 slope and peak VO2. Eur Heart J 2000;21:154–61.
7. Moore B, Brubaker PH, Stewart KP, et al. VE/VCO2 slope in older heart failure patients with normal versus reduced ejection fraction compared with age-matched healthy controls. J Card Fail 2007; 13(4):259–62.
8. Maldonado-Martin S, Brubaker PH, Kaminsky LA, et al. The relationship of a 6-min walk to VO(2 peak) and VT in older heart failure patients. Med Sci Sports Exerc 2006;38(6):1047–53.
9. Higginbotham MB, Morris KG, Williams RS, et al. Regulation of stroke volume during submaximal and maximal upright exercise in normal man. Circ Res 1986;58:281–91.
10. Higginbotham MB, Morris KG, Williams RS, et al. Physiologic basis for the age-related decline in aerobic work capacity. Am J Cardiol 1986;57: 1374–9.
11. Sullivan M, Knight JD, Higginbotham MB, et al. Relation between central and peripheral hemodynamics during exercise in patients with chronic heart failure: muscle blood flow is reduced with maintenance of arterial perfusion pressure. Circulation 1989;80:769–81.
12. Higginbotham MB, Sullivan M, Coleman RE, et al. Regulation of stroke volume during exercise in patients with severe left ventricular dysfunction: importance of Starling mechanism. J Am Coll Cardiol 1987;9:58A.
13. Kitzman DW, Sullivan M, Cobb FR, et al. Exercise cardiac output declines with advancing age in normal subjects. J Am Coll Cardiol 1989;13(2): 241A.
14. Sullivan M, Cobb FR, Knight JD, et al. Stroke volume increases by similar mechanisms in men and women. Am J Cardiol 1991;67:1405–12.
15. Kitzman DW, Higginbotham MB, Cobb FR, et al. Exercise intolerance in patients with heart failure and preserved left ventricular systolic function: failure of the Frank-Starling mechanism. J Am Coll Cardiol 1991;17:1065–72.
16. Sullivan M, Higginbotham MB, Cobb FR. Increased exercise ventilation in patients with chronic heart failure: intact ventilatory control despite hemodynamic and pulmonary abnormalities. Circulation 1988;77:552–9.
17. Sullivan M, Higginbotham MB, Cobb FR. Exercise training in patients with chronic heart failure delays ventilatory anaerobic threshold and improves submaximal exercise performance. Circulation 1989;79:324–9.
18. Sullivan M, Cobb FR. Central hemodynamic response to exercise in patients with chronic heart failure. Chest 1992;101:340S–6S.
19. Nagueh SF, Middleton KJ, Kopelen HA, et al. Doppler tissue imaging: a noninvasive technique for evaluation of left ventricular relaxation and estimation of filling pressures. J Am Coll Cardiol 1997; 30(6):1527–33.
20. Ommen SR, Nishimura RA, Appleton CP, et al. Clinical utility of Doppler echocardiography and tissue Doppler imaging in the estimation of left ventricular filling pressures: a comparative simultaneous Doppler-catheterization study. Circulation 2000; 102(15):1788–94.
21. Hadano Y, Murata K, Yamamoto T, et al. Usefulness of mitral annular velocity in predicting exercise tolerance in patients with impaired left ventricular systolic function. Am J Cardiol 2006;97(7):1025–8.
22. Skaluba SJ, Litwin SE. Mechanisms of exercise intolerance: insights from tissue Doppler imaging. Circulation 2004;109(8):972–7.
23. Ha JW, Oh JK, Pellikka PA, et al. Diastolic stress echocardiography: a novel noninvasive diagnostic test for diastolic dysfunction using supine bicycle exercise Doppler echocardiography. J Am Soc Echocardiogr 2005;18(1):63–8.
24. Kitzman DW, Sullivan M. Exercise intolerance in patients with heart failure: role of diastolic dysfunction. In: Grossman W, editor. Diastolic relaxation of the heart. Boston: Kluwer Academic Publishers; 1994. p. 295–302.
25. Brubaker PH, Joo KC, Stewart KP, et al. Chronotropic incompetence and its contribution to exercise intolerance in older heart failure patients. J Cardiopulm Rehabil 2006;26(2):86–9.
26. Borlaug BA, Melenovsky V, Russell SD, et al. Impaired chronotropic and vasodilator reserves limit exercise capacity in patients with heart failure and a preserved ejection fraction. Circulation 2006; 114(20):2138–47.
27. Kitzman DW, Gardin JM, Gottdiener JS, et al. Importance of heart failure with preserved systolic function in patients > or = 65 years of age. Cardiovascular Health Study Research Group. Am J Cardiol 2001;87(4):413–9.

28. Iriarte M, Murga N, Morillas M, et al. Congestive heart failure from left ventricular diastolic dysfunction in systemic hypertension. Am J Cardiol 1993; 71:308–12.
29. Iriarte MM, Perez OJ, Sagastagoitia D, et al. Congestive heart failure due to hypertensive ventricular diastolic dysfunction. Am J Cardiol 1995;76(13):43D–7D.
30. Little WC. Enhanced load dependence of relaxation in heart failure: clinical implications. Circulation 1992;85(6):2326–8.
31. Gelpi RJ. Changes in diastolic cardiac function in developing and stable perinephritic hypertension in conscious dogs. Circ Res 1991;68:555–67.
32. Shannon RP, Komamura K, Gelpi RJ, et al. Altered load: an important component of impaired diastolic function in hypertension and heart failure. In: Lorell BH, Grossman W, editors. Diastolic relaxation of the heart. Norwell (MA): Kluwer Academic Publishers; 1994. p. 177–85.
33. Little WC, Braunwald E. Assessment of cardiac performance. In: Braunwald E, editor. Heart disease. Philadelphia: W.B. Saunders Company; 1996. p. 421–44.
34. Hoit BD, Walsh RA. Diastolic dysfunction in hypertensive heart disease. In: Gaasch WH, LeWinter MM, editors. Left ventricular diastolic dysfunction and heart failure. Philadelphia: Lea & Febiger; 1994. p. 354–72.
35. Little WC, Ohno M, Kitzman DW, et al. Determination of left ventricular chamber stiffness from the time for deceleration of early left ventricular filling. Circulation 1995;92:1933–9.
36. Lakatta E. Cardiovascular aging research: the next horizons. J Am Geriatr Soc 1999;47:613–25.
37. Lakatta EG, Levy D. Arterial and cardiac aging: major shareholders in cardiovascular disease enterprises: part I: aging arteries: a "set up" for vascular disease. Circulation 2003;107(1): 139–46.
38. Hundley WG, Kitzman DW, Morgan TM, et al. Cardiac cycle dependent changes in aortic area and aortic distensibility are reduced in older patients with isolated diastolic heart failure and correlate with exercise intolerance. J Am Coll Cardiol 2001;38(3):796–802.
39. Rerkpattanapipat P, Hundley WG, Link KM, et al. Relation of aortic distensibility determine by magnetic resonance imaging in patients = 60 years of age to systolic heart failure and exercise capacity. Am J Cardiol 2002;90(11):1221–5.
40. Drexler H, Hayoz D, Monzel T, et al. Endothelial function in chronic congestive heart failure. Am J Cardiol 1992;69:1596–601.
41. Hayoz D, Drexler H, Munzel T, et al. Flow-mediated arterial dilation is abnormal in congestive heart failure. Circulation 1993;87:VII-92–6.
42. Hornig B, Maier V, Drexler H. Physical training improves endothelial function in patients with chronic heart failure. Circulation 1996;93(2):210–4.
43. Hornig B, Arakawa N, Haussmann D, et al. Differential effects of quinaprilat and enalaprilat on endothelial function of conduit arteries in patients with chronic heart failure. Circulation 1998;98(25):2842–8.
44. Hundley WG, Bayram E, Hamilton CA, et al. Leg flow-mediated arterial dilation in elderly patients with heart failure and normal left ventricular ejection fraction. Am J Physiol Heart Circ Physiol 2007; 292(3):H1427–34.
45. Myers J, Froelicher V. Hemodynamic determinants of exercise capacity in chronic heart failure. Ann Intern Med 1991;115:377–86.
46. Franciosa JA. Role of ventricular function in determining exercise capacity in patients with chronic left ventricular failure. Adv Cardiol 1986;34:170–8.
47. Wilson JR, Rayos G, Yeoh TK, et al. Dissociation between exertional symptoms and circulatory function in patients with heart failure. Circulation 1995; 92(1):47–53, Ref Type: Journal (Full).
48. Clark AL, Sparrow JL, Coats AJ. Muscle fatigue and dyspnoea in chronic heart failure: two sides of the same coin? Eur Heart J 1995;16(1):49–52.
49. Fink LI, Wilson JR, Ferraro N. Exercise ventilation and pulmonary artery wedge pressure in chronic stable congestive heart failure. Am J Cardiol 1966; 57:249–53.
50. Sullivan M, Cobb FR. The anaerobic threshold in chronic heart failure. Circulation 1990;81:II-47–58.
51. Green HJ. Manifestations and sites of neuromuscular fatigue. Biochem Exercise 1990;VII:13–35.
52. Brucks S, Little WC, Chao T, et al. Relation of anemia to diastolic heart failure and the effect on outcome. Am J Cardiol 2004;93(8):1055–7.
53. Deedwania PC, Gottlieb S, Ghali JK, et al. Efficacy, safety and tolerability of beta-adrenergic blockade with metoprolol CR/XL in elderly patients with heart failure. Eur Heart J 2004;25(15):1300–9.
54. Sanders P, Kistler PM, Morton JB, et al. Remodeling of sinus node function in patients with congestive heart failure: reduction in sinus node reserve. Circulation 2004;110(8):897–903.
55. Nagaya N, Moriya J, Yasumura Y, et al. Effects of ghrelin administration on left ventricular function, exercise capacity, and muscle wasting in patients with chronic heart failure. Circulation 2004;110(24): 3674–9.
56. Sullivan JJ, Green HJ, Cobb FR. Skeletal muscle biochemistry and histology in ambulatory patients with long-term heart failure. Circulation 1990;81: 518–27.
57. Adamopoulos S, Coats A, Brunotte F, et al. Physical training improves skeletal muscle metabolism in patients with chronic heart failure. J Am Coll Cardiol 1993;21:1101–6.

58. Stratton J, Dunn JF, Adamopoulos S, et al. Training partially reverses skeletal muscle metabolic abnormalities during exercise in heart failure. J Appl Physiol 1994;76:1575–82.
59. Kouba EJ, Hundley WG, Brubaker PH, et al. Skeletal muscle remodeling and exercise intolerance in elderly patients with diastolic heart failure [abstract]. Am J Geriatr Cardiol 2003;12(2):135.
60. Felker GM, Adams KF Jr, Gattis WA, et al. Anemia as a risk factor and therapeutic target in heart failure. J Am Coll Cardiol 2004;44(5):959–66.
61. Adams V, Jiang H, Yu J, et al. Apoptosis in skeletal myocytes of patients with chronic heart failure is associated with exercise intolerance. J Am Coll Cardiol 1999;33(4):959–65.
62. Wilson JR, Fink L, Maris J, et al. Evaluation of energy metabolism in skeletal muscle of patients with heart failure with gated phosphorus-31 nuclear magnetic resonance. Circulation 1985;71(1): 57–62.
63. Minotti JR, Johnson EC, Hudson TL, et al. Skeletal muscle response to exercise training in congestive heart failure. J Clin Invest 1990;86:751–8.
64. Minotti JR, Christoph I, Oka R, et al. Impaired skeletal muscle function in patients with congestive heart failure. J Clin Invest 1991;88:2077–82.
65. Mancini DM, Walter G, Reichek N, et al. Contribution of skeletal muscle atrophy to exercise intolerance and altered muscle metabolism in heart failure. Circulation 1992;85:1364–73.
66. Minotti JR, Christoph I, Massie BM. Skeletal muscle function, morphology, and metabolism in patients with congestive heart failure. Chest 1992;101: 333S–9S.
67. Wilson JR, Mancini DM. Skeletal muscle metabolic dysfunction. Implications for exercise intolerance in heart failure. Circulation 1993;87:VII-104–9.
68. Minotti JR, Pillay P, Oka R, et al. Skeletal muscle size: relationship to muscle function in heart failure. J Appl Physiol 1993;75(1):373–81.
69. Kao W, Helpern JA, Goldstein S, et al. Abnormalities of skeletal muscle metabolism during nerve stimulation determined by 31P nuclear magnetic resonance spectroscopy in severe congestive heart failure. Am J Cardiol 1995;76(8):606–9.
70. Lang CC, Chomsky DB, Rayos G, et al. Skeletal muscle mass and exercise performance in stable ambulatory patients with heart failure. J Appl Physiol 1997;82:257–61.
71. Harrington D, Anker SD, Chua TP, et al. Skeletal muscle function and its relation to exercise tolerance in chronic heart failure. J Am Coll Cardiol 1997;30(7):1758–64.
72. Peters DG, Mitchell HL, McCune SA, et al. Skeletal muscle sarcoplasmic reticulum Ca(2+)-ATPase gene expression in congestive heart failure. Circ Res 1997;81(5):703–10.
73. Vescovo G, Volterrani M, Zennaro R, et al. Apoptosis in the skeletal muscle of patients with heart failure: investigation of clinical and biochemical changes [see comments]. Heart 2000;84(4): 431–7.
74. Grimby G. Physical activity and effects of muscle training in the elderly. Ann Clin Res 1988;20:62–6.
75. Fleg JL, Lakatta EG. Role of muscle loss in the age-associated reduction in VO2 max. J Appl Physiol 1988;65(3):1147–51.
76. Rice CL, Cunningham DA, Paterson DH, et al. Arm and leg composition determined by computed tomography in young and elderly men. Clin Physiol 1989;9(3):207–20.
77. Kallman DA, Plato CC, Tobin JD. The role of muscle loss in the age-related decline of grip strength: cross-sectional and longitudinal perspectives. J Gerontol 1990;45:M82–8.
78. Buchner D, deLateur B. The importance of skeletal muscle strength to physical function in older adults. Ann Behav Med 1991;13:4206–14.
79. Menshikova EV, Ritov VB, Toledo FGS, et al. Effects of weight loss and physical activity on skeletal muscle mitochondrial function in obesity. Am J Physiol Endocrinol Metab 2005;288(4):E818–25.
80. Warner JG, Metzger C, Kitzman DW, et al. Losartan improves exercise tolerance in patients with diastolic dysfunction and a hypertensive response to exercise. J Am Coll Cardiol 1999;33:1567–72.
81. Aronow WS, Kronzon I. Effect of enalapril on congestive heart failure treated with diuretics in elderly patients with prior myocardial infarction and normal left ventricular ejection fraction. Am J Cardiol 1993;71:602–4.
82. Vandenberg VF, Rath LS, Stuhlmuller P, et al. Estimation of left ventricular cavity area with on-line, semiautomated echocardiographic edge detection system. Circulation 1992;86:159–66.
83. Bonow RO, Leon MB, Rosing DR, et al. Effects of verapamil and propranolol on left ventricular systolic function and diastolic filling in patients with coronary artery disease: radionuclide angiographic studies at rest and during exercise. Circulation 1981;65:1337–50.
84. Bonow RO, Dilsizian V, Rosing DR, et al. Verapamil-induced improvement in left ventricular diastolic filling and increased exercise tolerance in patients with hypertrophic cardiomyopathy: short- and long-term effects. Circulation 1985;72:853–64.
85. Udelson J, Bonow RO. Left ventricular diastolic function and calcium channel blockers in hypertrophic cardiomyopathy. In: Gaasch WH, editor. Left ventricular diastolic dysfunction and heart failure. Malvern, Pennsylvania: Lea & Febiger; 1996. p. 465–89.
86. Chen CH, Nakayama M, Talbot M, et al. Verapamil acutely reduces ventricular-vascular stiffening and

improves aerobic exercise performance in elderly individuals. J Am Coll Cardiol 1999;33:1602–9.
87. Serizawa T, Shin-Ichi M, Nagai Y, et al. Diastolic abnormalities in low-flow and pacing tachycardia-induced ischemia in isolated rat hearts-modification by calcium antagonists. In: Lorell BH, Grossman W, editors. Diastolic relaxation of the heart. Norwell (MA): Kluwer Academic Publishers; 1996. p. 266–74.
88. Cheng CP, Pettersson K, Little WC. Effects of felodipine on left ventricular systolic and diastolic performance in congestive heart failure. J Pharma and Exper Thera 1994;271:1409–17.
89. Cheng CP, Noda T, Ohno M, et al. Differential effects of enalaprilat and felodipine on diastolic function during exercise in dogs with congestive heart failure [abstract]. Circulation 1993;88(4): I-294.
90. Little WC, Cheng CP, Elvelin L, et al. Vascular selective calcium entry blockers in the treatment of cardiovascular disorders: focus on felodipine. Cardiovasc Drugs Ther 1995;9(5):657–63.
91. Ten Cate FJ, Serruys PW, Mey S, et al. Effects of short-term administration of verapamil on left ventricular filling dynamics measured by a combined hemodynamic-ultrasonic technique in patients with hypertrophic cardiomyopathy. Circulation 1983;68(6):1274–9.
92. Hess OM, Murakami T, Krayenbuehl HP. Does verapamil improve left ventricular relaxation in patients with myocardial hypertrophy? Circulation 1996;74:530–43.
93. Brutsaert DL, Rademakers F, Sys SU, et al. Analysis of relaxation in the evaluation of ventricular function of the heart. Prog Cardiovasc Dis 1985; 28:143–63.
94. Brutsaert DL, Sys SU, Gillebert TC. Diastolic failure: pathophysiology and therapeutic implications. J Am Coll Cardiol 1993;22:318–25.
95. Setaro JF, Zaret BL, Schulman DS, et al. Usefulness of verapamil for congestive heart failure associated with abnormal left ventricular diastolic filling and normal left ventricular systolic performance. Am J Cardiol 1990;66:981–6.
96. Little WC, Wesley-Farrington DJ, Hoyle J, et al. Effect of candesartan and verapamil on exercise tolerance in diastolic dysfunction. J Cardiovasc Pharmacol 2004;43(2):288–93.
97. Little WC, Zile MR, Klein AL, et al. Effect of losartan and hydrochlorothiazide on exercise tolerance in exertional hypertension and diastolic dysfunction. Am J Cardiol 2006;98(3):383–5.
98. Pitt B, Reichek N, Willenbrock R, et al. Effects of eplerenone, enalapril, and eplerenone/enalapril in patients with essential hypertension and left ventricular hypertrophy: the 4E-left ventricular hypertrophy study. Circulation 2003;108(15):1831–8.
99. Rajagopalan S, Pitt B. Aldosterone as a target in congestive heart failure. Med Clin North Am 2003; 87(2):441–57.
100. Zannad F, Alla F, Dousset B, et al. Limitation of excessive extracellular matrix turnover may contribute to survival benefit of spironolactone therapy in patients with congestive heart failure: insights from the randomized Aldactone evaluation study (RALES). Rales Investigators. Circulation 2000;102(22):2700–6.
101. Daniel KR, Wells GL, Fray B, et al. The effect of spironolactone on exercise tolerance and quality of life in elderly women with diastolic heart failure [abstract]. Am J Geriatr Cardiol 2003; 12(2):131.
102. Mottram PM, Haluska B, Leano R, et al. Effect of aldosterone antagonism on myocardial dysfunction in hypertensive patients with diastolic heart failure. Circulation 2004;110(5):558–65.
103. Little WC, Zile MR, Kitzman DW, et al. The effect of alagebrium chloride (ALT-711), a novel glucose cross-link breaker, in the treatment of elderly patients with diastolic heart failure. J Card Fail 2005;11(3):191–5.
104. Kass DA, Chen CH, Talbot MW, et al. Ventricular pacing with premature excitation for treatment of hypertensive-cardiac hypertrophy with cavity-obliteration. Circulation 1999;100(8):807–12.
105. Packer M, Carver JR, Chesebro J, et al. Effect of oral milrinone on mortality in severe chronic heart failure: The Prospective Randomized Milrinone Survival Evaluation (PROMISE). N Engl J Med 1991;325:1468–75.
106. Creager MA, Massie BM, Faxon DP, et al. Acute and long-term effects of enalapril on the cardiovascular response to exercise and exercise tolerance in patients with congestive heart failure. J Am Coll Cardiol 1985;6(1):163–73.
107. Sullivan M. Role of exercise conditioning in patients with severe systolic left ventricular dysfunction. In: Fletcher GF, editor. Cardiovascular response to exercise. Mount Kisco: Futura Publishing Company; 1994. p. 359–72.
108. Vaitkevicius PV, Fleg J, Engel JH, et al. Effects of age and aerobic capacity on arterial stiffness in healthy adults. Circulation 1993;88(5):1456–62.
109. Pina IL, Apstein CS, Balady GJ, et al. Exercise and heart failure: a statement from the American Heart Association Committee on exercise, rehabilitation, and prevention. Circulation 2003;107(8): 1210–25.
110. Coats A, Adamopoulos S, Radaelli A, et al. Controlled trial of physical training in chronic heart failure. Circulation 1992;85:2119–31.
111. Arbab-Zadeh A, Dijk E, Prasad A, et al. Effect of aging and physical activity on left ventricular compliance. Circulation 2004;110(13):1799–805.

112. Kitzman DW, Brubaker PH, Abdelahmed A, et al. Effect of exercise training on exercise capacity, quality of life, and flow-mediated arterial dilation in elderly patients with diastolic heart failure [abstract]. J Am Coll Cardiol 2004;110(17):III-558.

113. Smart N, Haluska B, Jeffriess L, et al. Exercise training in systolic and diastolic dysfunction: effects on cardiac function, functional capacity, and quality of life. Am Heart J 2007;153(4): 530–6.

# Index

*Note:* Page numbers of article titles are in **boldface** type.




Cardiol Clin 29 (2011) 479–483
doi:10.1016/S0733-8651(11)00060-9

## D



## E

S



T



U



V



W

Printed and bound by CPI Group (UK) Ltd, Croydon, CR0 4YY
03/10/2024
01040359-0008